GYNECOLOGIC ENDOSCOPY:
Principles In Practice

GYNECOLOGIC ENDOSCOPY:
Principles In Practice

Michael J. Sammarco, M.D.
Clinical Assistant Professor
Department of Obstetrics and Gynecology
University of Illinois School of Medicine
Chicago, Illinois

Thomas G. Stovall, M.D.
Associate Professor and Head
Gynecology Section
Bowman Gray School of Medicine of
Wake Forest University
Winston-Salem, North Carolina

John F. Steege, M.D.
Chief, Division of Gynecology
University of North Carolina School of Medicine
Chapel Hill, North Carolina

Illustrated By:
Joyce Lavery

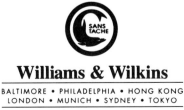

Williams & Wilkins
BALTIMORE • PHILADELPHIA • HONG KONG
LONDON • MUNICH • SYDNEY • TOKYO

A WAVERLY COMPANY

Editor: Charles W. Mitchell
Managing Editor: Marjorie Kidd Keating
Production Coordinator: Kim Nawrozki and Anne Stewart Seitz
Copy Editor: Margaret D. Hanson, R.N.
Illustration Planner: Raymond Lowman
Typesetter: Graphic Sciences Corporation
Designer: Rita Baker-Schmidt

Copyright © 1996 Williams and Wilkins

351 West Camden Street
Baltimore, Maryland 21201-2436 USA

Rose Tree Corporate Center
1400 North Providence Road
Building II, Suite 5025
Media, Pennsylvania 19063-2043 USA

All rights reserved. This book is protected by copyright. No part of this book may be reproduced in any form or by any means, including photocopying, or utilized by any information storage and retrieval system without written permission from the copyright owner.

Accurate indications, adverse reactions and dosage schedules for drugs are provided in this book, but it is possible that they may change. The reader is urged to review the package information data of the manufacturers of the medications mentioned.

Printed in the United States of America

First Edition

Library of Congress Cataloging-in-Publication Data

Gynecologic endoscopy : principles in practice / [edited by] Michael
  J. Sammarco, Thomas G. Stovall, John F. Steege : Illustrated by
  Joyce Lavery.
     p.   cm.
  Includes bibliographical references and index.
  ISBN 0-683-07509-8
   1. Generative organs, Female—Endoscopic surgery. 2. Laparoscopic
surgery. I. Sammarco, Michael J.   II. Stovall, Thomas G.
III. Steege, John F.
   [DNLM: 1. Surgery, Laparoscopic. 2. Genital Diseases, Female-
—surgery. 3. Hysteroscopy. WP 141 G9964 1996]
RG104.7.G96   1996
618.1'059—dc20
DNLM/DLC
for Library of Congress   95-17585
                                                              CIP

The publishers have made every effort to trace the copyright holders for borrowed material. If they have inadvertently overlooked any, they will be pleased to make the necessary arrangements at the first opportunity.

96 97 98 99 00
1 2 3 4 5 6 7 8 9 10

Reprints of chapters may be purchased from Williams & Wilkins in quantities of 100 or more. Call Isabella Wise, Special Sales Department, (800) 358-3583.

PREFACE

For decades, gynecologists have used endoscopy to minimize the need for more invasive and potentially morbid surgeries. Although initially felt to be primarily diagnostic techniques, both laparoscopy and hysteroscopy are widely used to perform practically every intrauterine and intraperitoneal gynecological procedure. The technology necessary to perform operative endoscopy places additional challenges before the surgeon. The surgeon must not only master the eye-hand coordination skills to perform surgery via a two-dimensional monitor, but also must be familiar with the functions and foibles of the accessory equipment and instruments. For the novice or unprepared surgeon, this may be quite overwhelming.

The purpose of this text is to teach the fundamentals necessary to perform safe and efficient endoscopic surgery. It is our feeling that learning to perform endoscopic surgery requires a different approach than that used to learn open techniques. We also feel that endoscopic techniques cannot be learned well by simply viewing a video, reading a text, or observing an actual surgical case. The techniques are best learned by combining all of these modalities. Unfortunately, the availability of teaching centers and qualified instructors is not universal. This text's major focus is to provide in detail not only the "what needs to be known" but the "how to do it" and the "how to learn it" aspects of endoscopic surgery.

The text is organized in both a problem and procedure oriented fashion. Although the individual chapter authors may note a preference for a particular approach, instrument, or piece of equipment, every effort has been made to provide the reader with objective information in a concise manner. Procedures are described in detail to include every aspect of the surgery, including preoperative preparation, intraoperative decision making, and postoperative care. Where applicable, the chapters include a description of the models and the exercises available to aid in the development of the skills needed for that particular procedure. A separate chapter has been included that deals solely with the preparation and usage of tissue models. These exercises and models have been found to be very effective in teaching residents and practicing physicians. The models and exercises have been developed through the cooperation of many of the authors as well as those that were so instrumental in the development and presentation of the CREOG endoscopic workshops.

It is always difficult to give adequate recognition to all of those responsible for the completion of this text. We give our special thanks to all of the authors who generously gave us their time and effort. We also thank Joyce Lavery for her time, patience, and expertise in preparing the illustrations.

Michael J. Sammarco, M.D.
Thomas G. Stovall, M.D.
John F. Steege, M.D.

CONTRIBUTORS

Alan H. DeCherney, M.D. *Louis E. Phaneuf Professor and Chairman, Department of Obstetrics and Gynecology, Tufts University School of Medicine and New England Medical Center, Boston, Massachusetts*

Frank DeLeon, M.D. *Director, Reproductive Endocrinology and Fertility, John Peter Smith Hospital, Associate Clinical Professor, Department of Obstetrics and Gynecology, Southwestern University, Fort Worth, Texas*

Edward G. Evantash, M.D. *Assistant Professor, Department of Obstetrics and Gynecology, Tufts University School of Medicine and New England Medical Center, Boston, Massachusetts*

Richard J. Gimpelson, M.D. *Assistant Clinical Professor, St. Louis University School of Medicine, St. Louis, Missouri, Private Practice, Chesterfield, Missouri*

Verda J. Hunter, M.D. *Associate Professor and Director, Division of Gynecologic Oncology, University of Missouri, Kansas City, Kansas City, Missouri*

D. Alan Johns, M.D. *Director, Gyn Laparoscopy Center, Harris Methodist Fort Worth Hospital, Fort Worth, Texas, Associate Clinical Professor, Department of Obstetrics and Gynecology, The University of Texas Southwestern Medical Center, Dallas, Texas*

Gary H. Lipscomb, M.D. *Assistant Professor, Department of Obstetrics and Gynecology, University of Tennessee, Memphis, Tennessee*

Charles M. March, M.D. *Professor, Department of Obstetrics and Gynecology, University of Southern California, School of Medicine, Los Angeles, California*

Malcolm G. Munro, M.D. *Professor and Associate Chair, Department of Obstetrics and Gynecology, Division of Gynecology, UCLA School of Medicine, Los Angeles, California*

Michael J. Sammarco, M.D. *Clinical Assistant Professor, Department of Obstetrics and Gynecology, University of Illinois School of Medicine, Chicago, Illinois*

Richard M. Soderstrom, M.D. *Clinical Professor, Department of Obstetrics and Gynecology, University of Washington School of Medicine, Seattle, Washington*

John F. Steege, M.D. *Chief, Division of Gynecology, Department of Obstetrics and Gynecology, University of North Carolina School at Chapel Hill, Chapel Hill, North Carolina*

Thomas G. Stovall, M.D. *Associate Professor and Head, Section of Gynecology, Bowman Gray School of Medicine, Wake Forest University, Winston-Salem, North Carolina*

Robert L. Summitt, Jr., M.D. *Associate Professor and Chief, Section of Urogynecology, Department of Obstetrics and Gynecology, University of Tennessee, Memphis, Memphis, Tennessee*

CONTENTS

Preface v
Contributors vii
Introduction–Laparoscopy versus Laparotomy: Is There a Difference?
    Edward G. Evantash and Alan H. DeCherney xi

1. **Laparoscopic Management of the Ectopic Pregnancy**
   Michael J. Sammarco and Thomas G. Stovall 1
2. **Pelvic Mass: Preoperative and Intraoperative Decision Making**
   Verda J. Hunter and Michael J. Sammarco 25
3. **Laparoscopic Treatment of the Adnexal Mass**
   D. Alan Johns 37
4. **Office Hysteroscopy—The Basics**
   Charles M. March 51
5. **Operative Hysteroscopy—Myomas, Septums, and Synechiae**
   Richard J. Gimpelson 61
6. **Operative Hysteroscopy—Endometrial Ablation**
   Frank DeLeon 75
7. **Laparoscopically Assisted Vaginal Hysterectomy**
   Robert L. Summitt, Jr. 97
8. **Laparoscopic Sterilization**
   Gary H. Lipscomb 117
9. **Learning Operative Endoscopy**
   Michael J. Sammarco and Thomas G. Stovall 135
10. **Principles of Electrosurgery During Endoscopy**
    Richard M. Soderstrom 179
11. **Laparoscopic Suturing Techniques**
    Malcolm G. Munro 193
12. **Complications of Laparoscopy**
    Malcolm G. Munro 245
13. **Chronic Pelvic Pain: Assessment and Treatment Guidelines for the Laparoscopic Surgeon**
    John F. Steege 279
14. **Laparoscopic Pelvic Denervation Procedures**
    John F. Steege 293

    Appendix 305
    Index 341

INTRODUCTION
Laparoscopy versus Laparotomy: Is There a Difference?
Edward G. Evantash and
Alan H. DeCherney

Since Jacobaeus first reported visualizing the human peritoneal cavity with an optical instrument in 1910, contributions from various fields of science have had a significant impact on gynecological surgery (1). Arguably, the most important was the introduction of fiber optics in 1952 by Hopkins and Kapany (2). This advancement led to the first tubal fulguration in the human reported by Palmer in 1962 (3).

In the 1970s a few investigators found new uses for the laparoscope beyond sterilization and diagnostics. Kurt Semm of Germany is attributed with the development of new laparoscopic instruments that could be used for operative purposes (2). Procedures such as salpingectomy, oophorectomy, and myomectomy could now be safely performed without a laparotomy.

With the availability of new instruments, videoscopic pictures, and laser technology, more surgical techniques will most likely be accomplished through the laparoscope. The safety, efficacy, and cost-effectiveness of the uses for operative laparoscopy have not been thoroughly defined. Nonetheless, there appears to be an important role for laparoscopy where the laparotomy was once required.

COSMESIS

The most obvious benefit of the use of the laparoscope is cosmesis. Multiple trochar puncture sites on the abdomen ranging from 5–12 cm are aesthetically preferable to the Pfannenstiel or midline incision of laparotomy. This reduces the associated wound complications, such as infection and dehiscence. Since a great deal of laparoscopic surgery is for women of reproductive age, improving the cosmetic appearance has clear advantages for the patient.

HOSPITAL STAY AND RECUPERATION TIME

It would seem that with less invasive techniques, the laparoscopic approach would reduce hospitalization stay and patient recuperation time. Azziz et al. studied 90 patients undergoing a total of 92 endoscopic procedures, and determined that even the most radical endoscopic procedure requires considerably less recuperation time when compared with laparotomy (4).

For treatment of the ectopic pregnancy, studies have shown that the hospital stay and patient recovery period are significantly reduced in those patients managed by laparoscopic salpingostomy than after laparotomy. In a nonrandomized comparative study, Brumstead reported an average hospital stay of 1.34 days for those patients with ectopic gestation treated laparoscopically, compared to 3.92 days for those with laparotomy (5). This resulted in a significantly shorter convalescent period and reduced need for postoperative analgesia.

In 60 patients with unruptured ectopic gestations of 5 cm or smaller randomized to laparoscopy or laparotomy, Vermesh et al. reported an average length of stay of 1.4 days for laparoscopy, significantly less than the 3.3 days after laparotomy (6). Follow-up studies on these patients showed no significant difference regarding reproductive outcome and tubal patency. These results were similar to those of Silva, who found an average hospital stay of 1.1 days in 22 patients treated for ectopic pregnancy by laparoscopy (7). Most patients were released for work in 1–2 weeks.

ADHESION FORMATION

Infertility is often a result of periadnexal adhesions (8). It has been suggested that laparoscopy may cause less peritoneal damage and therefore be preferable to laparotomy (9). The laparotomy often requires retractors, bowel packs, and exposure of large surfaces of peritoneum to talc, manipulation, and an open-air environment. All of these factors may contribute to adhesion formation.

By working in a closed environment, laparoscopy avoids the dehydration of pelvic organs and the peritoneal membrane, thereby decreasing adhesion formation. By magnifying the operative field, there is little need for bowel packs or large retractors. Additionally, the magnification allows for better visualization of lesions, thus preventing excessive cauterization that may irritate the peritoneal surface.

Diamond et al. performed second-look laparoscopy on 161 women 1–12 weeks after laparotomy for reproductive pelvic surgery. In addition to adhesion reformation, they found that more than 50% of these women had de novo adhesion formation at second-look laparoscopy (10). A multicenter collaborative study then examined the frequency and severity of postoperative adhesion development after operative laparoscopy, as assessed by early second-look laparoscopy. They found that de novo adhesion formation occurred in only 8 of 68 (12%) women (11). This was consistent with a report by Nezhat, who described the total absence of de novo adhesion formation among 157 women who underwent operative laparoscopy followed by second-look laparoscopy 4–18 months later because of persistent infertility, recurrence of pelvic pain, ectopic pregnancy, or electively at the time of dilatation and curettage for spontaneous abortions (12).

Lundorff et al. found that in those patients who underwent second-look laparoscopy after treatment of ectopic pregnancy, there were significantly fewer adhesions on the affected side in those managed by laparoscopy than those who were managed by laparotomy (13). Mecke et al. determined that laparoscopic management of the ectopic gestation with concomitant pelvic adhesiolysis greatly reduces the severity of adhesion recurrence (14).

COSTS

Decreasing hospital stay, patient recovery time, and postoperative morbidity translate to a clear economic benefit. This is a strong consideration in modern medicine when the benefits to cost are nearly as important as the benefits to clinical outcome. Not only does the reduced hospital cost result in savings to the insurance company, but by returning the patient to work earlier, there is a savings in wage loss and productivity, affecting the overall economy.

A comparative cost analysis between laparotomy and laparoscopy for lysis of adhesions and fulguration of endometrial implants showed savings of $1174.00; for resection of ovaries, lysis of adhesions, and salpingostomy, it was $1581.00; and for salpingo-oophorectomy, oophorectomy, salpingectomy, and myomectomy, $1007.00 (15). This represents a 49% reduction in overall hospital costs for endoscopic surgery. These significant savings are primarily due to a 79% reduction in costs for drugs and medical supplies, and a 69% reduction in costs for postoperative hospitalization.

The average savings for a patient with ectopic pregnancy treated by laparoscopy is $1500.00 compared to laparotomy (5). With 70,000 ectopic gestations reported each year, a savings of over 50 million dollars would be possible if only half of those patients had been treated with laparoscopy. This does not take into account the savings to the employer for sick pay, to the patient for child- care costs, and to the relatives for work absence.

It is important to realize, however, that the start-up costs for laparoscopic equipment and the need for continuous maintenance do add to the overall costs for endoscopic surgery. Many of the newer laparoscopic instruments are disposable, adding great costs to each procedure. As technology advances, new instruments will be made available in a highly competitive industry with strategic marketing directed at both the physician and the patient, leading to higher costs for updating equipment. This does not include the costs for retraining physicians and attending educational programs in order to stay current.

Defining newer techniques that can be done by laparoscopy may add to costs in operating room time that could be more quickly and cheaply performed by laparotomy. As Gant suggested, ". . . there can be no advantage in performing a 8-hour laparoscopic marathon to ablate endometriosis that might just as well have been completed 5 hours earlier through a mini-laparotomy incision at the same cost in dollars and post-operative recovery time and with better results and fewer complications" (16).

As the surgeon becomes more adept at applying these techniques, operative time will surely decrease. Thus, it is imperative that we view the emerging technology in the field of operative laparoscopy with a critical eye to determine not only its short-term cost savings, but its overall long-term economic impact.

QUALITY ASSURANCE

In the litigious environment in which we currently practice medicine, a procedure that allows for improved documentation offers an advantage over the procedure that can only be described in a postoperative dictation. Laparoscopy, with the use of video technology, provides the surgeon with photographic documentation of normal and abnormal pelvic anatomy during diagnostic evaluation. Operative endoscopy can be recorded on video, still photos, or computer floppy disks that will provide a visual image of what was accomplished during surgery (17).

Credentialing the laparoscopic surgeon has not as yet become standardized, which remains a problem (18). The process of determining what skills the gynecologist must possess prior to performing a difficult endoscopic procedure differs between institutions. We have requirements for board certification in fields within obstetrics and gynecology, but we have no way of assuring that complex surgery is not being attempted by the novice who believes that anything can be done through the laparoscope. The American Association of Gynecologic Laparoscopists reported in 1988 that 36,928 operative laparoscopy procedures were performed by members that responded to a survey (19). As these procedures become even more popular, we must develop better appropriate credentialing criteria.

THE FUTURE

Has the obituary of laparotomy been written and published as predicted in the mid-1980s? (20). Critics would claim that until randomized, controlled studies are performed, there is no solid evidence that laparoscopy is preferable to other surgical techniques (21). However, a study of surgical procedure, unlike pharmaceuticals, is subject to significant shortcomings that would require long periods of analysis before conclusions could be attained.

The thousands of laparoscopies that have been done to date provide us now with an understanding of the benefits, and also point out the weaknesses. A laparoscopic vaginal hysterectomy requiring 120 minutes that could have been done with similar results in half the time is clearly without benefit. But the abdominal hysterectomy converted to a vaginal procedure by laparoscopic assistance offers great rewards in terms of patient satisfaction and cost savings (22).

Not all that can be done abdominally should be performed laparoscopically. The surgeon's bravado to attempt anything through the laparoscope obscures the true role of operative laparoscopy in gynecologic surgery. The imagination of the surgeon must be tempered with skepticism, and always with an eye toward achieving what is in the patient's best interest.

There are clear advantages to operative laparoscopy with respect to laparotomy. Pelvic endoscopy can offer decreased hospital stay and recuperation period, less adhesion formation, substantial cost savings, and overall improved patient satisfaction. What remains to be written is the future of operative laparoscopy.

REFERENCES

1. Jacobaeus HC. Ueber die Moglichkeit, die Zystoskopie bei Untersuchung seroser Hohlungen anzuwenden. Munich Med Wochenshr 1910;57:2090–2092.
2. Gomel V. Operative laparoscopy: time for acceptance. Fertil Steril 1989;52:1–11.
3. Palmer R. Essais de sterilisation tubaire celioscopique par electrocoagulation istmique. Bull Fed Soc Gynecol Obstet Lang Fr. 1962;14:298.
4. Azziz R, Steinkampf MP, Murphy A. Postoperative recuperation: relation to the extent of endoscopic surgery. Fertil Steril 1989;51:1061–1064.
5. Brumsted J, Kessler C, Gibson C, Nakajima S, Riddick DH, Gibson M. A comparison of laparoscopy and laparotomy for the treatment of ectopic pregnancy. Obstet Gynecol 1988;71:889–892.
6. Vermesh M, Silva PD, Rosen GF, Stein AL, Fossum GT, Sauer MV. Management of unruptured ectopic gestation by linear salpingostomy: a prospective randomized clinical trial of laparoscopy versus laparotomy. Obstet Gynecol 1989;73:440–444.
7. Silva PD. A laparoscopic approach can be applied to most cases of ectopic pregnancy. Obstet Gynecol 1988;72:944.

8. Caspi E, Halperin Y, Bukovsky I. The importance of periadnexal adhesions in tubal reconstructive surgery for infertility. Fertil Steril 1979;131:296–298.
9. Filmar S, Gomel V, McComb PF. Operative laparoscopy versus open abdominal surgery: a comparative study on postoperative adhesion formation in the rat model. Fertil Steril 1987;48: 486–489.
10. Diamond MP, Daniell JF, Feste J, Surrey MW, McLaughlin DS, Friedman S, Vaughn WK, Martin DC. Adhesion formation and de novo adhesion formation after reproductive pelvic surgery. Fertil Steril 1987;47:864–866.
11. Operative Laparoscopy Group. Postoperative adhesion development after operative laparoscopy: evaluation at early second-look procedures. Fertil Steril 1991;55:700.
12. Nezhat CR, Nezhat FR, Metzger DA, Luciano AA. Adhesion reformation after reproductive surgery by videolaseroscopy. Fertil Steril 1990;53:1008–1010.
13. Lundorff P, Thorburn J, Hahlin M, Lindblom B, Kallfelt B. Adhesion formation after laparoscopic surgery in tubal pregnancy: a randomized trial versus laparotomy. Fertil Steril 1991;55:911–915.
14. Mecke H, Semm K, Freys I, Argiriou C, Gent H. Incidence of adhesions in the true pelvis after pelviscopic operative treatment of tubal pregnancy. Gynecol Obstet Invest 1989;28:202–204.
15. Levine RL. Economic impact of pelviscopic surgery. J Reprod Med 1985;30:655–659.
16. Gant NF. Infertility and endometriosis: comparison of pregnancy outcomes with laparotomy versus laparoscopic techniques. Am J Obstet Gynecol 1992;166:1072–1081.
17. Tadir Y, Fisch B. Operative laparoscopy: a challenge for general gynecology? Am J Obstet Gynecol 1993;169:7–12.
18. Pitkin RM. Operative laparoscopy: surgical advance or technical gimmick? Obstet Gynecol 1992;79:441–442.
19. Peterson HB, Hulka JF, Phillips JM. American Association of Gynecologic Laparoscopists' 1988 membership survey on operative laparoscopy. J Reprod Med 1990;35:587–589.
20. DeCherney AH. "The leader of the band is tired . . ." Fertil Steril 1985;44:299–302.
21. Grimes DA. Frontiers of operative laparoscopy: a review and critique of the evidence. Am J Obstet Gynecol 1992;166:1062–1067.
22. Nezhat F, Nezhat C, Gordon S, Wilkins E. Laparoscopic versus abdominal hysterectomy. J Reprod Med 1992;37:247–250.

Chapter 1

Laparoscopic Management of the Ectopic Pregnancy

Michael J. Sammarco and Thomas G. Stovall

The purpose of this chapter is to present the preoperative and intraoperative factors important for determining the proper surgical procedure. The attention given to detail is specifically offered to emphasize the need for adequate preparation. Often, it is that aspect of the surgery that is the most taken for granted that becomes the most critical to the completion of the procedure.

The final portion of this chapter will present a variety of exercises that are developed to aid in acquisition of the laparoscopic skills necessary to perform these procedures.

Treatment Approaches

The traditional management of ectopic pregnancy has always been surgical, with more recent use of conservative surgical modalities, such as linear salpingostomy rather than salpingectomy. Sensitive and rapid β-hCG radioimmunoassay and high resolution ultrasound technology have made possible the earlier detection of ectopic pregnancy. As a result, the emphasis on treatment has shifted from an emergency surgical procedure to control hemorrhage to a greater concern for the patients' future reproductive potential. Thus, salpingostomy can often replace salpingectomy in the hope of better long-term reproductive outcome.

Recent clinical trials have demonstrated an effective medical alternative for selected patients with an unruptured ectopic pregnancy. Patients eligible for methotrexate treatment include those who:

1. Are hemodynamically stable,
2. Have an unruptured ectopic pregnancy <3.5 cm in the greatest dimension,
3. Desire future fertility,
4. Have no laboratory evidence of blood dyscrasia, renal or liver disease, and
5. No evidence of an intrauterine pregnancy, (*a*) either by a transvaginal ultrasound when the hCG titer is >2,000 mIU/mL or (*b*) by endometrial suction curettage when the hCG titer is <2,000 mIU/mL (1). Stovall et al. achieved an overall 95% success rate with medical therapy (1–6). In the presence of cardiac activity in the ectopic pregnancy, however, this success rate diminishes to 80–85%, making cardiac activity in the ectopic pregnancy a relative contraindication to medical therapy.

It appears that methotrexate treatment would be associated with substantial cost savings. Creinin and Washington reviewed the charts and billing statements of all ectopic pregnancies treated at the San Francisco General Hospital in 1991 (7). Fifteen of the 50 (30%) of the patients would have been eligible for methotrexate treatment. Their treatment would have resulted in a cost savings greater than $160,000 at this institution alone. On a national basis, the potential annual cost savings would be in excess of $280 million. Given these data, it seems reasonable to offer medical treatment if the ectopic pregnancy can be confirmed without laparoscopy, and the patient meets the above criteria.

In most institutions, diagnostic and operative laparoscopic procedures are commonplace. However, laparotomy is still required for ectopic pregnancy treatment if the patient is hemodynamically unstable, or if the operator lacks sufficient operative laparoscopic experience. At times, appropriate laparoscopic instrumentation, equipment, or ancillary training of the operating room personnel will make laparotomy the easier approach. Selecting the proper operative approach requires preoperative assessment of (*a*) the patient's status, (*b*) size of the ectopic pregnancy, (*c*) presence or absence of fetal cardiac activity, evidence of hemoperitoneum, (*d*) the patient's desire for future fertility, and (*e*) the patient's past surgical history. If the woman has had previous tubal surgery on the involved side, preserving that tube may not be in her best interest.

When should a laparoscopy rather than a laparotomy be performed in a patient with an ectopic pregnancy? The answer is best explained by reviewing the results of prospective and randomized clinical trials which have been completed comparing laparoscopic salpingostomy to salpingostomy performed at laparotomy. The choice of laparoscopy as the primary surgical approach should not compromise the patient's care, either by increasing the potential for morbidity or in the inability to perform the desired procedure.

Brumsted et al. performed a case control trial in which 25 patients undergoing laparoscopic management were compared with 25 patients treated by laparotomy, who were matched to minimize differences in preoperative morbidity and technical difficulty (8). Patients treated laparoscopically had significantly shorter mean hospital stays, shorter operating time, shorter convalescence, and reduced postoperative analgesia. In a separate trial, Vermesh et al. prospectively randomized 60 patients with an unruptured ectopic pregnancy measured laparoscopically to be less than 5 cm to salpingostomy by laparoscopy ($n = 30$), or laparotomy ($n = 30$) (9). In this trial, patients treated laparoscopically had less operative blood loss, and a shorter hospital stay. A postoperative hysterosalpingogram demonstrated tubal patency in the involved side in 16/20 (80%), and 17/19 (89%) of the patients in the laparoscopic and laparotomy groups, respectively. Subsequent pregnancy rates were 10/18 (56%) and 11/19 (58%) in the two groups. Following salpingostomy, there was incidence of persistent trophoblastic tissue detected by persistently elevated hCG levels in 3.3% in both groups. Vermesh also found that the salpingostomy success rate decreased significantly when the gestational size was greater than 4 cm.

Murphy et al. in 1992 reported a series of patients that were prospectively allocated on alternative months to laparoscopy ($n = 26$) or laparotomy ($n = 37$) (10). In this trial, the mean intraoperative blood loss was significantly lower in the laparoscopy group. Perioperative complications were similar in both groups, as was the operative time. As noted in the previous studies, analgesic requirement, length of hospital stay, and time to resume normal activity were significantly shorter in the laparoscopy group. The intrauterine and recurrent ectopic rates were similar in both groups.

Lundorff et al. studied 105 women with a tubal ectopic pregnancy (11). Patients were prospectively randomized to laparoscopy or laparotomy. In 73 patients with a desire for pregnancy (laparoscopy $n = 31$; laparotomy $n = 42$), a second-look laparoscopy was performed 12 weeks (1–29) after the primary surgery. Patients in the previous laparotomy group developed significantly more adhesions at the operative site than those patients in the previous laparoscopy group. There was no difference in the tubal patency between the two groups.

When taken together, these studies provide evidence that laparoscopic surgical management of the unruptured ectopic pregnancy offers distinct advantages over laparotomy; including decreased blood loss, shorter hospital stay and recovery time, decreased adhesion formation, and reduced cost. Based on these prospective studies, it seems that if surgery is required, a laparoscopic approach offers advantages over laparotomy.

PREOPERATIVE PREPARATION

The key to the success of any endoscopic surgery is adequate preparation. A standard set of operative laparoscopic instruments and equipment is generally adequate except when one expects to encounter a large hemoperitoneum, or when a segmental tubal resection is chosen. In these situations, additional equipment is suggested.

In addition to an adequate light source, camera and monitor, rapid insufflator (>6 L/minute), multiple ports and reducers, there must be the ability to evacuate large amounts of blood, remove tissue, and the ability to place ligatures or suture. Standard trumpet valved 5-mm aspirating/irrigating cannulae will not efficiently remove large volumes of fluid or blood clots (Fig. 1.1). The ability to evacuate the blood, locate the source of bleeding, and control it is essential whenever a hemoperitoneum is encountered. A large diameter aspirator (10 or 11 mm) is the most efficient for this purpose. Alternatively, any straight cannula without valves or a standard wall suction tubing with a bevel cut in the end and a notch placed approximately 18 inches from the end will function well (Fig. 1.2).

A uterine manipulator with the ability to inject fluid or dye is also needed in

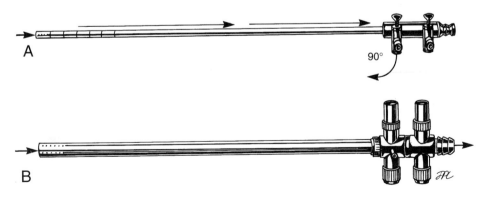

Figure 1.1. **A.** 5-mm trumpet valved irrigator/aspirator. Material must turn 90° before exiting. **B.** 10-mm irrigator/aspirator. Material directly exits.

4   GYNECOLOGIC ENDOSCOPY: Principles in Practice

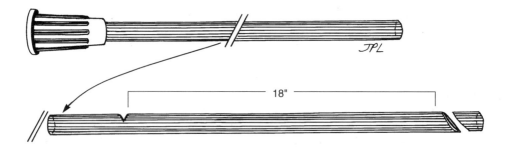

Figure 1.2. Commonly used ribbed suction tubing altered to be used for an aspirator during laparoscopy.

case the patency of the unaffected tube is in question. This information may be helpful in deciding whether a conservative or radical (salpingectomy) procedure is necessary.

A bipolar forceps is needed for the control of large bleeders. Any of the bipolar forceps commonly used for tubal sterilization can be used, but those with directly compressible tips are preferable to those that are dependent upon a spring mechanism (Fig. 1.3). Directly compressible tip instruments tend to slip off edematous and friable tissue less frequently, and more reliably compress and control bleeding points.

A needle-tipped electrode can be used for either a cutting tool or to fulgu-

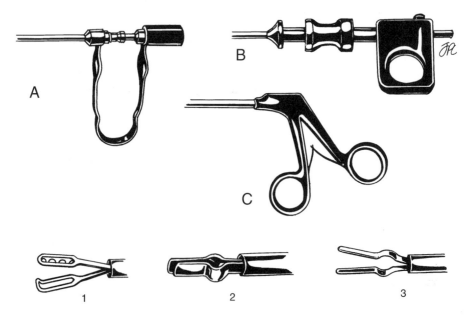

Figure 1.3. Shown are examples of 3 types of bipolar forceps. **A.** spring-handled, **B.** inline compressible, and **C.** pistol-handled. The available tip configuration (1, 2, 3) may not be available with each handle configuration.

rate small bleeding points. The electrode chosen should have a fine point to reduce the peripheral tissue damage, and should be examined prior to each case for carbonization and, if present, thoroughly cleaned. The finer the point, the more concentrated the current will be, hence the lower the current required, causing the least amount of peripheral tissue damage. The ability to use a foot switch rather than a hand control offers more precise control.

Several atraumatic graspers designed for manipulating the tube are needed and are more useful if equipped with a spring handle (Fig. 1.4). At least two 5-mm instruments should be available. A 10- or 11-mm spoon forceps is optimal for tissue removal. Endoscopic bag systems can be used, but offer no proven advantage over morcellation techniques, and add additional expense to the case.

Although needed infrequently, laparoscopic needle drivers, knot sliders, and sutures should be available. Recently developed bipolar electrosurgical microscissors are often used for a linear salpingostomy but are not essential unless this technique is to be used.

CHOICE OF PROCEDURE

The first criterion to consider in choosing an operative procedure is based initially on the patient's desire for future fertility. If the patient has no desire for future pregnancy, a salpingectomy should be performed and the contralateral tube can be occluded or removed at the same time. Since ectopic pregnancies have been reported after tubal ligation, a bilateral salpingectomy should be performed in any patient who has had a previous tubal ligation and subsequently has an ectopic pregnancy (12, 13). Removing the fallopian tubes allows for both the histologic assessment in the case of a failed tubal ligation and decreases the risk of a recurrent tubal pregnancy (14).

Although rarely indicated, a hysterectomy may be appropriate in those patients who have an ectopic pregnancy secondary to a uteroperitoneal fistula, or in the patient who has an ectopic pregnancy and has a separate indication for

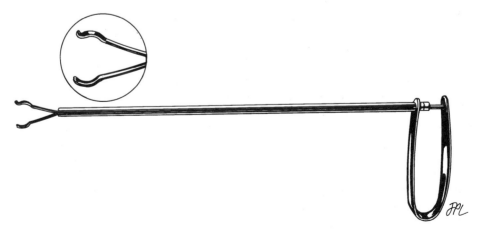

Figure 1.4. An example of an atraumatic, self-retaining grasping forcep. Note the smooth lining of the tip.

hysterectomy (15). Given the reported rates of morbidity and mortality after elective hysterectomy, it is difficult to advocate this procedure solely for the treatment of an ectopic pregnancy (16).

If a woman without a previous tubal ligation is having her first ectopic pregnancy and the patient has no desire for future pregnancy, the choice is between performing either a ligation procedure or a salpingectomy on the uninvolved tube. Although bilateral salpingectomy has not been directly compared to tubal occlusion, laparoscopic procedures for tubal ligation have a recognized failure rate (17). Ovarian and abdominal pregnancy rates following tubal occlusion are 1/7000 and 1/7269, respectively (18, 19). There are no reported rates for ovarian or abdominal pregnancies after bilateral salpingectomy, but it is doubtful that the incidence would be increased. Both of these rates are lower than the reported failure rates of 2–5/1000 for tubal occlusion methods with up to 50% of those resulting in ectopic pregnancies (20).

When an implantation site cannot be found, the choice may be not to proceed with any additional procedure other than the diagnostic laparoscopy. If there is no obvious tubal pregnancy, a thorough inspection of the entire abdominal cavity should be undertaken to rule out an abdominal or ovarian pregnancy. Omental pregnancies are easily resectable, whereas peritoneal implantations can be more challenging. If there is no apparent site of implantation, an interstitial pregnancy most be considered.

Early tubal pregnancies are often difficult to visualize. Performing a random salpingostomy to locate a suspected tubal pregnancy is discouraged, as this leads to tubal damage. Tubal patency confirmed by hydrotubation does not exclude the presence of a tubal pregnancy since the implantation may be extraluminal. If there is no evidence of an ectopic pregnancy and a hemoperitoneum is not present, terminating the laparoscopy and following the patient with serial quantitative hCG levels and vaginal sonography should be strongly considered.

SALPINGECTOMY (FIG. 1.5)

Salpingectomy is the procedure of choice in all cases of tubal pregnancy when future fertility is not desired or when the tube is unsalvageable. Several methods can be used, including electrosurgery, staples, or suture. The simplest technique is to employ bipolar forceps. Using a pure cutting current of 30–50 watts, the tube is desiccated just distal to the tubo-uterine junction. The mesosalpinx is successively desiccated and then cut until the tube is excised. A similar technique can be applied with a thermal coagulator.

In the case of the very large ectopic pregnancy (>5 cm), it often is easier to first evacuate the ectopic pregnancy by linear salpingostomy prior to proceeding with the salpingectomy. When tubo-ovarian adhesions are present, these should be lysed and the anatomy normalized prior to salpingectomy. These steps reduce the amount of peripheral tissue damage and possible compromise of the ovarian vascular supply or damage to other contiguous structures. An alternative technique is to utilize pretied ligatures to ligate the mesosalpingeal pedicle once the proximal portion of the tube is severed from the uterus. This is particularly useful in the cases of severe adhesive disease when tubal mobility is limited. Care must always be taken to completely occlude the artery contained in the fimbria

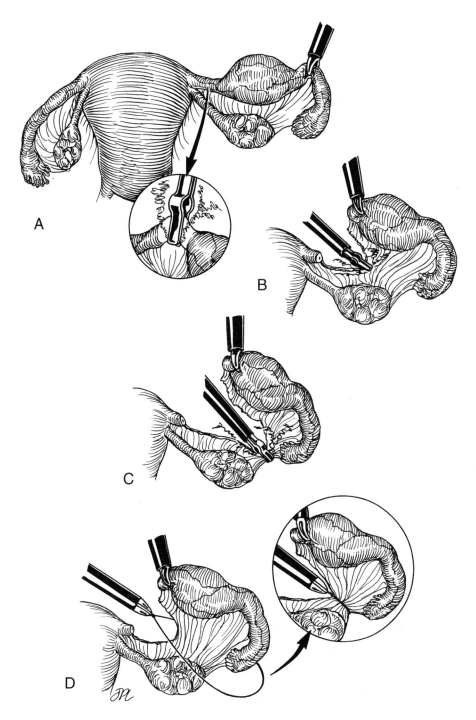

Figure 1.5. **A.** Desiccation of proximal portion of the tube and underlying mesosalpingeal vessel. **B.** Desiccation of the mesosalpinx while traction is placed on the tube. After desiccation, the mesosalpinx is cut. **C.** Desiccation of the fimbria ovarica. **D.** Alternative technique utilizing a pretied endoscopic ligature. After desiccation of the proximal portion of the tube and underlying mesosalpinx, the remaining mesosalpinx is ligated.

ovarica. The second site of concern is the tubo-uterine junction. The initial desiccation should not be placed too closely to the uterus. Desiccation in this area is often incomplete and when incised can result in remarkable bleeding. This bleeding is difficult to control. Sutures or further desiccation can be effective but it is best to avoid this area initially.

The excised tube can then be morcellated intraperitoneally and removed through a 10–12-mm port with a spoon forceps. Unless the tube was unruptured and the specimen is removed entirely intact, the patient must have weekly hCG levels until negative to detect the development of peritoneal and omental implants.

When the ovary is involved or ovarian pathology is encountered, a salpingo-oophorectomy may be necessary, although not routinely recommended. This can be done laparoscopically, but requires more advanced skills secondary to the potential for bleeding. To reduce to potential for severe hemorrhage, the infundibulopelvic ligament should be ligated prior to ligating the ovarian or tubo-uterine junction. This helps control the bleeding, is usually more accessible, and offers more mobility of the tube and ovary than other approaches.

CONSERVATIVE PROCEDURES

Patients who desire future fertility and have an unruptured tubal pregnancy are candidates for conservative surgery. Relative contraindications to performing a linear salpingostomy include (21):

- Ectopic pregnancy >6 cm,
- Presence of fetal heart activity,
- Quantitative hCG greater than 20,000 mIU/mL,
- Previous tubal surgery on involved tube,
- Isthmic implantation,
- Unreliable follow-up.

These are all relative and are largely dependent upon operator skill and the surgeon's intraoperative assessment. Each of these conditions places the patient at a higher risk of the procedure failing or leaving the tube with compromised function. Linear salpingostomy is the procedure of choice only when it is reasonably certain that a minimally damaged tube will remain and the contralateral tube has been assessed.

No benefit of a salpingostomy has been shown when compared to salpingectomy in the absence of additional infertility factors or contralateral tubal disease (22). Ory et al. retrospectively reviewed the charts of 88 patients surgically treated at the time of laparotomy for their first tubal pregnancy and reported on their pregnancy rates over the subsequent 12 years (23). The patients were divided into those that were treated conservatively (38) i.e., salpingostomy, salpingotomy and fimbrial expression, and those treated with a radical procedure (50) i.e., partial or complete salpingectomy. They found that the most significant factor for future fertility was the presence of infertility prior to the procedure. The choice of surgical procedure had no influence on the patient's future fertility if there was a history of infertility (11% versus 25% subsequent pregnancy, $p = .405$). Conversely, if there was no prior history of infertility, both conservative and radical procedures offered similarly good subsequent fertility rates (50% versus 58%).

Although a linear salpingostomy can be performed regardless of size or location of the ectopic pregnancy, the final result must always be considered. In those cases that are uncertain, a salpingectomy should be done in the presence of a normal, patent, contralateral tube.

Hemorrhage into the mesosalpinx or rupture through the tubal serosa are two situations that require special attention. In each of these cases, the entire thickness of the tubal wall is involved. By enlarging the site of the serosal rupture or performing a linear salpingostomy over the area of mesosalpingeal hemorrhage, the trophoblastic tissue can be removed. This is a high risk situation for persistent trophoblastic tissue and subsequent hemorrhage. In this case, a segmental resection may be more appropriate.

Isthmic and infundibular implantations also present special situations. Since the isthmic portion of the tube has a thicker muscular wall, complete removal of all of the trophoblasts is more difficult. Control of bleeding in this area often results in scarification. Implantations in the infundibulum can also be associated with bleeding that is difficult to control.

Fimbrial expression, i.e., "milking" the tissue from the tube, can be effective but also carries the risk of retained trophoblastic tissue (21). Splaying the distal portion of the tube can be attempted but caution must be used to control thermal damage to the fimbria (Fig. 1.6). If the contralateral tube is normal in appearance and patent, a salpingectomy should be strongly considered in each of these situations.

A linear salpingostomy is accomplished as follows. First stabilize the tube with one or two atraumatic graspers. Then make an incision on the antimesenteric border over the ectopic pregnancy. This can be done by sharp dissection, laser, unipolar electrode, or bipolar scissors (Fig. 1.7). The key to success is control of peripheral tubal damage. Control of bleeding points should be precise. Sharp dissection with a microscissors causes minimal tissue damage, but its effectiveness may be negated by the overzealous use of unipolar or bipolar coagulation to control bleeding.

Injection of a dilute vasopressin solution (0.05–0.5 units/mL) into the mesosalpinx directly beneath the ectopic pregnancy prior to incision has been found beneficial by some (Fig. 1.8) (24). This procedure should be done as atraumatically as possible and is best performed with a 22-gauge needle. The use of vasopressin has been associated with cardiac arrhythmias and carries the theoretical increased risk of delayed hemorrhage (25).

The ectopic pregnancy should be allowed to deliver itself. Probing or blindly grasping tissue often leads to additional bleeding. If the trophoblastic tissue is adherent, hydrodissection can be helpful, but this often means that there is deep invasion into the tubal wall. This may necessitate a segmental resection or salpingectomy. Prior to terminating the procedure, all bleeding points must be controlled. Closure of the incision has not been found to be necessary (26).

Postoperatively, hCG titers are monitored weekly until negative to make certain that no viable trophoblastic tissue remains. Rates of persistent trophoblasts that require treatment have ranged from 4.8% to 20%, but is currently felt to be approximately 7% (27–29). Persistent trophoblastic tissue may require reoperation, but can usually be managed with methotrexate. In a group of 157 women with unruptured ampullary ectopic pregnancy, Seifer et al. compared 103 women who had laparoscopic salpingostomy with 54 who had salpingostomy

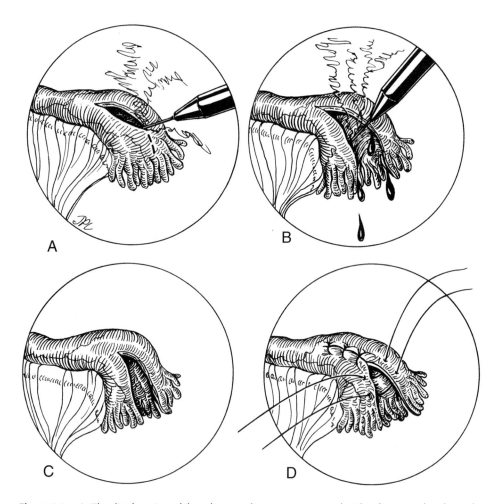

Figure 1.6. **A.** The distal portion of the tube over the ectopic is incised with a fine unipolar electrode. **B.** The bleeding points are electrocoagulated. **C.** Adequate hemostasis of the incisional edge and tubal epithelium is verified. **D.** The incision is closed with a monofilament or fine braided suture in an interrupted fashion to minimize anatomical distortion.

via laparotomy (30). Of the women undergoing a laparoscopic salpingostomy, 16/103 (15.5%) were treated for persistent ectopic pregnancy, in contrast to one of 54 women (1.8%) who had a laparotomy. In this report, factors associated with persistence were a laparoscopic approach, smaller ectopic pregnancy size, and fewer days of amenorrhea.

Even though the majority of patients with an ectopic pregnancy who are hemodynamically stable can safely undergo laparoscopy, this technology must be critically evaluated, for it is not without both potential and real pitfalls. For example, no study has yet to report the number of "failed" laparoscopic salpingostomy procedures; that is, the situation in which the surgeon begins a salpingostomy and ultimately must perform a salpingectomy secondary to hemorrhage or inability to complete the procedure by laparoscopy. Although one of the advantages of the laparoscopic approach is a decreased cost, if the Seifer et al. (30)

Chapter 1: Laparoscopic Management of the Ectopic Pregnancy 11

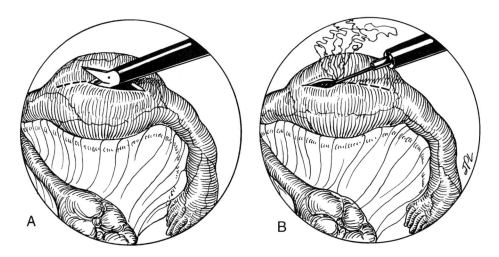

Figure 1.7. A linear salpingostomy is performed using **A.** microscissors and **B.** unipolar needle electrode.

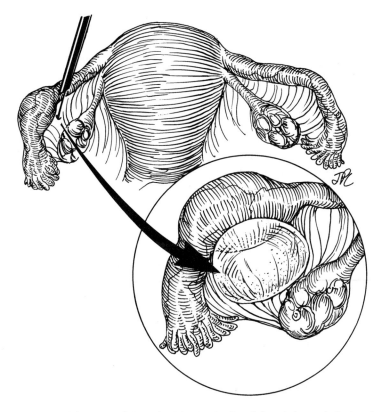

Figure 1.8. Injection of the mesosalpinx. The injection is placed directly beneath the involved portion of the tube.

report accurately reflects the true incidence of persistence after laparoscopic salpingostomy, the cost of laparotomy would be less given that 15% of patients would require additional medical or surgical treatment.

Injection of prostaglandins, methotrexate and hyperosmolar glucose have all been used to treat the unruptured tubal pregnancy (31–33). These methods are attractive for those patients that the surgical removal of the pregnancy may cause excessive tubal damage. There are no large, long-term studies available to determine possible sequelae.

More information is available on the use of systemic methotrexate. Systemic methotrexate should be considered in lieu of surgical excision in the presence of:

- Small (<2 cm) tubal pregnancy when the opposite tube is occluded, absent or severely diseased;
- Small (<2 cm) cornual pregnancy when opposite tube is occluded or severely damaged.

SEGMENTAL RESECTION

Segmental resection is appropriate for those patients desiring future fertility, who have a compromised opposite tube and are not candidates for a linear salpingostomy, or in whom attempted salpingostomy has not been successful. The major focus should be on the maximal tubal conservation. A minimum of 3 cm with a segment including the ampullary isthmic junction is the minimal requirement for tubal reconstruction. Optimally, a total length of at least 6 cm offers the best results (34). The procedure is appropriate only in those cases in which a future tubal reanastomosis is intended.

There are several available techniques. One of the simplest, although potentially more destructive, is desiccation of the tube immediately adjacent to the ectopic. This is most commonly accomplished with a bipolar forceps. Once desiccated, the involved tubal segment is excised and any remaining bleeding points are coagulated (Fig. 1.9). Though hemostatic, this technique may compromise the blood supply to the remaining tubal segment, resulting in less than the 3–6-cm segment needed for reanastomosis. If the ectopic is large or ruptured, removal of the intraluminal material by salpingostomy often allows for better visualization of segment to be resected.

Suture techniques using relatively nonreactive materials such as polydioxanone or polyglyconate will leave a maximal amount of viable tube intact (Fig. 1.10). Similarly, if the affected segment of tube is small, i.e., failed linear salpingostomy, the segment can be excised after ligation with a pretied ligature, similar to a Pomeroy tubal ligation. Alternatively, a Hulka clip can be applied on both sides of the ectopic for hemostasis followed by excision of the involved segment.

Regardless of the technique chosen, if the remaining tubal segment is unsatisfactory for future reanastomosis, a salpingectomy is probably more appropriate. Any patient undergoing a conservative surgery should return for an evaluation of tubal patency prior to attempting to conceive.

ABDOMINAL PREGNANCY

Fortunately, abdominal pregnancy rarely occurs, approximately 9.2/1000 ectopic pregnancies, but carries a maternal mortality rate of 0.5–18% (35). The pri-

Chapter 1: Laparoscopic Management of the Ectopic Pregnancy 13

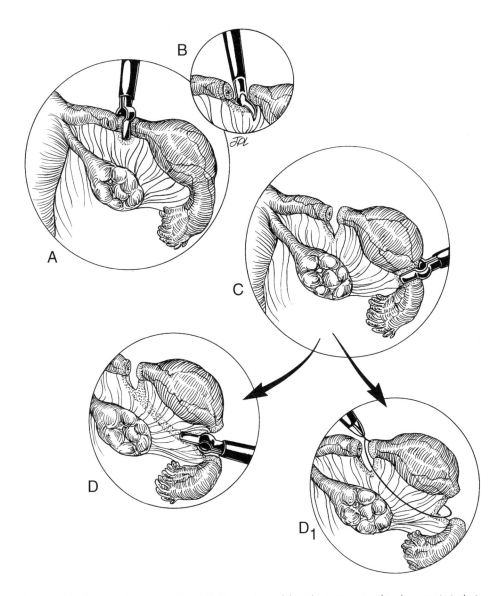

Figure 1.9. Segmental resection. **A** and **B.** The portion of the tube just proximal to the ectopic is desiccated with a bipolar forceps and incised. **C.** The portion of the tube distal to the ectopic is desiccated and incised. The involved portion of the tube can be removed using desiccation and excision (**D**) or by a ligature technique (**D$_1$**).

mary approach for the management of this situation is by laparotomy (29). Adjunctive management with selective embolization of the retained placenta and the use of methotrexate has also been described and may be useful in selected cases (36–38).

There is one confirmed case of an abdominal pregnancy managed successfully laparoscopically (Brill A. Laparoscopic treatment of an abdominal pregnancy. [Personal communication] Chicago: University of Illinois, 1994). With only

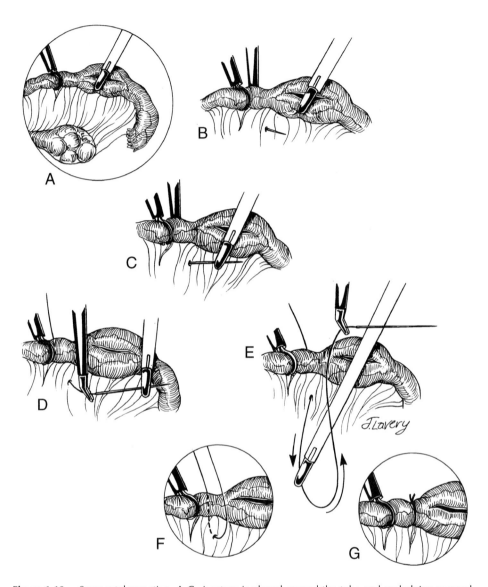

Figure 1.10. Segmental resection. **A-C.** A suture is placed around the tube and underlying mesosalpingeal artery just proximal to the involved portion of the tube. Either a straight or curved needle can be used. **D-F.** Once the needle has been placed through the tissue, the suture is grasped just distal to the needle and atraumatically pulled through the tissue. **G.** An extracorporeal knot is tied into place. **H.** The tube is incised and the incision is extended into the mesosalpinx. **I-K.** The involved portion of the tube and underlying mesosalpinx is ligated and excised.

limited experience, laparoscopy should be used only for diagnosis until more data are available.

OVARIAN PREGNANCY

Ovarian pregnancy is also infrequently encountered. It represents only 0.5–1% of all ectopic pregnancies and has an incidence of 1/7000 deliveries (18,

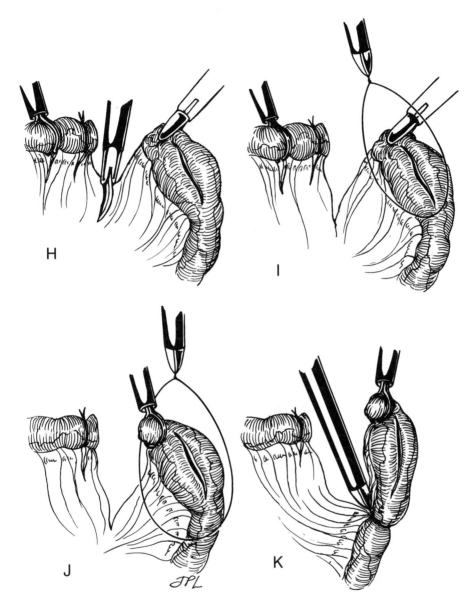

Figure 1.10. *continued*

19). If the ovary is unsalvageable, an oophorectomy is indicated, and can generally be accomplished laparoscopically. In this procedure, it is best to ligate the infundibulopelvic ligament first.

Successful management of ovarian pregnancy without oophorectomy has been reported (39, 40), including ovarian wedge resection or cystectomy (41). Others have successfully used systemic methotrexate and local injection of prostaglandins (42–44). All of these options should be considered at the time of diagnosis to offer the patient the best outcome.

If a conservative management is chosen, guaranteed patient follow-up is an absolute necessity. If this is not possible, definitive treatment (oophorectomy) should be employed.

INTERSTITIAL PREGNANCY

The management of interstitial pregnancies is a challenging surgical situation. Depending upon the size and specific location, a variety of surgical and medical options are available (45). These options include systemic methotrexate, local injection of methotrexate, hysteroscopic removal, laparoscopically guided intrauterine curettage and laparoscopic resection and suture repair. In general, few data exist regarding these approaches and subsequent reproductive performance.

RISKS

Morbidity associated with the laparoscopic management of ectopic pregnancy is usually related to the ability to control hemorrhage at the time of surgery and the ability to complete the appropriate procedure. This is dependent upon the expertise and skill of the surgeon along with the nuances of the particular case. Laparotomy to control hemorrhage has been reported infrequently in several large series (8).

While authors have reported similar rates of persistent ectopics with procedures performed at laparotomy and laparoscopically, there is a concern that there may be an increased incidence of persistent ectopic pregnancies at the time of laparoscopic linear salpingostomy (30, 46). Therefore, careful follow-up with weekly hCG titers until negative is required whenever a conservative procedure is done, whether by laparoscopy or laparotomy (47). The choice of procedure should not be influenced by choice of the surgical approach. Although these outcomes are difficult to measure, the majority of studies to date have not demonstrated a difference between laparoscopic and laparotomy approaches in future fertility or intraoperative morbidity (29, 48).

CONCLUSION

With very few exceptions, patients with the diagnosis of ectopic pregnancy should be primarily addressed by laparoscopy. The major limitations to this approach are operator dependent. Special consideration should be given to the choice of the procedure and technique employed to offer the patient the best results in terms of future fertility or prevention of recurrence. Familiarity with several surgical techniques will allow the surgeon more options in treatment and subsequent good patient outcome.

LABORATORY EXERCISES FOR PROFICIENCY DEVELOPMENT

Exercises designed to aid in the development of the skills needed to laparoscopically manage an ectopic pregnancy focus on gentle tissue handling and applications of various energy sources. It is not necessary to be totally versatile with each technique but there should be a general understanding of each. The exercises presented will highlight the pertinent clinical applications.

Materials needed:

uterine/ectopic model with 2 ectopic pregnancies/side
(1) 10-mm sleeve
(2) 5-mm sleeves
(1) 10/12-mm sleeve
(2) 5-mm atraumatic spring handled graspers
(1) 5-mm scissors
(1) Unipolar fine-tipped needle electrode, 3 or 5 mm, with cord
(1) 5-mm bipolar coagulating forceps, with cord
(2) 5-mm graspers, one that is self-retaining
(1) 5-mm laparoscopic needle holder
3-0 and 4-0 monofilament suture
Pretied endoscopic ligature systems
(1) 4-mm reducing sleeve to introduce ligature systems
Reducing caps and/or sleeves
(1) 7-inch 22-gauge needle
(1) 18-gauge spinal needle
(1) 12-mL syringe
Laser (optional)

General considerations: The objectives of the exercises are to:

1. Develop a familiarity with the presented techniques.
2. Learn to handle the tissues gently.
3. Develop an appreciation for proper trocar placement and proper positioning of the tissue.
4. Practice with new instrumentation
5. Review the available irrigation/aspirating systems.
6. Review the proper assembly and disassembly of the commonly used reusable instrumentation.

If a laser is to be used, review the proper setup, energy settings, safety checklist and assembly of the specific instrumentation required. Review the available instrumentation and equipment in a standard operative laparoscopic tray to determine if any additional instrumentation may be required for the management of an ectopic pregnancy. The exercises are best performed several times.

Exercise #1 Injection of the mesosalpinx (Fig. 1.11)

1. Position the uterine model with the ectopic pregnancies within the pelvic trainer. The model should be properly grounded.
2. If a laser is to be used, moisten the surrounding towels and sheets.
3. Place two 5-mm sleeves in the lower lateral ports and a 10-mm sleeve for the laparoscope either through the top or the end of the pelvic trainer.
4. Position all of the light, camera and electrical cables prior to starting the exercises.
5. Properly white set the camera and have all of the necessary instrumentation available.

By repeatedly preparing for performing these exercises in a similar manner as preparing for surgery, adequate preparation will become habit.

6. Grasp the tube on each side of the ectopic with two atraumatic graspers. Introduce the 18-gauge spinal needle immediately above the ectopic. Attach the 22-gauge needle to

18 GYNECOLOGIC ENDOSCOPY: Principles in Practice

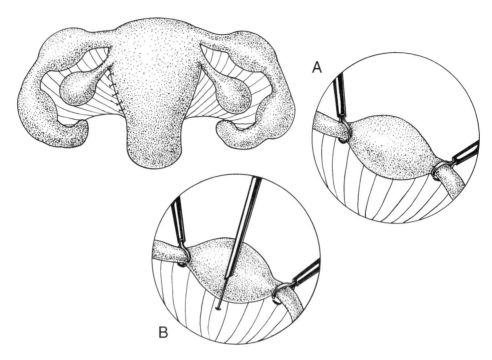

Figure 1.11. **A.** The model is positioned and the ectopics are visualized. **B.** The ectopic is stabilized with two atraumatic graspers. The mesosalpinx is injected.

a water-filled 12-mL syringe and introduce this into the 18-gauge needle after the stylette is withdrawn. Using the 18-gauge needle as a guide, angle the 22-gauge needle toward the mesosalpinx. Advance the needle and inject. Notice the wheal that is raised.

This technique can be used prior to or after a linear salpingostomy is performed to control bleeding. The spinal needle helps direct and stabilize the 22-gauge needle. With this technique, any portion of the abdominal wall can be used as an entry site.

Exercise #2 Linear salpingostomy (Fig. 1.12)

After completing exercise #1:

1. Place a 10/12-mm sleeve in the lower, middle port. Reduce the port sleeve size to 3 or 5 mm with a reducing cap or sleeve.
2. Introduce a 3- or 5-mm unipolar needle electrode.
3. Set the electrical generator to 50 watts of pure cutting current.
4. Perform a linear salpingostomy. Attempt to produce a single linear incision on the antimesenteric side of the tube. Notice that the tissue is cut more effectively, with less peripheral charring, when the current is on prior to contacting the tissue. Control the depth the needle is advanced into the tissue. It is the electrical spark that actually cuts the tissue and therefore incises more effectively when no contact is made. If there is an incision on the ectopic itself, then the needle was too deep.
5. Attempt to make the incision in the midportion of the ectopic pregnancy and remove the ectopic through the smallest incision possible.
6. Remove the ectopic pregnancy with a spoon forceps through the middle port.

Chapter 1: Laparoscopic Management of the Ectopic Pregnancy   19

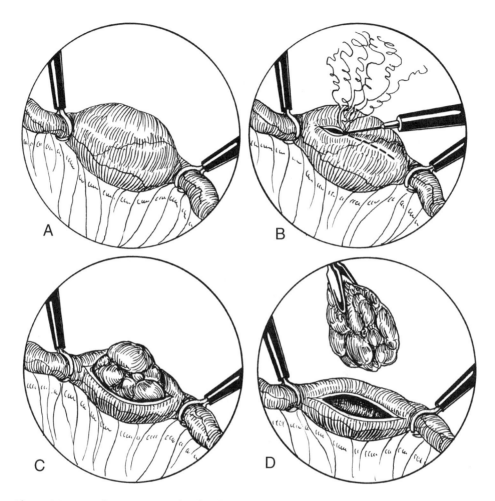

Figure 1.12. **A.** The ectopic is isolated with two atraumatic graspers. **B.** An incision is made with a unipolar needle electrode. **C.** The ectopic protrudes through the incision. **D.** The ectopic is removed with a spoon forceps.

This procedure can then be repeated on the remaining ectopics using a laser, an alternative unipolar needle or knife or with microscissors. The purpose is to gain an appreciation for the instrumentation and positioning of the instruments.

Exercise #3 Segmental resection (Fig. 1.13)

After completing the linear salpingostomy:

1. Replace the distal atraumatic grasper with a 5-mm self-retaining grasper.
2. Grasp the tube at the site of the linear salpingostomy. Move the atraumatic grasper more proximal to the uterus.
3. Introduce a 3-0 monofilament suture through the middle port.
4. Place the needle through the mesosalpinx immediately beneath the proximal edge of the linear salpingostomy.
5. Release the self-retaining grasper and grasp the end of the needle and pull the remainder of the needle through the mesosalpinx.

20 GYNECOLOGIC ENDOSCOPY: Principles in Practice

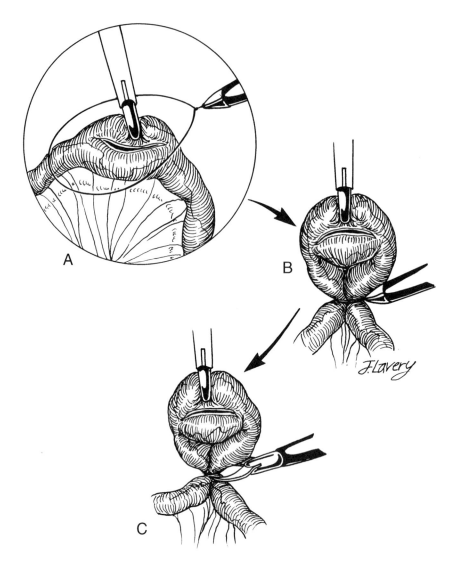

Figure 1.13. **A.** The involved portion of the tube is grasped. **B.** A pretied loop is placed and tied around the knuckle of tube formed. **C.** The ligated portion of the tube is excised.

6. Grasp the suture immediately behind the needle with the needle holder, release the self-retaining grasper. Use the self-retaining grasper to pull additional suture into the pelvic trainer. Once an adequate amount of suture has been introduced, withdraw the needle. Use a knot-pusher or other instrument as a pulley, to avoid "sawing through" the tissue with the suture.
7. Tie an extracorporeal knot and tighten it down.
8. Cut the suture with a scissors through the middle port.
9. Re-grasp the linear salpingostomy site and place the tube on traction laterally.
10. Using a unipolar needle or scissors, incise the mesosalpinx immediately adjacent to the tube. Once the tubal segment has been entirely freed, remove the unipolar needle or scissors.

11. Introduce a pretied endoloop system through the middle port and place the loop over the grasper.
12. Release the proximal portion of tube and grasp the freed tubal segment by placing the atraumatic grasper through the loop. Release the self-retaining grasper.
13. Tie the loop down around the distal edge of the tubal segment.
14. Remove the pushrod and introduce a scissors through the middle port and excise the tubal segment, then cut the suture.
15. Remove the excised tubal segment with a spoon forceps through the middle port.

Once this procedure has been accomplished several times, modifications can be developed to improve efficiency. This procedure can also be performed using Hulka clips. Alternatively, a single suture can be applied as a loop (Fig. 1.13) if the linear salpingostomy site is small. This technique can sometimes be applied to a small ruptured or unruptured ectopic if there remains an adequate amount of normal tube.

Exercise #4 Salpingectomy (Fig. 1.5)

This procedure can be accomplished by two techniques. Each begins with the same initial step. Since the tube is to be removed, there is little need for atraumatic instruments.

1. Grasp the tube just distal to the ectopic.
2. Introduce the bipolar forceps through the middle port. Desiccate the tubal-uterine junction and cut the area that has been desiccated.
3. Repeat this procedure until the mesosalpinx is incised to the area just above the ovarian ligament.
4. The proximal portion of the tube is then grasped and placed on gentle traction.
5. The mesosalpinx is then successively desiccated and incised until the entire tube is removed.

Alternatively, the mesosalpinx is incised only to the point that a pedicle is formed by the distal portion of the mesosalpinx. A pretied ligature loop is then introduced and placed over the proximal portion of the tube. The grasper is released and regrasps the proximal portion of the tube through the loop. A second grasper is then used to position the loop around the entire pedicle. Once this has been accomplished, the loop is tightened and cut. A second loop is placed in a similar manner. The suture is cut. The formed pedicle is then cut and the tube removed. If the ectopic is large, the specimen will need to be morcellated or placed within a bag for removal.

REFERENCES

1. Stovall TG, Ling FW, Buster JE. Outpatient chemotherapy of unruptured ectopic pregnancy. Fertil Steril 1989;51:435–438.
2. Stovall TG, Ling FW, Buster JE. Reproductive performance after methotrexate treatment of ectopic pregnancy. Am J Obstet Gynecol 1990;162:1620–1624.
3. Stovall TG, Ling FW, Gray LA, et al. Methotrexate treatment of ectopic pregnancy: a report of 100 cases. Obstet Gynecol 1991;77:954–956.
4. Stovall TG, Ling FW, Gray LA. Single dose methotrexate for treatment of ectopic pregnancy. Obstet Gynecol 1991;77:754–757.
5. Stovall TG, Ling FW, Gray LA. Single dose methotrexate: an expanded clinical trial. Am J Obstet Gynecol 1993;168:1759–1765.
6. Stovall TG, Ling FW. Ectopic pregnancy: diagnostic and therapeutic algorithms minimizing surgical intervention. J Reprod Med 1993;38:807–812.
7. Creinin MD, Washington AE. Cost of ectopic pregnancy management: surgery versus methotrexate. Fertil Steril 1993;60:963–969.
8. Brumsted J, Kessler C, Gibson C, et al. A comparison of laparoscopy and laparotomy for the treatment of ectopic pregnancy. Obstet Gynecol 1988;71:889–892.

9. Vermesh M, Silva PD, Rosen GF, et al. Management of unruptured ectopic gestation by linear salpingostomy: prospective randomized clinical trial of laparoscopy versus laparotomy. Obstet Gynecol 1989;73:400–404.
10. Murphy AA, Nager CW, Wujek JJ, et al. Operative laparoscopy versus laparotomy for the management of ectopic pregnancy: a prospective trial. Fertil Steril 1992;57:1180–1185.
11. Lundorff P, Hahlin M, Kallfelt B, et al. Adhesion formation after laparoscopic surgery in tubal pregnancy: a randomized trial versus laparotomy. Fertil Steril 1991;55:911–915.
12. Greisman, B. Ectopic pregnancy in women with previous tubal sterilizations at a Canadian hospital. J Reprod Med 1991;36(3):206–209.
13. Stock RJ. The changing spectrum of ectopic pregnancy. Obstet Gynecol 1988;71:885.
14. Soderstrom RM. Sterilization failures and their causes. Am J Obstet Gynecol 1985;152:395–403.
15. McCausland A. Endosalpingosis ("endosalpingoblastosis") following laparoscopic tubal coagulation as an etiologic factor of ectopic pregnancy. Am J Obstet Gynecol 1982;143:12–24.
16. Bachmann GA. Hysterectomy—A critical review. J Reprod Med 1990;35(9):839–862.
17. American College of Obstetrics and Gynecology. Sterilization. ACOG technical bulletin no. 113, 1988.
18. Grimes HG, Nosal RA, Gallagher JC. Ovarian pregnancy: a series of 34 cases. Obstet Gynecol 1983;61:174.
19. Stafford JC, Ragan WD. Abdominal pregnancy: a review of current management. Obstet Gynecol 1977;50:548.
20. McCann MF, Kessel E. International experience with laparoscopic sterilization: follow-up of 8500 women. Adv Planned Parent 1978;12:199.
21. Bruhat MA, Mage G, Pouly JL, Manhes H, Canis M, Wattiez A. Operative laparoscopy. 1st Ed. New York: McGraw-Hill, 1992:150–153.
22. Silva PD, Schaper AM, Rooney B. Reproductive outcome after 143 laparoscopic procedures for ectopic pregnancy. Obstet Gynecol 1993;81:710–715.
23. Ory SJ, Nnadi E, Herrman R, et al. Fertility after ectopic pregnancy. Fertil Steril 1993;60:231–235.
24. Silva PD. Laparoscopic approach can be applied to most cases of ectopic pregnancy. Obstet Gynecol 1988;72:944–946.
25. Townsend DE. Vasopressin pack for treatment of bleeding after myoma resection. Am J Obstet Gynecol 1991;165:1405–1407.
26. Tulandi T, Guralnick M. Treatment of ectopic pregnancy by salpingotomy with or without tubal suturing and salpingectomy. Fertil Steril 1991;55:53–55.
27. DiMarchi JM, Kosasa TS, Kobara TY, et al. Persistent ectopic pregnancy. Obstet Gynecol 1987;70:555–561.
28. Mecke H, Semm K, Lehmann-Weillenbrock E. Results of operative pelviscopy in 202 cases of ectopic pregnancy. Int J Fertil 1989;34:93–100.
29. Sanfilippo JS, Woodworth SH. Ectopic pregnancy (suppl). In: Thompson JD, Rock JA, eds. Te Linde's Operative gynecology. 7th Ed. Philadelphia: JB Lippincott, 1993:1–14.
30. Seifer DB, Gutmann JN, Grant WD, et al. Comparison of persistent ectopic pregnancy after laparoscopic salpingostomy verses salpingostomy at laparotomy for ectopic pregnancy. Obstet Gynecol 1993;81:378–382.
31. Lang PF, Tamussino K, Honig W, et al. Treatment of unruptured tubal pregnancy by laparoscopic instillation of hyperosmolar glucose solution. Am J Obstet Gynecol 1992;166:1378–1381.
32. Pansky M, Bukovsky J, Golan A, et al. Reproductive outcome after laparoscopic local injection for tubal pregnancy. Fertil Steril 1993;60:85–87.
33. Lindblom B, Kallfelt B, Hahlin M, et al. Local prostaglandin F_2 injection for termination of ectopic pregnancy. Lancet 1987;1:776–777.
34. Silber SJ, Cohen R. Microsurgical reversal of female sterilization: the role of tubal length. Fertil Steril 1980;33:598.
35. Atrash HK, Friede A, Hogue CJR. Abdominal pregnancy in the United States: frequency and maternal mortality. Obstet Gynecol 1987;69:333–337.
36. Martin JN, Sessums JK, Martin RW, et al. Abdominal pregnancy: current concepts of management. Obstet Gynecol 1988;71:549–557.
37. Kivikoski AI, Martin C, Weyman P, et al. Angiographic arterial embolization to control hemorrhage in abdominal pregnancy: a case report. Obstet Gynecol 1988;71:456–459.

38. Lathrop JC, Bowles GE. Methotrexate in abdominal pregnancy. Report of a case. Obstet Gynecol 1968;32:81–85.
39. Van Coevering RJ, Risher JE. Laparoscopic management of ovarian pregnancy: a case report. J Reprod Med 1988;33:774–776.
40. Hage PS, Arnouk IF, Zarou DM, et al. Laparoscopic management of ectopic pregnancy. J of AAGL 1994;1:283–285.
41. Rock JA. Ectopic pregnancy. In: Thompson JD, Rock JA, eds. Te Lindes Operative Gynecology. 7th Ed. Philadelphia: JB Lippincott, 1993.
42. Shamma FN, Schwartz LB. Primary ovarian pregnancy successfully treated with methotrexate. Am J Obstet Gynecol 1992;167:1307–1308.
43. Henig I, Prough SG. Methotrexate treatment of ovarian pregnancy. Am J Gynecol Health 1991;5:30–31.
44. Koike H, Chuganji Y, Watanabe H, et al. Conservative treatment of ovarian pregnancy by local prostaglandin F_{2a} injection [letter]. Am J Obstet Gynecol 1990;163:696.
45. Budnick SG, Jacobs SL, Nulsen JC, et al. Conservative management of interstitial pregnancy. Obstet Gynecol Surv 1993;48:694–698.
46. Lundorff P, Hahlin M, Sjoblom P, et al. Persistent trophoblast after conservative treatment of tubal pregnancy: prediction and detection. Obstet Gynecol 1991;77:129–133.
47. Dumesic D, Hafez R. Delayed hemorrhage of a persistent ectopic pregnancy following laparoscopic salpingostomy and methotrexate therapy. Obstet Gynecol 1991;78:960–962.
48. Sultana CH, Easley K, Collins RL. Outcome of laparoscopic versus. traditional surgery for ectopic pregnancies. Fertil Steril 1992;57:285–289.

Chapter 2

Pelvic Mass

Preoperative and Intraoperative Decision Making

Verda J. Hunter and Michael J. Sammarco

The practice of medicine is founded in the trilogy of education, research, and patient care. Most modern medical knowledge and practice has developed under a "scientific-model" influence where new treatments and techniques are first researched and compared to "standards" prior to public health application. The explosive development of laparoscopic surgical techniques has not followed traditional research and development standards. Physicians have developed the technique for the laparoscopic approach to the pelvic mass without the benefit of scientific data to indicate the best surgical alternative. The purpose of this chapter is to review the current literature and to make cautious preliminary recommendations for a laparoscopic approach to the ovarian mass despite the lack of prospective randomized studies.

DIFFERENTIAL DIAGNOSIS OF PELVIC MASS

For the purpose of this discussion, a 4–5-cm ovarian cyst will be considered within normal functional range for premenopausal-aged women. Normal ovarian stroma adds approximately 2 cm. Thus, an ovarian mass greater than 6–7 cm is considered an abnormal finding. For postmenopausal women, a 1.5 × 1.0 × 0.5-cm ovary is considered normal size. Any palpable pelvic finding (other than the uterus) is abnormal and has the potential to be malignant and require evaluation (1, 2).

A pelvic mass is diagnosed at physical examination or as an incidental finding following a routine screening or diagnostic study (Table 2.1). Patient signs and

Table 2.1. Differential Diagnosis of a Pelvic Mass

Right-Sided	Left-Sided	Central
Functional ovarian cyst	Functional ovarian cyst	Ovarian cancer
Ovarian tumor/torsion	Ovarian tumor/torsion	Fibroid uterus
Leiomyoma	Leiomyoma	Uterine sarcoma
Cecal carcinoma	Sigmoid carcinoma	Stool
Appendiceal abscess	Diverticulitis	
Pelvic kidney	Pelvic kidney	Distended bladder
Ectopic pregnancy	Ectopic pregnancy	Intrauterine pregnancy
Tubo-ovarian abscess	Tubo-ovarian abscess	

symptoms will vary depending on the etiology. A thorough history and physical examination are always required. Additional risks, i.e., family history and previous surgeries, must always be considered when developing a differential diagnosis.

DIAGNOSTIC EVALUATION OF A PELVIC MASS

Traditional pelvic mass workup includes history and physical examination and laboratory and radiologic studies. Often, the initial examination of the patient may narrow the differential diagnosis. The remainder of this discussion will focus on the evaluation and management of the pelvic mass of possible ovarian origin.

Laboratory studies to be attained are: a CBC with differential, chemistry panel with electrolytes, liver function studies, and tumor markers, as indicated. Any abnormal findings on history and physical examination or laboratory studies should be further evaluated as possible indicators of malignant spread of a pelvic primary or as an unassociated additional medical problem. CA-125 is often obtained to assist in the differential diagnosis, but other markers, such as hCG and AFP, need to be obtained in adolescents since germ cell tumors are more frequently seen in this age group.

Commonly, an intravenous pyelogram (IVP) and barium enema (BE) are recommended as diagnostic tests for pelvic mass. These tests should be reserved if the etiology of the mass is in question or if the patient is symptomatic. The IVP is useful to rule out pelvic kidney, ureteral obstruction or deviation, which may indicate a retroperitoneal process. Many large pelvic masses will create a "mass effect" on bladder or ureter. The mass effect can be ignored unless marked hydronephrosis is present. The BE is useful to rule out a bowel etiology and to screen the patient for a concurrent bowel-related problem that may need to be addressed during surgery, i.e., diverticulitis, diverticulosis, or inflammatory bowel disease. This test is probably not indicated in a patient less than 35 years of age without bowel symptoms with a negative stool guaiac. Extrinsic compression of the sigmoid colon by a pelvic mass is not significant.

Ultrasound of the pelvis should be routinely obtained in the workup for a pelvic mass, especially if a laparoscopic approach is anticipated. In the past, gynecologists felt that an ultrasound was unnecessary because the findings were not used to alter the surgery planned for evaluation and treatment of the mass. With advancing ultrasound technology, improved resolution has provided increased diagnostic information to help delineate a benign from a malignant process. If a CT scan has been obtained, an IVP is not necessary to evaluate the urinary tract and retroperitoneum. For any woman without a palpable pelvic mass, neither abdominal nor transvaginal ultrasound should be obtained as a routine screening test to "rule out an ovarian cancer" (3–6). Ultrasound is recommended in the following cases: (*a*) as an adjunct to pelvic examination when pelvic mass is detected, (*b*) when pelvic examination is difficult secondary to obesity, and (*c*) when cancer can not be ruled out because the patient presents with vague abdominal complaints, irregular bleeding, possible leiomyomata, or other unclear symptoms or findings (3–7).

CT scans of the abdomen and pelvis are not routinely indicated to evaluate a pelvic mass, unless malignancy is near certain. Then, CT scan may be helpful, but not required, to provide additional information as to the extent of disease.

RISK FACTORS FOR MALIGNANCY

The primary focus in the evaluation of a pelvic mass of probable ovarian origin is to determine the risk of malignancy. The following are the significant factors to be considered:

1. Patient age
2. Size of the mass
3. Ultrasound characteristics
4. Serum tumor markers

Age of Patient

There is an age-dependent risk to the malignant pelvic mass (Table 2.2). Koonings et al. (8) reported on the 10 year experience at a single institution. Their data represent the risk that an ovarian neoplasm is malignant by age group. The data were obtained by reviewing all of the records of patients that carried a discharge histologic diagnosis of an ovarian neoplasm. This is in contrast to the report of Killackey et al. (9) who reviewed all of the charts of patients that carried a preoperative diagnosis of "pelvic mass/uterine leiomyomata." These data present a more realistic view of clinical risk of malignancy as it relates to age at the time of patient presentation. Both of these reports demonstrate the relative histologic frequency of the various ovarian neoplasms. Germ cell malignancies are most common in the 2nd decade of life, benign conditions predominate during the main reproductive years, and malignancies resurface as a significant etiology of pelvic masses after menopause.

Size of Mass

The size of an adnexal mass is also associated with the risk of malignancy (Table 2.3). In a study of 180 patients of all ages, Granberg et al. (10) found 1% of masses <5 cm and 11% of masses 5–10 cm were malignant. Of masses >10 cm, 72% were found malignant. Similar results were reported by Rulin and Preston (11) in a study of 150 postmenopausal (PM) patients. In a transvaginal sonography evaluation of women of all ages (mean age 41), Sassone et al. (12) found similar results for masses <5 cm or between 5–10 cm. Their values for patients >10 cm are difficult to evaluate as they had only 8 patients with one malignancy in that group. Miller et al. (1) reported on 20 postmenopausal women with palpable ovaries less than 5 cm. They found malignancy in 1 of 11 patients (9%) with ovar-

Table 2.2. Risk of Malignancy by Age

Age (yr)	Killackey (9) n	(%)	Koonings (8) n	(%)
<19	10	(20)	61	(8.2)
20–29	72	(0)	294	(4.1)
30–39	179	(1.7)	171	(14)
40–49	192	(5.7)	128	(35.2)
50–59	37	(18.9)	104	(46.2)
60–69	31	(38.7)	79	(49.4)
>70	19	(47.4)	24	(29.2)

Table 2.3. Risk of Malignancy versus Size of Adnexal Mass

Study	(Ref.)	Age	Mass Size[a] (% Malignant)		
			<5 cm	5–10 cm	>10 cm
Rulin	(11)	PM[b]	3	11	63
Andolf	(13)	PM	1	19	—
Granberg	(10)	All	1	11	72
Sassone	(12)	All	3	7	13
Miller	(1)	PM	9	22	—
Luxman	(14)	PM	14	36	38

[a]size determined by ultrasound
[b]PM = postmenopausal

ian size <5 cm and in 2 of 9 patients (22%) with size 5–10 cm. Andolf (13) similarly found a low rate of malignancy in those patients with masses less than 5 cm; the 3 of 801 patients that were found to have cancer in a totally anechoic mass had masses that were greater than 10 cm. Luxman et al. (14) found an overall rate of 28% malignancy in a series of 102 postmenopausal patients (42–90 years of age). Only 2 of the 33 patients with unilocular cysts were found to have cancer; both had cysts less than 5 cm.

It is clear from these reports that size alone is inadequate for separating benign from malignant tumors. The reports are difficult to compare since different ultrasound techniques were employed. These reports exemplify the need for caution when addressing any ovarian mass, regardless of size. Particular caution is needed for the menopausal patient.

Ultrasound Characteristics of Mass

There is no single accepted ultrasound scoring index to predict malignancy. Many authors have identified features usually characteristic of benign versus malignant neoplasms. Collated data from recent studies of ultrasound accuracy in prediction of malignancy have an average positive predictive value of 74% and average sensitivity of 88% (Table 2.4). The accuracy may be improved with the

Table 2.4. Comparison of Ultrasound Performance Characteristics in Differentiating Benign from Malignant Ovarian Lesions[a]

Author(s)	No. of patients	Prevalence of disease (%)	Positive predictive value (%)	Negative predictive value (%)	Sensitivity (%)	Specificity (%)
Kobayashi, 1976	406	15	31	93	71	73
Meire et al., 1978	51	35	83	91	83	91
Pussell et al., 1980	25	48	83	91	83	84
Herrmann, 1987[b]	241	21	75	95	82	93
Finkler, 1988	102	36	88	81	62	95
Benacerraf, 1990	100	30	72	91	80	87
Granberg, 1990	180	21.5	74	95	82	92
Sassone, 1991	143	10	37	100	100	83

[a]Calculated including borderline tumors as malignancies
[b]Second-look representations
From Sassone AM, Timor-Tritsch IE, Arthur A, et al. Transvaginal sonographic characterization of ovarian disease: evaluation of a new scoring system to predict ovarian malignancy. Obstet Gynecol 1991;78:70–76. Used with permission from Elsevier Science Publishing Co.

use of a transvaginal probe in conjunction with Doppler flow studies (Table 2.5). The use of Doppler flow continues to be studied. The most accurate indices and critical cutoff values are still under investigation. Currently, Doppler flow does not appear superior to high resolution ultrasound studies (18, 20, 21).

There are limited data on ultrasound accuracy specific to women in menopause. Most of the available studies do not separately report on postmenopausal women and it is difficult to draw any conclusions. Luxman, in his study of postmenopausal women, found a sensitivity of 93%, but a positive predictive value and specificity of 39% and 42%, respectively (14). This is much lower than the aforementioned collected ultrasound data.

Kawai et al. have recently summarized ovarian ultrasound findings according to malignant risk (17). These guidelines are not "official", but they encompass many similar findings of current authors. These findings are based on the use of a transvaginal probe (Table 2.6).

Tumor Markers

CA-125 can be used as a tumor marker, but not as a general population screening test. CA-125 is a tumor-associated antigen recognized by the monoclonal antibody OC-125 and expressed by approximately 80% of patients with epithelial ovarian cancer. Many benign gynecologic conditions, i.e., pregnancy, leiomyomata, pelvic inflammatory disease, and endometriosis, are associated

Table 2.5. TVUS-Color Doppler Performance Characteristics in Differentiating Benign from Malignant Ovarian Lesions

Author	(Ref.)	n	Sensitivity	(%)	Specificity	(%)
Fleischer	(15)	63	13/15	(87)	39/42	(93)
Weiner	(16)	52	15/16	(94)	35/36	(97)
Kawai	(17)	24	8/8	(88)	9/15	(60)
Kurjak	(18)	174	37/38	(97)	136/136	(100)
Kurjak	(19)	254	37/38	(97)	167/216	(77)
Total			110/115	(96)	386/445	(87)

Table 2.6. Ultrasound Characteristics of Ovarian Neoplasms

Benign Pattern
1. Simple cyst without internal echo
2. Simple cyst with scattered echoes
3. Polycystic echo
4. Sessile or polypoid smooth mural echoes
5. Central dense round echoes
6. Thin or thick multiple linear echoes
7. Thin or thick multiple linear echoes with dense part
8. Polycystic echoes with thick septum

Malignant pattern
9. Cystic echoes with papillary or indented mural part
10. Polycystic echoes with irregularly thick septum and solid part
11. Solid pattern (solid part >50%) heterogeneous component with irregular cystic part
12. Completely solid with homogeneous component

Adapted from Kawai M, Kano T, Kikkawa F, et al. Transvaginal Doppler ultrasound with color flow imaging in the diagnosis of ovarian cancer. Obstet Gynecol 1992;79:163–167.

with an elevated CA-125. Patients with Stage III and IV endometriosis were found to have mean levels of CA-125 of 33.8 U/mL and 68.7 U/mL at the time of menses, respectively (22). Even the phase of the menstrual cycle has been shown to affect CA-125 levels, with the values highest at the time of menses (23–25).

Non-gynecologic conditions also affect CA-125 results. Involvement of the pleura or peritoneum by non-gynecologic tumors can increase CA-125 levels as well as benign conditions which result in ascites, such as cirrhosis of the liver or congestive heart failure.

Menopausal patients have lower baseline values of CA-125 when compared to premenopausal women (26–28). Grover found that the 95th percentile for CA-125 in pre and perimenopausal women was 50 U/mL as compared to 34 U/mL for postmenopausal women. Other factors that were found to significantly lower CA-125 levels were a history of hysterectomy and a history of postmenopausal hormonal replacement. Factors that had no influence on the CA-125 levels were parity, history of unilateral oophorectomy, oral contraceptive use, and a family history of ovarian cancer (29). When using the CA-125 level to evaluate an ovarian mass, all of these factors must be considered to determine the significance of the finding.

CA-125 levels can be used to differentiate benign from malignant conditions in patients who present with a pelvic mass (Table 2.7). Since menopausal women have fewer gynecologic conditions that give rise to false positive elevations of CA-125, the test is more sensitive and specific in the menopause (31, 32). Several authors have demonstrated that a panel of assays can improve the sensitivity and specificity of detecting ovarian malignancies (32, 33). For example, Soper and others demonstrated 100% specificity and positive predictive value for CA-125 with TAG 72 or CA-15-3 (32).

LITERATURE REVIEW ON LAPAROSCOPIC APPROACH TO PELVIC MASS

Over the last decade, laparoscopy has been used by gynecologists with increasing frequency to evaluate patients who present with pelvic masses. As of 1990, no official guidelines for use of laparoscopy as a diagnostic and therapeutic technique had been established by the American College of Obstetrics and Gynecology (ACOG), but a need for such guidelines was addressed at an ACOG retreat (34).

Seltzer further addressed the need for such guidelines at the Society of Gynecologic Oncologists (SGO) in February, 1991. She reported on an SGO sur-

Table 2.7. CA-125 Accuracy in Predicting Malignancy in Women Presenting with Pelvic Masses

Author	(Ref.)	Sensitivity	Specificity	PPV[a] (%)	NPV[b] (%)
Einhorn	(30)	—	78	93	—
Malkasian	(31)	78	97	98	72
Soper	(32)	85	70	77	80

[a]Positive predictive value
[b]Negative predictive value

vey of 156 respondents who had identified 42 cases of malignancies that were initially diagnosed at the time of laparoscopy (35). Although 71% of these patients ultimately had definitive staging surgery, the average delay to this surgery was 4.8 weeks. Twelve percent of the patients never underwent definitive surgery. It was concluded that the role of laparoscopy in the treatment of ovarian masses remains to be defined.

Hulka et al. reported on the survey of the American Association of Gynecologic Laparoscopists (AAGL) (36). In this survey of 13,739 laparoscopies performed for persistent ovarian masses, an overall incidence of ovarian malignancy in a benign-appearing cyst removed laparoscopically was 3.8/1000 cases. A subsequent 1991 AAGL survey reported on 56,536 laparoscopic procedures (37). A total of 24 cases of ovarian cancer were identified with an incidence of 3.2/1000 cases. These findings were based on a 20% and 17% membership response rate, respectively, and obviously gave a different view of laparoscopy in the assessment and treatment of an ovarian mass than that presented by Seltzer et al. (34).

There are increasing numbers of reports supporting the laparoscopic management of the pelvic mass (Table 2.8). The largest series to date is from Nezhat et al. (38): in an analysis of 1209 masses in 1011 patients, there was only a 0.4% incidence of an ovarian malignancy. The four patients found to have cancer underwent laparotomy 3–60 days after the initial procedure. This is in comparison to the four other reports in which all the patients found to have cancer were accurately diagnosed at laparoscopy and underwent an immediate laparotomy (39–42). All of these reports emphasize the relatively low incidence of ovarian cancer that is being reported at the time of laparoscopic surgery for an ovarian mass. Several other aspects of these studies are noteworthy. It is difficult to overlook that of 1209 masses reported, 35.2% (358) were functional cysts; 48% (172) of these were <5 cm. Additionally, although all 19 patients with an ovarian malignancy were accurately identified at the time of surgery, 10 masses were purposely ruptured intraperitoneally to make the diagnosis and an additional 27 patients underwent a laparotomy for a benign process.

Reports confined to menopausal patients are less frequent. Parker and Berek reported in 1990 on 25 menopausal patients with adnexal masses who were correctly predicted to have benign masses based on the following criteria: (a) <10 cm, (b) ultrasound findings with distinct borders, no evidence of irregular or solid parts, thick septa, ascites or matted bowel, and (c) normal CA-125 (43). A more recent study by Shalav used similar criteria, but had no size criteria; they found no malignancies in 55 patients (44). Mann and Reich reported on 44 postmenopausal patients; one patient was found to have cancer and underwent immediate laparotomy (45). These authors felt that only ". . . ascites and apparent

Table 2.8. Laparoscopic Management of Women of All Ages With Adnexal Masses

Study	(Ref.)	Patients (n)	Ovarian Mass (n)	CA (n)	[%]
Mage	(39)	481	508	9	[1.7]
Nezhat	(38)	1011	1209	4	[0.4]
Mecke	(40)	773	773	2	[0.3]
Mettler	(41)	490	490	2	[0.4]
Canis	(42)	757	819	19	[2.3]

intraperitoneal disease are relative contraindications to laparoscopy . . ." (45). Such a cavalier approach is difficult to condone and presently not supported by the literature.

At the 1994 National Institute of Health Consensus Development Conference on ovarian cancer, the following recommendation was made:

Although laparoscopic management of the ovarian mass is being utilized, there is no current evidence that if the mass is malignant the patient's opportunity for cure is comparable to that with a more traditional approach. Studies shall be done to evaluate the risks and benefits of laparoscopic surgery for these women (46).

Until such studies are completed, laparoscopic management of a potentially malignant ovarian mass will remain a controversial topic.

TUMOR SPILL IN APPARENT STAGE I OVARIAN MALIGNANCY

There are no randomized studies on the effect of intraoperative tumor rupture for surgically staged, Stage I ovarian cancer patients. Current practices are strongly influenced by the individual surgeon's bias from review of literature and training.

The International Federation of Gynecology and Obstetrics changed the classification of Stage I ovarian tumors in 1985 (47). The classification IC is for patients with tumor confined to one or both ovaries with ruptured capsule, or ascites containing malignant cells, or with positive peritoneal washings. The rationale for the subdivision of Stage I tumors is based on retrospective univariate analyses, which demonstrate different survival for the different subgroups: a 1990 FIGO report confirms a survival rate of 82.3%, 74.9%, and 67.7% for Stages IA, B, and C, respectively (48).

Reviewing ovarian cancer literature is difficult, as studies reported often evaluate patients who are incompletely staged. In 1970 Parker et al. (49) reported on the Duke University experience of patients diagnosed with ovarian cancer between 1951 and 1968. Stage I patients with intraoperative rupture ($n = 20$) had similar survival to those whose ovaries were removed intact ($n = 27$). However, most patients with rupture were treated with chemotherapy or radiation therapy. Patients with adhesions to viscera ($n = 6$) or excrescences ($n = 3$) had worse survival. Webb et al. (50) reported the Mayo clinic experience for 271 patients from 1950 to 1966. Patients with ruptured masses ($n = 53$) had a 56% 5-year survival compared to 90% for patients with intracystic lesions ($n = 111$). The patients with presence of ovarian adhesions ($n = 28$) had similar survival as those with tumor rupture (51). Most patients in the Mayo series were given postoperative radiation. In 1974 the University of Iowa experience for management of peritoneal cytology in gynecologic malignancies was reported. The 5-year survival of 42.8% was found for Stage I patients with ruptured cyst at surgery or presence of ascites; this was in contrast to a survival of 72.7% for similar patients treated with radioactive gold (52). Sainz de la Cuesta (53) reported the experience at Massachusetts General Hospital from 1975 to 1990 on patients with Stage I ovarian cancer. They noted a 20% versus a 3% risk of recurrence and death in women with I-C ruptured tumors and I-A tumors, respectively. This was in spite of 55% of the IC patients receiving postoperative treatment with chemotherapy, P-32, or chemotherapy and radiation therapy.

Other studies identify grade of tumor to be the most significant prognostic variable in early stage disease (54–56). No impact upon survival was found for tumor rupture, excrescences, or bilaterality. All patients in these studies were not completely staged and most patients received adjuvant therapy. Ascites has been noted to be a prognostic finding when present in volume greater than 250 mL (54, 55, 57). The authors agree with a recently published statement by E. Partridge in the 1994 SGO Handbook: "The independent significance of rupture, excrescences, bilaterality and positive peritoneal fluid remains controversial and perhaps unanswered" (57).

An additional consideration is the rate of spill when an attempt is made to prevent rupture. Many studies report the incidence of spill but do not specify whether or not it was intentional. The authors are aware of only one report from the literature for risk of intraoperative rupture during laparoscopy. This study by Hunter et al. noted a 58% spill rate of adnexal masses attempted to be removed intact (58). If spill is significant, this information would be an additional factor to consider when choosing an operative approach.

CONCLUSION

The driving force in evaluation of the pelvic mass is the risk of malignancy. The safest time to approach a pelvic mass laparoscopy is when there is considered to be no risk of malignancy. To approach the lowest risk possible for the patient based on current literature, the patient should have:

1. No physical findings suspicious for malignancy,
2. Reproductive age (premenopausal),
3. Mass size <5 cm,
4. Benign sonographic characteristics by a high resolution scan,
5. Normal tumor markers.

If only these masses were addressed, the expected rate of malignancy found at laparoscopy would be very low but the rate of laparotomy for benign disease would be expected to be relatively high. If these indications were expanded to include:

1. Unilocular cysts less than 10 cm in the reproductive age patients,
2. Sonographically benign cysts less than 5 cm in the menopausal patients,

the number of patients that would become candidates for a laparoscopic approach would increase; likewise, the number of patients requiring laparotomy would decrease.

Every attempt should be undertaken to prevent the intraperitoneal spill of any but the most benign appearing ovarian mass. It only makes sense that the patient should be prepared to undergo immediate exploratory laparotomy with surgical staging if an unsuspected ovarian malignancy is found. It is still appropriate to do the right operation on the right patient at the right time.

REFERENCES

1. Miller RC, Nash JD, Weiser EB, et al. The postmenopausal palpable ovary syndrome. A retrospective review with histopathologic correlates. J Reprod Med 1991;36:568–571.

2. Griffiths CT, Parker L. Cancer of the ovary. In: Knapp RL, Berkowitz RS, eds. Gynecologic Oncology. New York: Macmillan, 1986;362–363.
3. Andolf E, Jorgensen C, Astedt B. Ultrasound examination for detection of ovarian carcinoma in risk groups. Obstet Gynecol 1990;75:106–109.
4. Granberg S, Wikland M. A comparison between ultrasound and gynecologic examination for detection of enlarged ovaries in a group of women at risk for ovarian carcinoma. J Ultrasound Med 1988;7:59–64.
5. Campbell G, Bohan J, Roysten P, et al. Transabdominal ultrasound screening for early ovarian cancer. BMJ 1989;299:1363–1367.
6. Van Nagell JR, Higgins RV, Donaldson ES, et al. Transvaginal sonography as a screening method for ovarian cancer. A report of the first 1000 patients screened. Cancer 1990;65:573–577.
7. Spanks JM, Varner RE. Ovarian cancer screening. Obstet Gynecol 1991;77:787–792.
8. Koonings PP, Campbell K, Mishell DR, et al. Relative frequency of primary ovarian neoplasms: A 10 year review. Obstet Gynecol 1989;74:921–926.
9. Killackey MA, Neuwirth RS. Evaluation and management of the pelvic mass: a review of 540 cases. Obstet Gynecol 1988;71:319–322.
10. Granberg S, Wikland M, Jansson I. Macroscopic characterization of ovarian tumors and the relation to the histologic diagnosis: criteria to be used for ultrasound evaluation. Gynecol Oncol 1989;35:139.
11. Rulin M, Preston A. Adnexal masses in postmenopausal women. Obstet Gynecol 1987;70:578–581.
12. Sassone AM, Timor Tritsch IE, Artner A, et al. Transvaginal sonographic characterization of ovarian disease: evaluation of a new scoring system to predict ovarian malignancy. Obstet Gynecol 1991;78:70–76.
13. Andolf E, Jorgensen C. Cystic resins in elderly women, diagnosed by ultrasound. Br J Obstet Gynecol 1989;96:1076–1079.
14. Luxman D, Burgman A, Sagi J, et al. The post menopausal adnexal mass: correlation between ultrasonic and pathologic findings. Obstet Gynecol 1991;77:726–728.
15. Fleischer AC, Rodgers WH, Rao BK, Kepple DM, Worrell JA, Williams L, Jones HW. Assessment of ovarian tumor vascularity with transvaginal color Doppler sonography. J Ultrasound Med 1991;10:563–568.
16. Weiner Z, Thaler I, Beck D, Rottem S, Deutsch M, Brandes JM. Differentiating malignant from benign ovarian tumors with transvaginal color flow imaging. Obstet Gynecol 1992;79(2):159–162.
17. Kawai M, Kano T, Kikkawa F, et al. Transvaginal Doppler ultrasound with color flow imaging in the diagnosis of ovarian cancer. Obstet Gynecol 1992;79(2):163–167.
18. Kurjak A, Predanic M. New scoring system for prediction of ovarian malignancy based on transvaginal color Doppler sonography. J Ultrasound Med 1992;11:631–636.
19. Kurjak A, Predanic M, Kupesic-Urek S, Jukic S. Transvaginal color and pulsed Doppler assessment of adnexal tumor vascularity. Oncology 1993;50:3–9.
20. Carter J, Saltzman A, Hartenbach E, et al. Flow characteristics in benign and malignant gynecologic tumors using transvaginal color flow Doppler. Obstet Gynecol 1994;83:125–130.
21. Lerner JP, Timor-Tritsch LE, Federman A, et al. Transvaginal ultrasonographic characterization of ovarian masses with an improved, weighted scoring system. Am J Obstet Gynecol 1994;170:81–85.
22. O'Shaughnessy A, Check J, Nowroozi K, Lurie D. CA-125 levels measured in different phases of the menstrual cycle in screening for endometriosis. Obstet Gynecol 1993;81:99–103.
23. Mastropaolo W, Fernandez Z, Miller EL. Pronounced increases in the concentration of an ovarian tumour marker CA-125 in serum of a healthy subject during menstruation. Clin Chem 1989;32:2110–2111.
24. Pittaway DE, Fayez JA. Serum CA-125 antigen levels increase during menses. Am J Obstet Gynecol 1987;156:75–76.
25. Lehtovirta P, Apter D, Stenman UH. Serum CA-125 levels during the menstrual cycle. Br J Obstet Gynaecol 1990;97:930–933.
26. Helzisouer K, Bush T, Alberg A, et al. Prospective study of serum CA-125 levels as markers of ovarian cancer. JAMA 1993;269:1123–1126.
27. Haga Y, Sakamoto K, Egami H, et al. Evaluation of serum CA-125 values in healthy individuals and pregnant women. Am J Med Sci 1989;292:25–29.

28. Niloff JM, Knapp RC, Scaetzl E, et al. CA125 antigen levels in obstetric and gynecologic patients. Obstet Gynecol 1984;64:703–707.
29. Grover S, Quinn MA, Weideman P, et al. Factors influencing serum CA-125 levels in normal women. Obstet Gynecol 1992;79:511–514.
30. Einhorn, Bast RC, Knepp CC, et al. Preoperative evaluation of serum CA-125 levels in patients with primary epithelial ovarian carcinoma. Obstet Gynecol 1986;67:414–416.
31. Malkasian GD Jr, Knapp RC, Levin PT, et al. Preoperative evaluation of serum CA-125 levels in premenopausal patients with pelvic masses: discrimination of benign from malignant disease. Am J Obstet Gynecol 1988;159:341–346.
32. Soper JT, Hunter VJ, Daly L, et al. Preoperative serum tumor associated antigen levels in women with pelvic masses. Obstet Gynecol 1990;75:249–254.
33. Gadducci A, Ferdeghini M, Prontera C, et al. The concomitant determination of different tumor markers in patients with epithelial ovarian cancer and benign ovarian masses: Relevance for differential diagnosis. Gynecol Oncol 1992;44:147–154.
34. Seltzer V, Maiman M, Boyce J, et al. Laparoscopic survey in the management of ovarian cysts. The Female Patient 1992;17:19–23.
35. Maiman M, Seltzer V, Boyce J. Laparoscopic excision of ovarian neoplasm subsequently found to be malignant. Obstet Gynecol 1991;77:563–565.
36. Hulka J, Parker W, Surrey M, Phillips J. Management of ovarian masses. AAGL 1990 Survey. J Reprod Med 1992;37:599–602.
37. Hulka JF, Peterson HB, Phillips JM, et al. Operative laparoscopy. American Association of Gynecologic Laparoscopists 1991 Membership Survey. J Reprod Med 1993;38:569–571.
38. Nezhat F, Nezhat C, Welander C, Benigno B. Four ovarian cancers diagnosed during laparoscopic management of 1011 women with adnexal masses. Am J Obstet Gynecol 1992;167:790–796.
39. Mage G, Canis M, Mankes H, et al. Laparoscopic management of adnexal masses. J Gynecol Surg 1990;6:71–79.
40. Mecke H, Lehmann-Willenbrock E, Ibrahim M, Semm K. Pelviscopic treatment of ovarian cysts in premenopausal women. Gynecol Obstet Invest 1992;34:36–42.
41. Mettler L, Irani S, Semm K. Ovarian surgery via pelviscopy. J Reprod Med 1993;38:130–132.
42. Canis M, Mage G, Pouly JL, Wattiez A, Manhes H, Bruhat MA. Laparoscopic diagnosis of adnexal cystic masses: a 12-year experience with long-term follow-up. Obstet Gynecol 1994;83(5):707–712.
43. Parker W, Berek J. Management of selected cystic adnexal masses in postmenopausal women by operative laparoscopy: a pilot study. Am J Obstet Gynecol 1990;163:1574–1577.
44. Shalve E, Eliyahu S, Peleg D, Tsabari A. Laparoscopic management of adnexal cystic masses in postmenopausal women. Obstet Gynecol 1994;83(4):594–596.
45. Mann WJ, Reich H. Laparoscopic Adnexectomy in postmenopausal women. J Reprod Med 1992;37:254–256.
46. Ovarian cancer: screening, treatment, and follow-up. NIH Consensus Development Conference Statement. Bethesda, MD: April 5–7, 1994, p. 18.
47. International Federation of Gynecology and Obstetrics Annual report on the results of treatment in gynecologic cancer. Int J Gynecol Obstet 1989;28:189–190.
48. Annual report on the results of treatment in gynecologic cancer (FIGO). Pattersson F, ed. Int J Gynecol Obstet Suppl 1991;21:11.
49. Parker RT, Parker CH, Wilbanks GD. Cancer of the ovary. Am J Obstet Gynecol 1970;108:878–888.
50. Webb MJ, Decker DG, Mussey E, Williams TJ. Factors influencing survival in Stage I ovarian cancer. Am J Obstet Gynecol 1973;116:222–226.
51. Keetel WC, Pixley EE, Buchsbaum HJ. Experience with peritoneal cytology in the management of gynecologic malignancies. Am J Obstet Gynecol 1974;120:174–182.
52. de la Cuesta RS, Goff BA. Prognostic importance of intraoperative rupture of malignant ovarian epithelial neoplasms. Obstet Gynecol 1994;84(1):1–7.
53. Finn CB, Luesley DM, Buxton EJ, et al. Is Stage I epithelial ovarian cancer overtreated both surgically and systemically? Results of a five-year cancer registry review. Br J Obstet Gynaecol 1992;99:54–58.
54. Dembo AJ, Davy M, Stenwig AE, et al. Prognostic factors in patients with Stage I epithelial ovarian cancer. Obstet Gynecol 1990;75:263–273.

55. Svelda P, Vavra N, Schemper M, Salzer H. Prognostic factors for survival in Stage I epithelial ovarian carcinoma. Cancer 1990;65:2349–2350.
56. Swenerton KD, Hislop TG, Spinelli J, et al. Ovarian carcinoma: A multivariate analysis of prognostic factors. Obstet Gynecol 1985;65(2):264.
57. Partridge EE (discussant). Carcinoma of the ovary. SGO Handbook. Staging of Gynecologic Malignancies, SGO, 1st Ed, January, 1994, p. 31.
58. Hunter V, Sammarco M, Mou S. Laparoscopic surgical approach to patients with a pelvic mass: a pilot study of indications, findings, and postoperative complications. Presented at the Annual Meeting of the Kansas City Chapter of American College of Surgeons, Kansas City, MO, September 25, 1993.

Chapter 3
Laparoscopic Treatment of the Adnexal Mass
D. Alan Johns

Once the decision has been made to surgically evaluate and treat an adnexal mass, the surgeon is charged with determining the safest and most cost-effective surgical approach. Many factors must be considered before proceeding to surgery, and these have been thoroughly discussed in Chapter 2.

Based on clinical circumstances, the appropriate procedure must be ascertained and discussed with the patient. These options include oophorocystectomy, oophorectomy, salpingo-oophorectomy, and hysterectomy, with concomitant removal of the mass. All can be accomplished via laparoscopy.

Laparoscopic puncture and drainage of an adnexal mass, although an option, should rarely be considered. Aspiration provides no meaningful specimen for pathologic diagnosis and many cysts so treated will quickly recur. If an aspirated ovarian mass does not recur, it likely did not require intervention. When simple cyst aspiration seems appropriate, however, it can be accomplished safely and inexpensively with transvaginal ultrasound guidance. Laparoscopy offers no advantage over this simple office procedure.

When the appropriate surgical procedure has been determined, it should be performed regardless of the surgical route (laparoscopy or laparotomy). The procedure always dictates the size of the skin incision, not the reverse. Whether a conservative (oophorocystectomy) or radical (salpingo-oophorectomy) procedure is indicated, it can be accomplished laparoscopically, if the surgeon is adequately trained and skilled in endoscopic surgery.

EQUIPMENT

Laparoscopic surgery is extremely "equipment dependent," however, possessing a wide variety of expensive laparoscopic equipment is much less desirable than having the correct equipment. Particularly, when dealing with more difficult laparoscopic procedures, the frustration associated with missing or inadequate equipment may needlessly prolong the operation, increase the risk of complications, or necessitate laparotomy. All are undesirable. There is an infinite variety of laparoscopic equipment from which to choose, and an infinite variety of surgeons (each with his or her preference). Therefore, no attempt will be made here to produce an "equipment list". Most adnexal masses can be safely treated by endoscopic techniques using a minimal number of instruments. These instruments will be discussed in general terms, leaving the surgeon to choose his or her preference.

Without question, electrosurgery is the most cost-effective energy source for endoscopic surgery. It can be used for conservative procedures (oophorocystectomy) or radical procedures (salpingo-oophorectomy). Cutting, superficial fulguration, and coaptation of large vessels are all quickly and safely accomplished using electrosurgical techniques (1). As with laser energy, however, proper use of electrosurgery requires the surgeon to be knowledgeable in the physics and tissue interaction of electrical energy. Once these principles are understood, electrosurgery becomes an invaluable tool in endoscopic surgery.

When electrical energy is clinically inappropriate, endoscopic suturing techniques provide quick and effective hemostasis in the hands of the experienced, skilled, gynecologic endoscopist. The combination of suturing and electrosurgery free the surgeon from dependence on stapling devices, enabling a more cost-effective approach to laparoscopic surgery.

A unipolar "needle" electrode is a versatile and inexpensive tool that can be used for cutting and fulguration. It can be used for oophorocystectomy, salpingo-oophorectomy, and colpotomy. As occurs with any monopolar instrument, electrical current in other instruments and sleeves can be induced, both in and out of the operative field (capacitance coupling) (1, 2). In order to use monopolar electrosurgical energy safely, the surgeon *must* understand the cause and prevention of capacitance coupling. Newer electrosurgical generators and instruments have been devised to minimize the risks associated with capacitance coupling and other electrosurgical problems unique to laparoscopy. The surgeon should be familiar with these problems, and their avoidance, when using unipolar electrosurgical energy.

For control of vascular pedicles, electrosurgical coaptation (3) and sutures both provide safe, quick, and inexpensive methods for hemostasis. As will be discussed further, both require skill in laparoscopic dissection techniques. Laparoscopic stapling devices are quick, simple to use, and require no dissection skills. Unfortunately, they are not applicable to every case, and the cost associated with these devices is difficult to justify (4).

If electrosurgery is used for hemostasis, the surgeon must be able to accurately determine the waveform and energy output of the electrosurgical generator. Newer ESU (electrosurgical units) allow selection of several "wave forms" (cutting, blended, or coagulation) current. Although these terms are commonly used, one should be familiar with the resulting tissue effects of each modality, and be able to choose the most appropriate output for a specific clinical situation.

When properly used, electrosurgical coaptation of vessels as large as the uterine artery is possible (3). Control of vessels comprising the "infundibulopelvic ligament" with electrosurgery has been well documented (4–6). A monitor (ammeter), measuring current flow through the vessel walls, aids in determining when the coaptation process has been completed; it should accompany each electrosurgical unit in an operating suite.

Most endoscopic surgeons operate while watching a video monitor. This allows the surgical assistant and scrub nurse to view the operation, thereby enhancing their ability to assist. Since the surgeon's view of the operative field totally depends on this video system, it should produce the highest quality image possible. Newer three-chip video cameras, coupled with high-resolution monitors and halogen light sources, produce an image with which any surgeon can operate, and should be in every operating room in which endoscopy is performed. The image with which the surgeon operates should never be compromised by antiquated or inferior video equipment.

The majority of laparoscopic procedures for adnexal masses can be completed using three ports: one 10-mm umbilical and two 5-mm suprapubic. Few circumstances require more than these three trochar sites. Because suturing may be necessary, trochar sleeves without trumpet valves or traps (either of which may ensnare needles or sutures) are preferable. Although disposable trochars are widely available, they offer no proven advantages over their more cost-efficient reusable counterparts.

Occasionally, 11-mm sleeves will be necessary for tissue removal. One or two should be available.

A blunt irrigation/dissection probe (often considered the most important instrument in operative laparoscopy) is mandatory. This probe is used for dissection, irrigation, aspiration, and traction. It should be hollow (for irrigation and aspiration) and have a rounded, smooth point for atraumatic dissection. As with trochars, disposable irrigation/dissection probes offer nothing but additional cost.

Grasping forceps and scissors finish the list of equipment necessary to complete most cases. Ideally, irrigation should be possible through these graspers and scissors. These options allow the surgeon to continually cleanse the operative field. Just as at laparotomy, rinsing of capillary bleeding away from the operative site allows the surgeon to proceed more efficiently and safely. Unfortunately, laparoscopic surgery done without this capability is often performed in a "pool" of blood.

THE OPERATIVE PROCEDURE

The potential necessity for laparotomy should *always* be discussed with every patient scheduled to undergo laparoscopic treatment of her adnexal mass. From a complication of trochar insertion to unexpected findings after the laparoscope is in place, laparotomy may become necessary. This eventuality should never be a shock to either the patient or surgeon.

As in a laparotomy, the surgeon must first assess the entire abdominal cavity. This should include visual inspection of the upper abdomen, omentum, liver surface, diaphragmatic surfaces, bowel serosa, all pelvic structures, and all visible peritoneal surfaces (both upper and lower abdomen). Peritoneal washings should be collected and saved for future evaluation should it become necessary. Any suspicious lesions are biopsied and evaluated by frozen section. If carcinoma is diagnosed, immediate laparotomy is performed if the surgeon possesses the skill and experience that is necessary to optimally treat the disease (including debulking, bowel resection, etc.). Otherwise, the laparoscopy is terminated and the patient referred for definitive surgical therapy.

Every preliminary procedure indicated at laparotomy must be done at laparoscopy prior to removal of the mass. The entire peritoneal cavity should be visually explored. The liver surface, both diaphragmatic surfaces, and the omentum should be inspected and peritoneal washings collected. The normal adnexa and all peritoneal surfaces should be thoroughly examined. When the preliminary evaluation has been completed and documented, the mass should be carefully inspected. Any evidence of malignancy should be noted to determine the appropriateness of the laparoscopic approach.

Once the decision is made to proceed with a laparoscopic approach, the appropriate procedure must be determined. The patient's age, desire for fertility, size of the mass, coexisting pathology, presumed diagnosis, and surgeon's skill and experience all must be considered before a radical (salpingo-oophorectomy) or conservative (oophorocystectomy) is chosen.

OOPHOROCYSTECTOMY

Laparoscopic oophorocystectomy is much more difficult and technically demanding than salpingo-oophorectomy. It should only be attempted by the experienced laparoscopic surgeon comfortable with dissection techniques.

Until the controversy surrounding the potential detrimental effects of spillage of the contents of a malignant ovarian mass is over, rupture of the mass should be avoided. Keep in mind the cyst walls rupture at laparotomy as well as at laparoscopy. Regardless of the size of the abdominal wall incisions, one should always take precautions to avoid spillage of the contents of an undiagnosed adnexal mass. Laparoscopic removal of an intact mass without intra-abdominal spillage will be discussed later in this chapter.

Initially, the ovary should be optimally positioned. The utero-ovarian ligament is grasped and the ovary (and mass) elevated. The uterus is retroverted, forming a "table" on which the ovary is placed. The uterus is maintained in this position with a uterine manipulator.

Ideally, the initial incision in the ovary should be made well away from its lateral surface (that surface lying against the pelvic side wall). It should be made parallel to the long axis of the ovary and be of sufficient length to allow dissection of the mass away from the base of the ovary without tearing of the ovarian cortex. Once the cyst has been removed, the ovary should fall together with the incision on the medial side of the ovary, away from the pelvic side wall. This technique will minimize the need for suturing of the ovary, thereby decreasing the potential for postoperative adhesions.

The initial incision should traverse the ovarian surface to (but not through) the cyst wall. Because electrosurgery or CO_2 laser energy can be precisely controlled, both are ideal for this incision.

Once the cyst wall is identified, the edge of the incision is grasped and the cyst wall carefully and slowly dissected free from surrounding ovarian stroma. Most nonmalignant masses (with the notable exception of endometriomas) will peel away from the surrounding tissue easily. This is accomplished by grasping the ovarian wall while dissecting the cyst wall from the ovary with a blunt irrigation/dissection probe (Fig. 3.1). Constant irrigation through the dissection probe often facilitates this dissection. Patience is mandatory.

Some ovarian surface should remain on the cyst after it has been enucleated. Since the cyst wall is often thin and friable, grasping it to maneuver the mass into a bag or the cul-de-sac might result in rupture and spillage. Ovarian tissue remaining attached to the enucleated mass can be used as a "handle" to manipulate the cyst, minimizing the risk of rupture.

After the mass has been enucleated, bleeding in the base of the ovarian wound is controlled with bipolar electrosurgery or unipolar "spray" fulguration. Either technique will control widespread surface capillary bleeding, a common problem at this point in the procedure. Fulguration produces very superficial injury and results in minimal damage to the remaining ovary and oocytes, and is, therefore, preferable.

Chapter 3: Laparoscopic Treatment of the Adnexal Mass   41

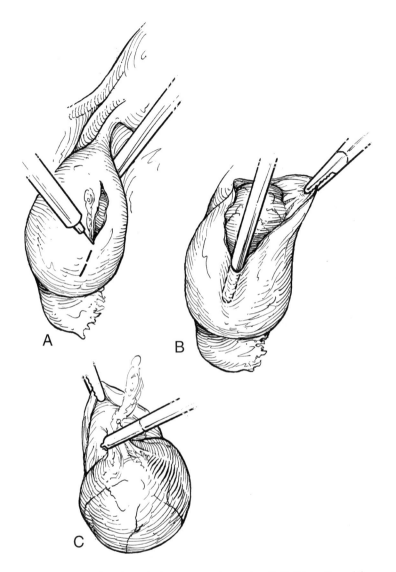

Figure 3.1. **A.** Linear incision through the ovary to the cyst wall. **B.** Dissection of the cyst from the ovary. **C.** Coagulation of vessels between the cyst and ovary.

If the initial ovarian incision was optimally placed, the remaining ovary should fall together in an anatomic position, the incision facing away from the lateral pelvic sidewall. Should closure of the ovarian wound be necessary, fine (5-0 to 7-0) monofilament, absorbable, minimally-reactive suture should be used. When possible, these sutures should be placed *within* the ovary, exposing little or none of the suture material. Most often, however, suturing will not be necessary.

Clearly, the technical aspects of oophorocystectomy at laparoscopy are no different than when the procedure is performed at laparotomy. Good surgical technique should never be dependent on the size of the abdominal incision.

ADNEXECTOMY

Oophorectomy or salpingo-oophorectomy are commonly required for surgical treatment of the adnexal mass. In most cases, both are technically feasible at laparoscopy. As noted above, the techniques used endoscopically should closely mimic those required at laparotomy.

The operative field is closely examined to determine the most appropriate surgical approach. If the ovary is adherent to adjacent structures (bowel or pelvic sidewall), the initial step should be dissection, isolation, and control of the ovarian artery and vein (the infundibulopelvic ligament). The ovary is then pulled medially and dissected free from other structures. If the uterus is present and to be retained, the vessels in the infundibulopelvic ligament should, in most cases, be controlled and transected before moving to the tube and utero-ovarian ligament.

Approaching the ovarian artery, ovarian vein, and ureter from the retroperitoneal space offers significant advantages. Rather than simply ligating, coaptating, or stapling the "infundibulopelvic ligament", the vessels that require control (the ovarian artery and vein) are isolated, skeletonized, and controlled well away from the pelvic sidewall and adjacent structures, minimizing risk of injury to these structures.

Entering the retroperitoneal space requires medial traction on the ovary and tube, stretching the peritoneum overlying the retroperitoneal space between the round and infundibulopelvic ligaments. The peritoneum is opened with scissors or unipolar electrosurgery (Fig. 3.2). The retroperitoneal space is dissected with a blunt irrigation/dissection probe or closed scissors. When performed correctly,

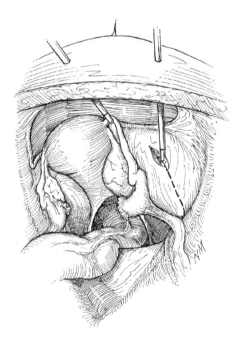

Figure 3.2. Placement of the peritoneal incision allowing access to the retroperitoneal space.

this dissection results in minimal bleeding and permits identification of structures in the retroperitoneal space (Fig. 3.3). Even in cases with dense cohesive adhesions between the ovary and pelvic sidewall the retroperitoneal approach allows simple identification of the ureter. The ovary is simply removed with the peritoneal sidewall still attached.

Once the retroperitoneal space has been dissected posterior to and below the ovary, the ovarian artery and vein (the infundibulopelvic ligament) are identified. Intact peritoneum transfers heat well; when electrosurgical coaptation is used, this "transferred" heat may damage adjacent structures (ureters). Therefore, when possible, peritoneum overlying the ovarian artery and vein should be incised, connective tissue and fat removed, and the vessels isolated. Skeletonization and dissection of these vessels then permit safe coaptation or ligation (Fig. 3.4).

Electrosurgical coaptation is safe, rapid, and effective for control of these vessels. The cutting waveform should be used, and an electrical endpoint monitor used to assure complete vessel desiccation and coaptation. In addition to minimizing lateral thermal injury, dissection and isolation of the vessels prior to coaptation assures more complete "welding" of the vessel walls by minimizing the volume of tissue to be desiccated by electrosurgical energy (Fig. 3.5).

Dissected and isolated vessels may also be controlled with sutures. An absorbable braided suture is passed around the vessels and both ends brought out through a suprapubic sleeve. Extracorporeal knotting techniques and a simple knot pusher can then be used to secure the pedicle. Both electrosurgical and suturing techniques are quick, safe, and inexpensive.

Devices are available that will simultaneously place two rows of surgical

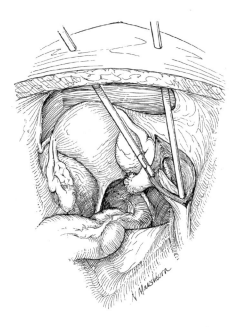

Figure 3.3. Dissection of the retroperitoneal space.

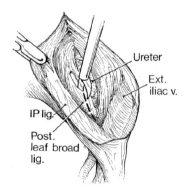

Figure 3.4. Skeletonization of the ovarian artery and vein (the infundibulopelvic ligament).

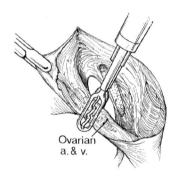

Figure 3.5. Coaptation of the skeletonized ovarian artery and vein with bipolar electrosurgery.

staples while simultaneously cutting between these rows. When these devices are used, the ovarian artery and vein should *not* be dissected and skeletonized prior to placement of the staples. Stapling devices provide hemostasis by crushing the vessels walls with surrounding connective tissue and fat. If this surrounding tissue is not present, bleeding will often occur around and through the staple line.

By using a blunt dissection/irrigation probe and medial traction, the intact ovary is then dissected from the pelvic sidewall and ureter. Remaining attachments to the uterus (tube and utero-ovarian ligament) or vaginal cuff (if the uterus is absent) are transected (Fig. 3.6). The intact ovary containing the mass is now free in the pelvis.

REMOVAL

Currently there is no consensus regarding the significance of intra-abdominal spillage of the contents of a malignant ovarian mass when there is no pre-existing spread of the tumor. Until the prognostic significance (or lack thereof) of this is ascertained, surgeons should avoid spillage of the contents of an undiagnosed ovarian mass. Several alternatives exist for removal of an adnexal mass without intra-abdominal contamination.

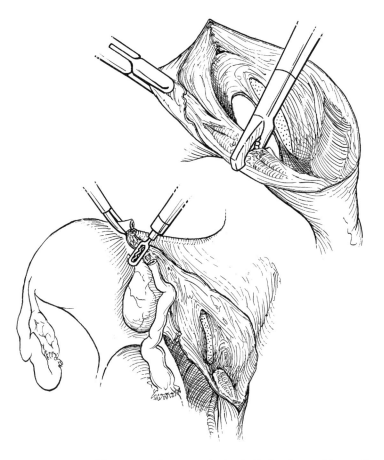

Figure 3.6. A. Transection of the coaptated artery and vein. **B.** Desiccation and transection of the fallopian tube and utero-ovarian ligament.

Laparoscopic "pouches" or "bags" have been designed to allow transabdominal decompression and removal of adnexal structures without intra-abdominal spillage. These bags are manufactured in varying sizes and designs, most of which require introduction through 10–12-mm laparoscopic sleeves.

The mass is placed into the appropriately sized bag. The laparoscopic sleeve is removed and the open end of the pouch is maneuvered through the suprapubic incisions. With the opening of the pouch exteriorized, the mass can be decompressed with suction or needle aspiration. Any contents leaking around the puncture site will be contained within the pouch. Once the mass is sufficiently collapsed, the pouch (with the decompressed mass inside) can be removed through the suprapubic incision (Fig. 3.7). Care must be exercised to avoid puncture of the bag with the instrument chosen for decompression and drainage. These devices are very useful for removal of smaller masses, but those larger than 7–8 cm in diameter may be difficult or impossible to insert into these devices.

The freed adnexal mass can also be removed through a colpotomy incision. To minimize the risk of bowel or ureteral injury, the cul-de-sac, uterosacral liga-

46 GYNECOLOGIC ENDOSCOPY: Principles in Practice

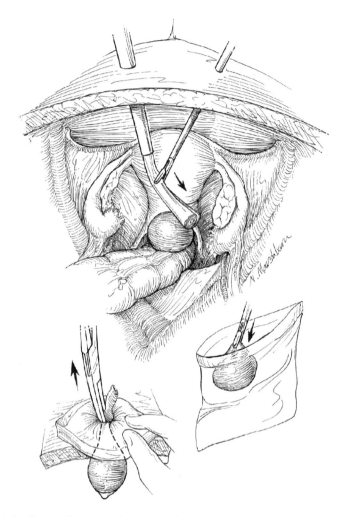

Figure 3.7. **A.** Sterile bag placed into the peritoneal cavity through an 11 mm sleeve. **B.** Positioning of the mass into the sterile bag. **C.** Open end of the bag is exteriorized, allowing decompression and removal of the mass.

ments, ureters, and rectum must be accurately identified. Then, any of the three following methods can be used to open the cul-de-sac.

The first method requires transvaginal identification of the uterosacral ligaments and cul-de-sac. An incision is created with scissors while applying traction on the cul-de-sac and cervix with forceps. This technique is identical to that used to enter the posterior cul-de-sac during vaginal hysterectomy or vaginal tubal ligation. Unfortunately, it requires "blind" entry into the peritoneal cavity and is often associated with significant bleeding.

A second technique requires the transvaginal placement of an 11- or 12-mm laparoscopic trochar through the posterior cul-de-sac under direct laparoscopic control. Laparoscopy allows precise placement of the trochar spike, thereby avoiding injury to the rectum or ureters. Once the trochar has been placed through the cul-de-sac and its spike removed, the sleeve provides easy transvaginal access to the peritoneal cavity (Fig. 3.8). This technique is quick and hemostatic, but produces the smallest incision through which the mass must be decompressed and removed.

The last method requires the colpotomy incision to be performed laparoscopically. Outward traction is applied to the cervix with a tenaculum while the cul-de-sac is identified and distended with a transvaginal sponge forcep. Viewed laparoscopically, the cul-de-sac, uterosacral ligaments, and rectum are readily apparent. An incision is made in the distended cul-de-sac with unipolar electrosurgery or CO_2 laser between the uterosacral ligaments and above the rectum. The sponge forcep distending the cul-de-sac prevents loss of pneumoperitoneum. This method is perhaps the most technically demanding, but minimizes the incision and should be the method of choice when large masses are encountered.

The mass is then seated into the cul-de-sac and the patient placed in reverse Trendelenburg position. Thus positioned, fluid leaking from the mass during decompression runs out the vagina and away from the peritoneal cavity. Depending on the size of the mass and the consistency of its contents, decompression is accomplished with wall suction or needle aspiration. Depending on the surgeon's preference, the colpotomy is closed vaginally or endoscopically (Fig. 3.9).

The abdomen is re-inflated and the operative field inspected. Blood and debris are removed by thorough irrigation of the entire peritoneal cavity. Residual bleeding is controlled with bipolar electrocautery.

Numerous studies have attested to the safety and efficacy of the laparoscopic approach to the adnexal mass (7–10). The current health care climate de-

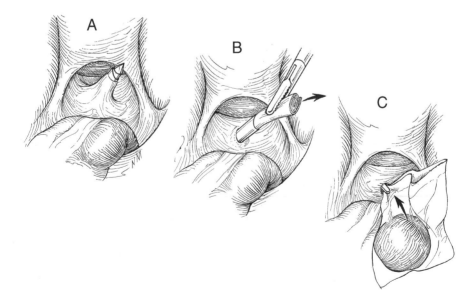

Figure 3.8. **A.** Transvaginal placement of an 11 mm laparoscopic trochar and sleeve. **B.** Sterile bag placed in the pelvis through the 11 mm sleeve. **C.** Open end of the bag is exteriorized into the vagina, allowing aspiration and removal.

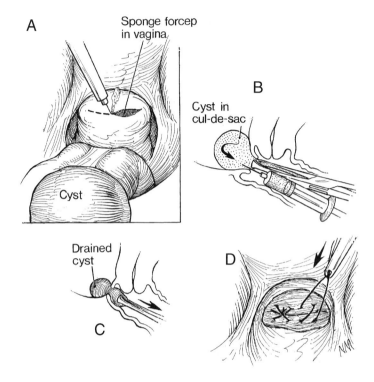

Figure 3.9. **A.** Distension of the cul-de-sac with a sponge forcep and laparoscopic colpotomy performed. **B.** Mass seated in the cul-de-sac and aspirated transvaginally. **C.** Collapsed cyst is removed through the colpotomy. **D.** Laparoscopic closure of the colpotomy.

mands the most cost-effective means for dealing with a surgical problem. Combining good surgical judgment, technique, and common sense will allow many patients requiring surgery for investigation and treatment of an adnexal mass to benefit from the endoscopic approach without additional risk.

REFERENCES

1. Odell R. Electrosurgery in laparoscopy. Infertil Reprod Med Clin North Am 1993;4:289–304.
2. Martin DC, Soderstrom RM, Hulka JF, Hasson HM, Luciano AA, Levy BS, Hunt RB, et al. Electrosurgical safety. AAGL Technical Bulletin, No. 1, January 1995.
3. Sigel B, Dunn MR. The mechanism of blood vessel closure by high frequency electrocoagulation. Surg Gynecol Obstet 1965;121:823–831.
4. Johns DA. The impact of laparoscopy on hysterectomy for benign disease in a large not-for-profit hospital. Presented at the annual meeting of the Central Association of Obstetricians and Gynecologists, Memphis, Tennessee, 1994.
5. Reich H, Johns DA, David G, Diamond MJ. Laparoscopic oophorectomy. J Reprod Med 1993;38: 497–501.
6. Johns DA. Laparoscopic-assisted vaginal hysterectomy: electrosurgical techniques. In: Diamond MP, Daniell JF, Jones HW III, eds. Hysterectomy. Cambridge, MA: Blackwell Science, 1995:45–58.
7. Shalev E, Eliyahu S, Peleg D, Tsabari A. Laparoscopic management of adnexal cystic masses in postmenopausal women. Obstet Gynecol 1994;83:594–596.

8. Pittaway DE, Takacs P, Bauguess P. Laparoscopic adnexectomy: a comparison with laparotomy. Am J Obstet Gynecol 1994;171:385–391.
9. Mage G, Canis M, Manies H, Pouly JL, Wattiez A, Bruhat MA. Laparoscopic management of adnexal cystic masses. J Gynecol Surg 1990;6:8–16.
10. Tucker SW. Advanced operative laparoscopy in the diagnosis and management of the pelvic mass. American Association of Gynecologic Laparoscopists 18th Annual Meeting Proceedings, Sante Fe Springs, CA. 1988:35–39.

Chapter 4
Office Hysteroscopy
The Basics

Charles M. March

For many decades, the value of hysteroscopy in diagnosing multiple types of intrauterine pathology has been proven to be superior to older, more traditional methods, such as curettage or hysterosalpingography (1–3). Moreover, operative hysteroscopy has been shown to be more efficacious, safer, and less costly than prior methods of treating submucosal leiomyomas, uterine septa, and intrauterine synechiae (4–7). Despite these data, recent surveys have indicated that few gynecologists perform hysteroscopy, and most of those physicians do so infrequently, and almost never in the office.

Old habits die slowly, but more than inertia has caused many gynecologists to remain skeptical about office hysteroscopy. Four misconceptions have prevailed: visualization is poor, the need for hysteroscopy is slight, the technique is difficult to learn, and office procedures are not tolerated by patients. Certainly the changing endometrial appearance and its fragility, together with uterine bleeding and the ready loss of uterine distension as medium passes out the fallopian tubes and/or a patulous cervix, can compromise hysteroscopic images. However, improvements in fiberoptic technology and the development of newer media and delivery systems have made hysteroscopy "user-friendly". Except in the most unusual circumstances, an adequate examination can be obtained in the office.

Intrauterine pathology is frequently detected in women with abnormal bleeding, infertility, and recurrent abortion. In some series, abnormalities have been found in up to 50% of cases (8–13). Although initially perceived as difficult to learn, hysteroscopy is simpler than laparoscopy. Courses, textbooks, and atlases abound. These facts, coupled with the demands of patients and third-party payors that care be provided more efficiently and outside hospitals as much as possible, have made office hysteroscopy a "must". Goldrath and Sherman estimated that office hysteroscopy and biopsy saved $1000 compared to a hospital curettage (14). Not only is hysteroscopy tolerated well by patients, but patients prefer the informal and familiar office setting to that of a hospital. They recover more quickly, have a diagnosis more rapidly, and spend less time away from family and work. Office surgery makes us more efficient and preserves patient safeguards. It is unlikely that future gynecologists will survive without offering this service to their patients.

INDICATIONS/CONTRAINDICATIONS

The most common indication for diagnostic hysteroscopy is abnormal uterine bleeding. In our experience and in that of others, more than one-fourth of these patients have been shown to have a submucosal myoma or an endometrial polyp (13; Kolton W, March CM, Personal communication). The frequency of these lesions is much higher in patients whose excessive bleeding is associated with ovulation and in those whose complaints have persisted for six months or more. Commonly, these lesions are not detected by curettage (1, 15). Other diagnostic tools such as hysterosalpingography or ultrasound can be used to detect intracavitary defects, but cannot differentiate one from the other with certainty, and often provide false positive results (16, 17). At the time of the patient's initial visit, appropriate medical or surgical treatment can be planned based upon definitive knowledge of the etiology of the uterine bleeding. Bleeding that occurs during hormone replacement therapy for menopausal patients alarms both the patients and their physicians, even if it occurs on a "scheduled" basis; that is, during a drug-free interval. If persistent, representative endometrial sampling or hysteroscopically-directed biopsy can be obtained. Focal endometrial hyperplasia can be diagnosed, and its response to medical treatment can be assessed.

Recurrent abortion may be caused by uterine cavity defects such as septa, myomas, or adhesions. If assessment of tubal patency is not necessary, hysteroscopy permits a diagnosis to be made with certainty, and can be used to verify the adequacy of the results following division of a septum, lysis of synechiae, or resection of one or more submucosal myomas. This precaution assures physician and patient that the uterine cavity is normal before the patient undertakes another pregnancy. Failure to verify that adhesiolysis has been complete has been associated with serious obstetrical problems, including repeated abortion, placental retention, uterine rupture, and postpartum hemorrhage (18, 19). Although unproven, it is likely that these patients had persistent disease. In our experience and that of Valle, none of these complications has occurred among women in whom post-treatment hysteroscopies or hysterograms were normal prior to conception (7, 20).

Retained intrauterine foreign bodies can be located and often removed in the office, thus reducing the need for multiple visits, complex imaging studies, and/or hospital procedures.

The three absolute contraindications to hysteroscopy are: an inexperienced operator, recent pelvic infection, and invasive cervical cancer. Multiple postgraduate courses are available to introduce physicians to hysteroscopy. Any smoldering infection could be exacerbated by the manipulation. Hysteroscopy cannot provide extra information about the diagnosis or staging of cervical cancer, and may spread disease. Endometrial cancer has been considered to be a relative contraindication. However, if a dry medium is used, the risk of disseminating disease is minimal. Endometrial cells have been found in the peritoneal cavity after 16% of hysteroscopies with carbon dioxide, and after 65% of hydrochromo pertubations (21). Data from Sweden indicate no worsening of prognosis among those who had undergone hysteroscopy prior to treatment. Because small or focal endometrial cancers may not be detected by curettage, possible endometrial cancer is more of an indication than contraindication to hysteroscopy. Pregnancy (no proven benefit and potential fetal loss), recent uterine perforation (inability to maintain uterine distension), and active bleeding (inadequate visualization), are relative contraindications to hysteroscopy.

The basic equipment for office hysteroscopy includes a 150-watt light source and hysteroscope with a 4.0–5.5-mm diagnostic sheath (Fig. 4.1), and an examining table that can be raised and tilted. The latter is essential for both patient and physician comfort. The telescope may have a 0° ("straight on") viewing

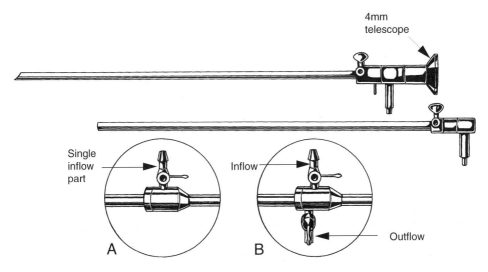

Figure 4.1. Diagnostic telescope with sheath. Diagnostic sheath may have one inflow port (**A**) or one inflow and one outflow port (**B**) for continuous flow capabilities.

angle, or be offset between 12° and 30° from the horizontal. Although any angle affords a good view of the endocervical canal, lower uterine segment, and upper fundus, the 30° telescope permits the surgeon to see even the most eccentrically placed tubal ostia (as occur in "T" shaped uteri). A liquid-filled light cable transmits light with minimal loss compared to standard cables. An insufflator that instills carbon dioxide under a high pressure (up to 200 mm Hg) and low rate of flow (up to 100 mL/minute) assures adequate uterine distension and patient safety (Fig. 4.2). Newer electronic models provide digital readouts of pressure and flow rate. Small disposable CO_2 cartridges are easier to use than large cylinders of CO_2, and may not require the use of filters to prevent contaminants from reaching the patient.

Recently, self-contained systems for the delivery of low-viscosity media have been developed. Media may be instilled by using gravity flow or delivered under pressure by wrapping the media bag in an infusion pump. Although low-viscosity media can be used with any type of hysteroscope, they are ideal when used with a continuous flow hysteroscope (Fig. 4.3). These instruments have multiple channels, which are isolated completely from one another. The medium flows into the uterus via one channel and then is returned via a second channel, and flows into a collection container. If the patient is bleeding, or if there is much cellular debris, these contaminants can be rinsed from the uterine cavity, thereby restoring a clear view.

After becoming familiar with hysteroscopy and convinced of its value, many physicians will add a video camera and monitor to complete their office setup. Usually a xenon light source is not required. For the occasional operative procedure, a 7–8-mm operating sheath and accessory instruments should be available (Fig. 4.4). These include aspirating catheters, grasping forceps, scissors, and biopsy forceps.

A "flexible" hysteroscope has a distal end that can be "steered" around a le-

54 GYNECOLOGIC ENDOSCOPY: Principles in Practice

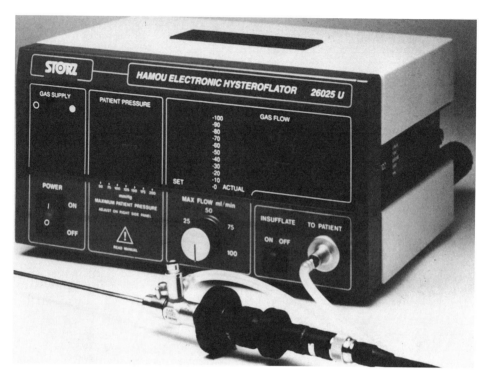

Figure 4.2. Example of a CO_2 insufflator. Units suitable for hysteroscopy have settings for maximum intrauterine pressure and maximum gas inflow.

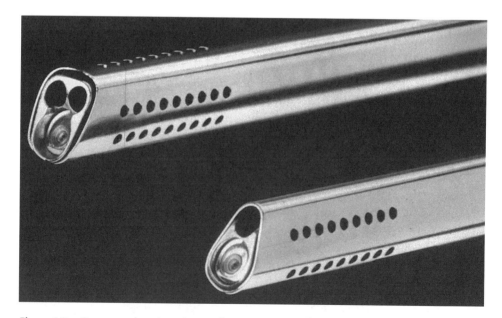

Figure 4.3. Two examples of continuous flow systems for fluid media (5.5 mm and 6.5 mm outer diameters).

Chapter 4: Office Hysteroscopy   55

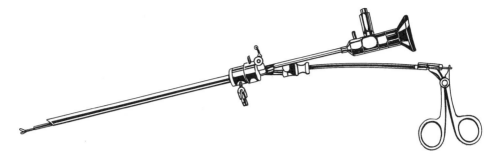

Figure 4.4. 30° panoramic hysteroscope with 7-mm sheath containing an operating channel and a 7 Fr flexible scissors.

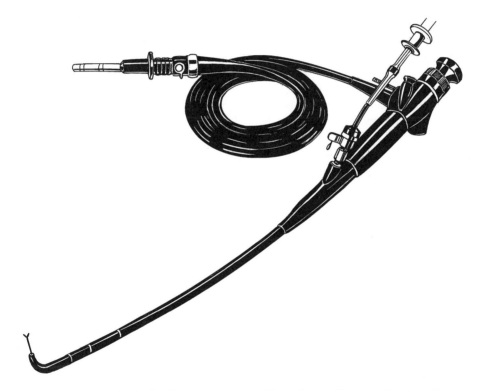

Figure 4.5. Example of a flexible hysteroscope and biopsy forceps. The outer diameter is 5 mm.

sion and can provide direct access to the tubal ostia (Fig. 4.5). The view is adequate but less clear than that provided by a rigid telescope. The greater cost and perhaps greater fragility have limited the acceptance of these instruments. If in-office hysteroscopic tubal occlusion becomes feasible, "flexible" instruments may become more popular. Carbon dioxide is used as a distending medium.

Hysteroscopy is performed with the patient on a standard power table. For diagnostic procedures, ordinary heel stirrups are used, but if a surgical procedure is planned, stirrups that provide support behind the knees are used. One mobile instrument cart contains sterile instruments, and another cart has the monitor, camera, light source, and CO_2 insufflator with tubing. If desired, a VCR and/or video printer can be used to document findings. This same instrument cart contains all emergency equipment, including an intravenous solution, airway, O_2, hand-operated ventilator, and appropriate drugs (adrenaline, atropine, diphenhydramine hydrochloride, etc.).

Hysteroscope sheaths, tenacula, small dilators (up to 8 mm), and a bivalve speculum with one side open are sterilized in the office. Telescopes are sterilized with ethylene oxide at a local hospital. This practice necessitates having an extra telescope (should a second procedure be performed on the same day), and therefore is more expensive than disinfection with alcohol or glutaraldehyde. However, it is convenient and obviates concerns about spores, other organisms, chemical residue, and the proper disposal of the disinfectant.

Carbon dioxide is the ideal medium for diagnostic hysteroscopy in the office. The tissue image is true-to-life and there is no magnification. CO_2 is not messy, as are wet media. If the patient is bleeding and if an aspirating catheter cannot clear the cavity of blood and cellular debris adequately, Hyskon is used. This very viscous solution of dextran (32% dextran of molecular weight 70,000 in 10% glucose in water) is not miscible with blood, and can be used for surgical procedures also. This "most forgiving" medium provides an impeccable view even if the patient is bleeding, and is ideal for surgical procedures. It is delivered via a 50-mL syringe attached to a wide-diameter tubing in intermittent 5–10-mL increments. If Hyskon is used, all equipment must be rinsed immediately with copious amounts of hot water to prevent caramelization.

TECHNIQUE

If hysteroscopy had not been explained to the patient at a prior visit, a brief explanation of the reason for the procedure and risks is provided. A written consent is not obtained. Ibuprofen, 600 mg or an equivalent medication is taken 20–45 minutes before hysteroscopy. Supplemental analgesia using 1–2 mg of butorphanol tartrate intranasally is both rapid in onset and highly effective. If an operative procedure is planned, a small dose of intravenous diazepam or midazolam may be used. If feasible, hysteroscopy should be performed early in the proliferative phase of the menstrual cycle, but any time except during menses is suitable. If there is any chance that the patient is pregnant, hysteroscopy should be deferred. No special preoperative studies or instructions are necessary other than avoiding a heavy meal just prior to hysteroscopy. Prophylactic antibiotics are not used.

Although analgesia and anesthesia are provided via medications, the consenting process, slow and precise movements and explanations by the physician during surgery, continual reassurance by an assistant and "distraction" by the video monitor, which permits the patient to view her uterine interior, are very helpful adjuncts and make almost every procedure, which lasts up to 30 minutes, acceptable to patients. A complete diagnostic procedure consumes less than 30 minutes, including anesthesia, surgery, recovery, and clean-up time.

The patient is assisted into stirrups. A pelvic examination determines the axis and size of the uterus and verifies that there is no uterine or adnexal tenderness. A speculum is introduced into the vagina and the cervix is visualized. If there is no evidence of vaginal or cervical inflammation, the cervix is "painted" with povidone-iodine, and grasped transversely with a single-tooth tenaculum. Using a 25-gauge spinal needle, the cervix is infiltrated with 1% chloroprocaine hydrochloride. A true paracervical block is not used. At least 5 minutes should elapse before further uterine manipulation. During this time, the hysteroscope, sheath, CO_2 tubing, and light cord are assembled. If the hysteroscope cannot be passed without cervical dilatation, small dilators (up to 5 mm) are used. Because a tight seal between cervix and hysteroscope reduces the loss of distending medium, laminaria are not used prior to hysteroscopy. The uterine cavity is not sounded and the dilators are not passed beyond the internal os so that the endometrium is not traumatized. The light source is turned on, the maximum pressure set at 200 mg Hg, the insufflation rate set at 60 mL/minute, and the hysteroscope is engaged in the endocervical canal. If a 0° telescope is used, it is kept in the center of the "black hole", which represents the upper endocervical canal and uterine fundus as the scope is advanced into the uterine cavity. If a 30° telescope is used, the black hole is kept at 6 o'clock (because the view is away from the horizontal) as the telescope is advanced. The uterus is explored in a systematic fashion beginning with the endocervical canal and proceeding to the right lateral wall, cornual recess and tubal ostium, top fundus, left ostium, cornual recess and side wall, anterior uterine surface, and then posterior fundus. If a 30° telescope is used, it is rotated counterclockwise as the right cornual recess is approached in order to see the tubal ostium, and in the opposite direction to view the left ostium. Slow, gentle movements are needed to reduce discomfort and bleeding (thereby obscuring the view). If uterine distension is inadequate, the flow rate is increased up to a maximum of 100 mL/minute. If bubbles, blood, or cellular debris obscure the view, patience will usually conquer these obstacles, as the offending elements pass out the fallopian tubes. If the view remains obscured by blood or debris, a larger operating sheath, which has an operating channel to accommodate an aspirating catheter, should be used. A 10-mL syringe attached to the catheter should remove any hindrance to a clear view. If the view is still poor, Hyskon replaces CO_2 as a uterine-distending medium. Glucose—5% in water—(or any other low-viscosity fluid) can also be used as a uterine distending medium if a continuous-flow hysteroscope is available. Gravity or pressure from a cuff placed around the infusion bag provides adequate pressure for uterine distension. If an operative procedure is to be done, the appropriate instrument is passed through the operating channel. After a brief rest period, the patient returns to the consultation room, where the results are explained and a treatment plan formulated. Any video tape or photographs are reviewed at that time. The patient may return home or to work immediately (unless a tranquilizer or narcotic was used—these patients need a driver to accompany them).

ENDOMETRIAL ANATOMY AND PATHOLOGY

The diagnosis of endometrial anatomy, both normal and abnormal, is based upon color, consistency, and vascular pattern. Proliferative endometrium is thin, pink, soft, and has very little vasculature. Immediately after menses the surface is uneven, with areas of denudation. As more estradiol is produced, the surface becomes covered by smooth, irregular folds. Secretory endometrium is 4–7-mm thick, lavender to reddish-brown, soft, somewhat mucoid, often adheres to the telescope, and has a well-developed, uniformly branching vascular pattern. It is fragile and bleeds on contact. Hyperplastic endometrium is thick and polypoid, pink to red, and often contains focal hemorrhage. The vascular pattern is elaborate and the vessels branch in an irregular fashion. As the histology becomes more abnormal, so does the vascular pattern, and there is more hemorrhage. Adenocarcinoma may be luminescent and may have raised, white patches in addition to bizarre vascularity. Adenomyosis is flat and has mosaicism with central perforations leading into the myometrium. Synechiae are avascular bridges, which join the anterior and posterior uterine walls. These bridges course in an irregular fashion. In contrast, the avascular fibers of a uterine septum run parallel to one another. Endometrial polyps are tan and soft. They may have a small central blood vessel, and the smaller ones can be transilluminated. Myomas are white or yellow, and firm. They cannot be transilluminated and usually have a complex but orderly network of vessels coursing over their surfaces.

COMPLICATIONS

Complications from diagnostic hysteroscopy are very rare. In our experience over the past 20 years none have occurred following diagnostic hysteroscopy, and even after operative hysteroscopy the incidence has been approximately 1%. Complications may include infection, uterine perforation, heavy bleeding (intrauterine or at the sites of tenaculum placement or anesthesia injections), drug allergy, or related to the media. Hypercarbia or gas embolization has not been reported if a proper insufflator was used, and fluid overload occurs only with the use of high volumes of liquid media. Vasovagal reactions are rare and usually resolve quickly without any intervention. Failure to dilate the cervix, failure to obtain an adequate view, and inability to complete an examination because of patient discomfort are rare.

Most diagnostic studies may be completed in a few minutes. If more time elapses and if one or both fallopian tube(s) is(are) patent, shoulder pain secondary to pneumoperitoneum may occur when the patient resumes the erect position, causing the CO_2 to contact the diaphragm. Patients are not told of this possibility before surgery because pain may not occur, and because they may become alarmed if it does not. Instead, my response to that complaint is one of encouragement: "That's great, it means that at least one of your fallopian tubes is open."

Occasionally, the cervix cannot be dilated because of stenosis—abandon the procedure, reschedule under general or regional anesthesia, and consider placing laminaria prior to surgery. To date, this has occurred only once in more than 7000 diagnostic and operative hysteroscopies. The sharply retroverted or anteverted uterus has not precluded an adequate examination to date, but probably will at some time in the future. A table that tilts and can be raised, dilators with an acute bend, and patience usually overcome marked uterine flexion or version.

If uterine distension is inadequate, check your system. Is there adequate gas in the tank? Is there a leak in the tubing itself, or between the insufflator and tubing, tubing and sheath, sheath and hysteroscope, or hysteroscope and cervix? Is the flow rate adequate? If no leak is detected and if an adequate volume of CO_2 is present, increase the flow rate. Withdraw the telescope to the region of the internal os. Has the uterus been perforated? If so, abandon the procedure. In our experience, uterine perforations have occurred only during operative hysteroscopy. In cases of central perforations we have not hospitalized the patient or followed the hematocrit. Antibiotics have not been prescribed. If uterine distension is adequate but the view is poor because of blood, cellular debris or bubbles, remember patience, an aspirating catheter and Hyskon. If the tubal ostia are obscured and the surgery was not timed for the early proliferative phase, do not be surprised. Failure to visualize the ostia may be because of overdeveloped endometrium, spasm or local lesions (polyps, adhesions). Proper timing and general anesthesia will overcome the former two problems, and appropriate instruments the latter.

If patient discomfort is extreme, desist immediately. Hysteroscopy should cause less discomfort than an HSG. Consider more analgesia or anesthesia. Perhaps the patient is not an appropriate candidate for an office procedure and should have a general or regional anesthesic in a day-surgery unit. This patient is the exception who proves the rule that hysteroscopy is an office procedure.

As with all new procedures, begin only after taking a course, reading some texts, and observing an accomplished surgeon. A short "how-to" text should be read prior to taking a course. Select a course that includes practice on inanimate (plastic uteri, squash, peppers, and liver) and animate (cow, rabbit) specimens. Next, observe an experienced operator. Finally, begin to do diagnostic procedures in the operating room under the watchful eye of an experienced proctor. After you have mastered the technique and can recognize most lesions, you are ready to begin diagnostic hysteroscopy in the office. This procedure will make more efficient use of your time, streamline patient evaluation, facilitate more precise treatment plans, and reduce patient costs. Every gynecologist needs a hysteroscope in the office, and the time is long overdue.

REFERENCES

1. Burnett JE. Hysteroscopy-controlled curettage for endometrial polyps. Obstet Gynecol 1964;24: 621–625.
2. Gimpelson RJ. Panoramic hysteroscopy with directed biopsies vs. dilatation and curettage for accurate diagnosis. J Reprod Med 1984;29:575–578.
3. Gimpelson RJ, Rappold HO. A comparative study between panoramic hysteroscopy with directed biopsies and dilatation and curettage. Am J Obstet Gynecol 1988;158:489–492.
4. Derman SG, Rehnstrom J, Neuwirth RS. The long-term effectiveness of hysteroscopic treatment of menorrhagia and leiomyomas. Obstet Gynecol 1991;77:591–594.
5. Neuwirth RS. Hysteroscopic management of symptomatic submucous fibroids. Obstet Gynecol 1983;62:509–511.
6. March CM, Israel R. Hysteroscopic management of recurrent abortion caused by septate uterus. Am J Obstet Gynecol 1987;156:834–842.
7. March CM, Israel R. Gestational outcome following hysteroscopic lysis of adhesions. Fertil Steril 1981;36:455–459.
8. Hamou J, Taylor PJ. Panoramic, contact and microcolpohysteroscopy in gynecologic practice. Curr Prob Obstet Gynecol 1982;6:2:1–75.
9. Loffer FD. Hysteroscopy with selective sampling compared with D&C for abnormal uterine bleeding: The value of a negative hysteroscopic view. Obstet Gynecol 1989;73:16–20.
10. March CM. Hysteroscopy as an aid to diagnosis in female infertility. Clin Obstet Gynecol 1983; 26:302–312.

11. Mencaglia L, Perino A, Hamou J. Hysteroscopy in perimenopausal and postmenopausal women with abnormal uterine bleeding. J Reprod Med 1987;32:577–582.
12. Valle RF. Hysteroscopic evaluation of patients with abnormal uterine bleeding. Surg Gynecol Obstet 1981;153:521–526.
13. Fraser IS. Hysteroscopy and laparoscopy in women with menorrhagia. Obstet Gynecol 1990;162:1264–1269.
14. Goldrath MH, Sherman AI. Office hysteroscopy and suction curettage. Can we eliminate the hospital diagnostic dilatation and curettage? Am J Obstet Gynecol 1985;152:220–229.
15. Ward B, Gravlee LC, Wideman GL: The fallacy of simple curettage. Obstet Gynecol 1958;12:642.
16. Frydman R, Eibschitz I, Fernadez IT, et al. Uterine evaluation by microhysteroscopy in IVF candidates. Hum Reprod 1987;2:481–485.
17. Fedele L. Transvaginal ultrasonography versus hysteroscopy in the diagnosis of uterine submucous myomas. Obstet Gynecol 1991;77:745–748.
18. Friedman A, DeFazio J, DeCherney A. Severe obstetric complications after aggressive treatment of Asherman's Syndrome. Obstet Gynecol 1986;67:864–867.
19. Jewelwicz R, Khalaf S, Neuwirth RS, et al. Obstetric complications after treatment of intrauterine synechiae (Asherman's Syndrome). Obstet Gynecol 1976;47:701.
20. Valle RF, Sciarra JJ. Intrauterine adhesions: hysteroscopic diagnosis, classification, treatment, and reproductive outcome. Am J Obstet Gynecol 1988;158:1459.
21. Ranta H, Aine R, Oksanen H, et al. Dissemination of endometrial cells during carbon dioxide hysteroscopy and chromotubation among infertile patients. Fertil Steril 1990;53:751.

Chapter 5

Operative Hysteroscopy
Myomas, Septums, and Synechiae

Richard J. Gimpelson

The hysteroscopic management of myomas, septums, and intrauterine synechiae can range from very simple procedures to extremely difficult ones, which should be managed by experienced hysteroscopists. Septums and synechiae will almost always require laparoscopic guidance; whereas myomas, in many circumstances, can be managed by hysteroscopy alone.

LEIOMYOMAS

Studies have shown that leiomyomas occur in 1.5% of the general fertile female population (1). Patients with infertility will have leiomyomas 2–6% of the time, whereas up to 17% of those women with abnormal uterine bleeding will have intrauterine leiomyomas (2–7).

Although a pelvic examination will reveal an enlarged uterus secondary to leiomyomas, there are many women with normal-to-borderline enlarged uteri with symptomatic submucous leiomyomas. In those women with abnormal bleeding, a transvaginal ultrasound will often reveal the size and amount of intramural component secondary to submucous leiomyomas (8). Leiomyomas in infertility patients will usually be diagnosed by hysterosalpingogram (9), but transvaginal ultrasound should still be utilized to evaluate the intramural component. Although magnetic resonance imaging (MRI) will give a remarkably clear picture of leiomyomas, its high cost prohibits its use in most cases (10). The definitive diagnosis of submucous leiomyomas is made by hysteroscopy. Once a leiomyoma is suspected as the cause of bleeding or infertility, hysteroscopy becomes the means to both diagnose and treat the condition. The method and location of treatment will vary depending on the skill of the operator and equipment available. Many submucous leiomyomas can be easily treated in an office setting, while others should be done only in an operating room under anesthesia, and at times, with laparoscopic guidance (11).

Leiomyomas that are 1 cm in diameter, regardless of the size of the intracavity component, can usually be resected in an office setting with a set of simple instruments and the equipment used for a routine diagnostic hysteroscopy (Table 5.1). Either CO_2 or normal saline can be used as the distension media. If the leiomyoma is on a stalk, it is simply grasped and removed. If the leiomyoma is mostly intramural (Fig. 5.1*A*), the capsule around the leiomyoma can be incised, causing the leiomyoma to rise into the cavity (Fig. 5.1*B*). At this point, the leiomyoma is grasped with the biopsy forceps (Fig. 5.1*C*), or the pituitary rongeur (Fig. 5.2). Either instrument can be inserted alongside the diagnostic sheath while keeping the cervical seal tight with the 4-toothed tenaculum (Fig. 5.3), (Richard Wolf Medical Instruments Company, Vernon Hills, IL, Patent #5,059,198). Using this technique, the myoma can be grasped and removed

62 GYNECOLOGIC ENDOSCOPY: Principles in Practice

Table 5.1. Additional Instruments for Myomectomy

Operating hysteroscope
Semi-rigid scissors and biopsy forceps
Pituitary rongeur
Corson myoma grasper
4-toothed cervical sealing tenaculum

under direct vision. Pedunculated myomas less than 2 cm in diameter can be similarly removed (Fig. 5.4).

Leiomyomas that are 2 to 3 cm in diameter and pedunculated are easily removed by using the Corson Myoma Grasper (Zinnanti Surgical Instruments, Inc., Chatsworth, CA (Fig. 5.5). The location of the myoma is visualized with the hysteroscope. The myoma grasper is inserted and the myoma is grasped. At this point, several rotations will assure separation of the myoma from its bed, and extraction is easily accomplished if the cervix has been adequately dilated. Once the myoma is removed, the uterine cavity should be hysteroscopically re-examined to verify complete removal and adequate hemostasis.

Myomas greater than 3 cm in diameter and that are over 50% intrauterine can be removed in the same manner as pedunculated myomas, once the capsule is incised to allow some migration out of the myometrium.

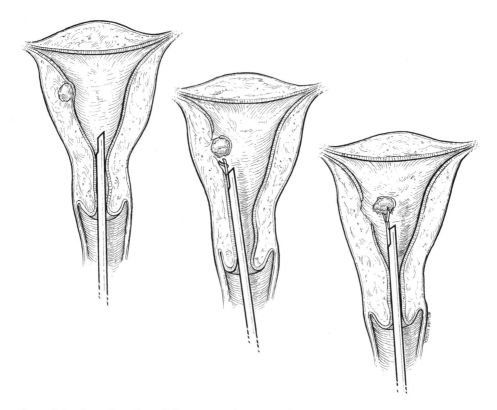

Figure 5.1. Resection of small leiomyoma that is mostly intramural. (From Isaacson K. Office Hysteroscopy. St. Louis: CV Mosby, 1994.)

Chapter 5: Myomas, Septums, and Synechiae   63

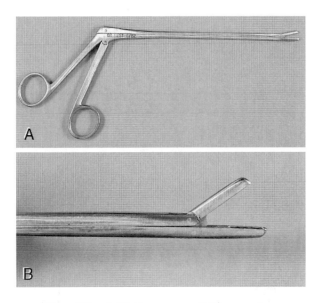

Figure 5.2. **A.** Pituitary rongeur. **B.** Close-up view.

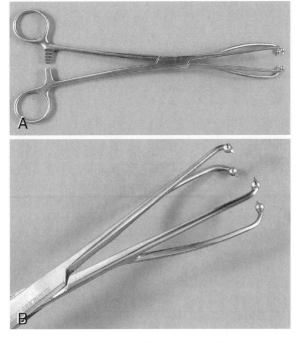

Figure 5.3. **A.** Four-toothed tenaculum. **B.** Close-up view.

64 GYNECOLOGIC ENDOSCOPY: Principles in Practice

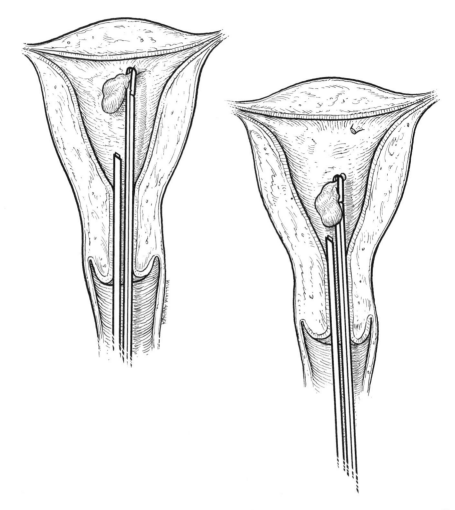

Figure 5.4. Removal of pedunculated leiomyoma with pituitary rongeur. (From Isaacson K. Office Hysteroscopy. St. Louis: CV Mosby, 1994.)

Sessile myomas of 2–3 cm in diameter, in which over 50% of the myoma is intramural, or myomas greater than 4 cm in diameter, are more easily removed with the resectoscope (Fig. 5.6A). The myoma is shaved until it is even with the myometrium (Fig 5.6B). At this point, after a few minutes, the contraction of the uterus will squeeze the myoma more into the uterine cavity, and resection can be continued (Fig. 5.6C). Occasionally, the myoma will not migrate into the uterine cavity during a single procedure. In this case, the patient can be brought back for a repeat procedure in 1 month. The myoma will often become largely intracavitary and more easily removed. It has been the author's experience that even a 3-stage procedure may be necessary. This was the case with a 6-cm myoma occupying the entire intramural space. If the myoma is reduced enough in size, the remaining portion can often be removed with the Corson Myoma Grasper, pituitary rongeur, or even with suction curettage (Fig. 5.6D). As with smaller my-

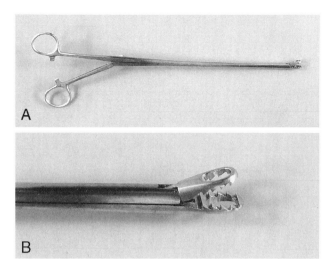

Figure 5.5. **A.** Corson Myoma Grasper. **B.** Close-up view.

omas, the hysteroscope should always be used to visualize the uterine cavity at the end of the procedure to verify complete removal of the leiomyoma, and check for perforations. If the myoma is of a size that it extends from submucous to subserous location, laparoscopic guidance may be used to reduce the risk of perforation or observe perforation immediately, if it occurs. When using the resectoscope, care should be taken not to resect below the level of the endometrial surface. This precaution will reduce the risk of perforation. Another problem encountered with the resectoscope is the management of the resected myoma fragments. If the size of the uterine cavity and the size and location of the leiomyoma allow the fragments to float away from the field of view, resection can be continued until visualization is compromised. At this point, the resection is stopped and the fragments will need to be removed. A polyp forceps, Corson Myoma Grasper, ring forceps, or suction curette, can be utilized to remove most of the fragments. The few remaining fragments can be removed by visualizing them with the resectoscope and trapping them between the loop and sheath, and then easily removed. If the myoma is in such a location, usually lower uterine segment, the view may be compromised by as little as one fragment. In this case, the resectoscope and its accompanying fragment should be removed with each stroke and the fragment then removed from the resectoscope and the resectoscope reinserted. Although this may seem tedious, it is the quickest and safest way to do a myomectomy when each fragment obscures the field of vision.

The resectoscope electrical generator is set at 80 watts (pure cut) and the power is increased as needed (usually not more than 90 watts). The resectoscopic loop should cut through the myoma without resistance. Although higher powers have been reported, it is rarely necessary (12). The resectoscope should only be powered during a withdrawal motion, and never during an insertion motion, to minimize the risk of perforation and other organ damage.

A paracervical block is given with up to 20 mL of 0.25% bupivacaine, containing 2 U pitressin, in each 10 mL of anesthetic. This paracervical block is given

66 GYNECOLOGIC ENDOSCOPY: Principles in Practice

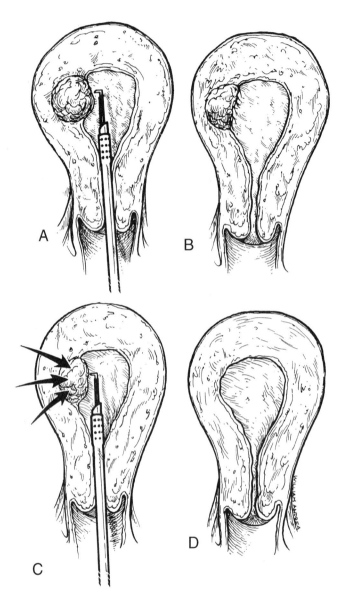

Figure 5.6. Excision of leiomyoma with resectoscope. (From Bieber E. Gynecologic Resectoscope. Cambridge, MA: Blackwell Scientific Publications.)

whether the patient is under general, regional, or local anesthesia. The block will provide postoperative comfort, allow easier insertion of the hysteroscope and resectoscope, and reduce the risk of bleeding and intravasation of distension media (13).

To reduce the risk of iatrogenic hyponatremia, CO_2 or conductive low-viscosity liquids (i.e., lactated Ringer's solution or normal saline) should be used when performing myomectomy with instruments other than a resectoscope. Fluid status should be monitored carefully. Preoperative electrolytes should be obtained and available to compare with intraoperative or postoperative levels, if needed.

Prophylactic antibiotics can be used at the time of myomectomy considering the number of insertions and removals that occur during this procedure. In those patients desiring fertility, a course of estrogen may be considered for one cycle following myomectomy to help the regeneration of any normal endometrium that may have been damaged.

Utilization of GnRH agonists may be a two-edged sword. In most cases, GnRH agonists will reduce bleeding and allow restoration of hemoglobin and hematocrit prior to myomectomy (14). Although heavy bleeding has been reported following the use of GnRH agonists with leiomyomas, this is rarely seen (15). GnRH agonists given over 3 to 4 months will generally reduce the myoma size over 25%. In this same time period, the uterus itself will shrink over 40% (16). Thus, GnRH agonists are utilized with myomas with a substantial intramural component, since the combined shrinkage of the uterus and myoma will often cause the myoma to migrate toward the uterine cavity, making removal or resection easier. However, in the case in which the myoma occupies at least 50% of the intrauterine cavity, after a course of a GnRH agonist the myoma may occupy nearly the entire cavity, and subsequently make the resection somewhat more tedious and difficult. The thinning of the endometrium secondary to the GnRH agonist's action does help with visualization during myoma resection. This same improved visualization is evident during the early to mid proliferative phase. Additionally, GnRH agonists appear to reduce the blood supply and bleeding that occur with myomectomy, as well as the amount of fluid absorption. Insertion of instruments may be slightly more difficult when GnRH agonists are secondary to the hypoestrogenic effect; therefore, care should be taken during cervical dilatation and insertion. GnRH agonist utilization has also resulted in the prolapsing of a myoma through the cervical canal. If this occurs, the myoma can be easily removed with a ring forceps. This reduces the risk of infection that can occur with prolapsed myomas. Usually only the stump remains and the myomectomy is essentially complete. Hysteroscopic examination should still be done to evaluate the uterine cavity for the presence of any other lesions, and to verify complete removal of the leiomyoma.

The Nd:YAG laser can also be used for myomectomy (16, 17). It can be used to incise the capsule, or, like a resectoscope, to slice the myoma into smaller pieces for removal. However, the author has found this method slower and with higher fluid absorption, especially if combined with endometrial ablation (18).

Bleeding is uncommon following hysteroscopic myomectomy by any method. However, if it does occur, a Foley catheter with a 30-mL bulb filled with 10–20 mL of saline can be used as tamponade. The catheter can be left in for 2 to 6 hours, then removed. This is effective in the majority of cases. If the bleeding continues, a catheter can be reinserted and left in overnight. If bleeding still persists, a repeat hysteroscopic examination with directed coagulation may be necessary.

SEPTUM

The treatment of the septate uterus has evolved from open metroplasty to a hysteroscopic procedure. In fact, today there is no reason to perform a metroplasty for uterine septum other than by hysteroscopy (19). As opposed to myomectomy when laparoscopic guidance is needed only under certain circumstances, laparoscopic guidance is essential for a hysteroscopic metroplasty. This is necessary to evaluate the uterine shape to rule out a bicornuate uterus, and to guide the metroplasty to minimize the risk and extent of perforation. Ultrasound and magnetic resonance imaging have been shown to be helpful in evaluating the type of mullerian fusion defect present, and to give an idea as to myometrial thickness and fundal deformity, but these evaluations are not replacements for laparoscopic evaluation, since other causes of infertility, such as endometriosis or adhesive disease, may be discovered and treated (20, 21). Compared to a myomectomy, scissors or fiber laser (Nd:YAG, argon, or KTP) are more easily utilized than the resectoscope. The scissors and laser fibers can be inserted through a 21 Fr operating hysteroscope when the resectoscope is 24 Fr or larger. This is especially important in the patient with a complete septum in which manipulation can be somewhat constricted.

Before a metroplasty is performed for infertility, a complete infertility workup should be performed. However, the patient does not have to demonstrate pregnancy loss prior to the procedure. Once a laparoscopy is indicated, a hysteroscopic metroplasty can be performed at the same time. Similarly, if a patient with abnormal bleeding has accompanying pelvic pain that warrants a laparoscopic and hysteroscopic assessment, a septum discovered at the time of hysteroscopy should be divided. A metroplasty, in this case, should be performed even if infertility has not been a problem, since it would be unfair to allow one or two pregnancy losses to occur in the future on this patient. The risk of laparoscopy is so much greater than that of hysteroscopy that there is no reason to delay the metroplasty to another time (22, 23).

Hysteroscopic metroplasty is best performed in early to mid-proliferative phase. As stated earlier, scissors or fiber lasers are preferred over electrosurgery secondary to the smaller operating sheaths required and the ability to use a balanced electrolyte solution for a distension medium. This reduces the additional risk of iatrogenic hyponatremia and fluid overload.

For a subseptate uterus, the septum is divided to the fundus. Caution should be exercised not to go too deep into the myometrium and cause a subsequent weakness. For a complete septum, the septum is divided to its midportion to allow a communication to occur between the two sides. This is done by inserting a sound or dilator on one side and pressing against the septum (Fig. 5.7A). The operating hysteroscope is inserted on the other side, and using either a scissors or fiber laser, the septum is divided at the bulge (Fig. 5.7B). Once an opening is created, the 4-toothed tenaculum or a small catheter is used to seal the side opposite the hysteroscope, and the septum is then divided toward the fundus in the same manner as the subseptate uterus. One must be careful near the tubal ostia when using the laser, since the free beam of the laser can cause thermal damage to the ostia. Any fiber laser can be used since the procedure is done with a dragging technique, resulting in thermal damage of 2-mm, whether an argon, KTP, or Nd:YAG laser is used (24). With a subseptate uterus, the septum is incised by dragging along each side, gradually thinning the septum (Fig. 5.8A) or incising across the septum, causing it to gradually shorten (Fig. 5.8B). With scissors, the shortening technique is optimal. With a complete septum, the lower uterine segment portion

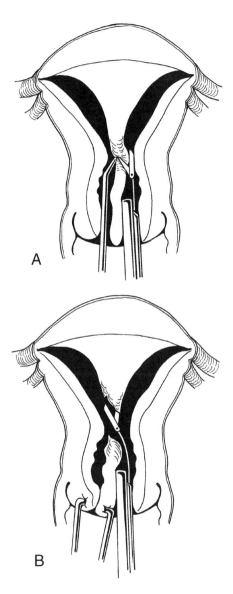

Figure 5.7. **A.** Hysteroscopic division of complete uterine septum with septate cervix. 1. A window is performed at level of internal cervical os. **B.** Hysteroscopic division of complete uterine septum with septate cervix. 2. The cervix not housing the hysteroscope is occluded and the corporeal uterine septum is divided.

is not divided if there is a double cervix. The general consensus is that this preserves the integrity of the cervix and reduces the risk of incompetence.

Following metroplasty, the patient is discharged on antibiotics and estrogen (22, 25, 26). There are many dosage regimens; however, the author prefers amoxicillin 250 mg three times daily for one week, and conjugated estrogen 2.5 mg daily for 20 days. Following the next menses, a diagnostic hysteroscopy or hysterogram should be performed. If there is residual septum or adhesions, these can

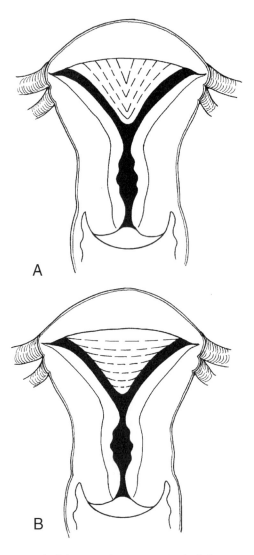

Figure 5.8. A. Gradual thinning of septum. **B.** Gradual shortening of septum.

easily be divided with scissors in an office setting (11). The success of hysteroscopic metroplasty is very high, and is the procedure of choice for septate uterus.

If a resectoscope with a loop electrode is used, the increased diameter of the sheath will sometimes make the procedure more difficult. However, a metroplasty can be performed with a horizontal loop or point electrode.

The technique is the same as that with the laser. The septum can be divided by either the thinning or shortening technique. If there is a complete septum, one side of the uterus must be occluded with a catheter or nonconductive probe to allow perforation of the septum. The resectoscope is more difficult to manipulate than a laser fiber or scissors, and additionally requires electrolyte-free distension media, which increases the operative risk of hyponatremia and the development of pulmonary edema. Since hyponatremia occurs at a lower volume of fluid intravasation than pulmonary edema, the use of electrical energy in this situation may increase the likelihood of stopping the surgery prematurely.

If either immediate or delayed bleeding is encountered following hysteroscopic metroplasty, the source is most likely small arteries (27). Hysteroscopic examination and selective coagulation of the bleeding source is the best treatment, rather than hormonal manipulation.

SYNECHIAE

Intrauterine adhesions can cause infertility or hematometra. Both of these conditions can be treated by operative hysteroscopy, usually accompanied by laparoscopic guidance. The author recommends the use of a hysteroscopic scissors, rather than using laser or electrical energy. Since patients with intrauterine adhesions already have areas of devitalized tissue, thermal damage caused by laser or electricity may create additional areas of devascularization.

A hysterosalpingogram should be done prior to intrauterine adhesiolysis to allow a preoperative mapping of the uterine cavity. If there is occlusion of the uterine cavity on hysterosalpingogram, a transvaginal ultrasound may give the operator an idea of the uterine size, myometrial thickness, and evidence of hematometra. If there is not obstructed entry into the uterus, the procedure will depend on the hystersalpingogram findings. Simple central adhesions can usually be divided easily without laparoscopic guidance, often in an office setting (11). If the adhesions are diffuse, especially if they occupy the lateral and cornual areas, laparoscopic guidance will reduce the risk and extent of perforation.

The consistency of the adhesions will give some guide to the prognosis of successful pregnancy outcome following adhesiolysis. Thin, filmy adhesions are easily divided and almost never recur. Fibromuscular adhesions when divided will usually not recur; however, thick avascular connective tissue adhesions may be divided, but frequently recur and may continue to cause infertility (28).

The best classification of adhesions involves location and aspect (Table 5.2) (29). Excellent results can be expected in terms of normal menses and pregnancy

Table 5.2. Classification According to the Location and the Aspect of the Adhesions

Degree	Location
I	Central adhesions (bridge-like adhesions)
	(a) Thin or filmy adhesions (endometrial adhesions)
	(b) Myofibrous or connective adhesions
II	Marginal adhesions (always myofibrous or connective)
	(a) Ledge-like projections
	(b) Obliteration of one horn
III	Uterine cavity absent on hystersalpingography
	(a) Occlusion of the internal os (upper cavity normal) (pseudo-Asherman's syndrome)
	(b) Extensive coaptation of the uterine walls (absence of uterine cavity) (true Asherman's syndrome)

From Donnez J, Nisolle M. Hysteroscopic lysis of intrauterine adhesions (Asherman's syndrome). In: Donnez J, Niselle M, eds. An Atlas of Laser Operative Laparoscopy and Hysterectomy. New York: Parthenon, 1994:305–312.

rates with adhesions classified as Ia, Ib, IIa, IIb, and IIIa. Adhesions classified as IIb and IIIb will usually recur and the prognosis for pregnancy is very poor.

The key to safe successful adhesiolysis is experience and patience. Lysis of adhesions can be tedious and not for the impatient operator. However, constant awareness of distension media balance and the possibility of fluid overload and subsequent pulmonary edema, is essential.

If the hysterosalpingogram does not demonstrate an entry into the uterine cavity, extreme caution should be exercised. Often, it is only the lower uterine segment that is occluded and once penetrated, the cavity is easily seen. Preoperative ultrasound is recommended. Once an adequate assessment of the uterine size, position, and presence or absence of hematometra is completed, the surgical procedure can be scheduled. This patient should be treated in the operating room under laparoscopic guidance. A smaller diameter telescope and sheath is often helpful to look into the small channels created. A specially designed dilator with measurements on it (Fig. 5.9) is very useful in probing into the adhesions and creating channels for the hysteroscope to enter. By not advancing this dilator beyond the premeasured uterine length, perforation is unlikely. By inserting the 4-mm telescope with 5-mm sheath into the cervical canal, and by gently advancing the hysteroscope, the adhesions can be viewed and divided. If the adhesions do not completely divide, the diagnostic sheath is replaced with an operative sheath; and using the scissors, the adhesions are carefully divided, or small channels can be probed under direct vision to avoid perforation. Eventually, the uterine cavity is entered, in most cases, when this technique is used. Once inside the cavity, any additional adhesions can be addressed. Just as with a uterine septum, the patient can be discharged on antibiotics for 1 week and conjugated estrogen for 20 days.

Occasionally, the procedure may need to be prematurely terminated secondary to uterine perforation, bleeding, or excess intravasation of distension media. In the case of perforation, it is necessary to wait 3 months to allow uterine healing prior to repeating the hystersalpingogram to decide if further lysis is

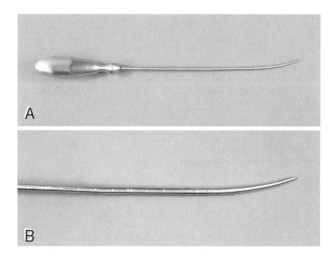

Figure 5.9. **A.** Sound dilator. **B.** Close-up view.

needed. If the procedure is terminated secondary to bleeding or fluid overload or hyponatremia, the hysterosalpingogram and hysteroscopy are repeated in 1 month. If significant adhesions re-form after subsequent procedures, any additional intrauterine surgery may serve only to create false hope and deplete financial resources.

REFERENCES

1. Cooper JM, Houck RM, Rigberg HS. The incidence of intrauterine abnormalities found at hysteroscopy in patients undergoing elective hysteroscopic sterilization. J Reprod Med 1983;28: 659–661.
2. Cohen MR, Dmowski WP. Modern hysteroscopy: Diagnostic and therapeutic potential. Fertil Steril 1973;24:905–911.
3. Mohr J, Lindemann HJ. Hysteroscopy in the infertile patient. J Reprod Med 1977;19:161–162.
4. Taylor PJ, Leader A, George RE. Combined laparoscopy and hysteroscopy in the investigation of infertility. In: Siegler AM, Lindemann HJ, eds. Hysteroscopy: principles and practices. Philadelphia: JB Lippincott, 1984:207–210.
5. Siegler AM, Kenmann E, Gentile GP. Hysteroscopic procedures in 257 patients. Fertil Steril 1976;27:1267–1273.
6. Sciarra JJ, Valle RF. Hysteroscopy: a clinical experience with 320 patients. Am J Obstet Gynecol 1977;127:340–348.
7. Valle RF. Hysteroscopic evaluation of patients with abnormal uterine bleeding. Surg Gynecol Obstet 1981;153:521–526.
8. Batzer FR. Vaginosonographic evaluation of the nonpregnant uterus. Am J Gynecol Health 1992;6(2):28–31.
9. Donnez J, Schrurs B, Gillerot S, Sandow J, Clerckx F. Treatment of uterine fibroids with implants of gonadotropin-releasing hormone agonist: assessment by hysterography. Fertil Steril 1989;51: 947–950.
10. Hricak H, Tscholakoff D, Heinrichs L, Fisher MR, Dooms GC, Rinhold C, Jaffe RB. Uterine leiomyomas: correlation of MR, histopathologic findings and symptoms. Radiology 1986;158: 385–391.
11. Gimpelson, RJ. Office hysteroscopy. Clin Obstet Gynecol 1992;35(2):270–281.
12. Townsend DE, Fields G, McCausland A, Kauffman K. Diagnostic and operative hysteroscopy in the management of persistent post-menopausal bleeding. Obstet Gynecol 1993;82:419–421.
13. Corson SL, Brooks PG, Serden SP, Batzer FR, Gocial B. Effects of vasopressin administration during hysteroscopic surgery. J Reprod Med 1994;39:419–423.
14. Friedman AJ, Barbieri RL, Benacerraf BR, Schiff I. Treatment of leiomyomata with intranasal or subcutaneous leuprolide, a gonadotropin-releasing hormone agonist. Fertil Steril 1987;48: 560–564.
15. Indman PD. Hysteroscopic treatment of menorrhagia associated with uterine leiomyomas. Obstet Gynecol 1993;81:716–720.
16. Donnez J, Gillerot S, Bourgonjon D, Clerckx F, Nisolle M. Neodymium:YAG laser hysteroscopy in large submucous fibroids. Fertil Steril 1990;54:999–1003.
17. Baggish MS, Barbot J, Valle RF. Operative hysteroscopy I. In: Baggish MS, Barbot J, Valle RF, eds. Diagnostic and operative hysteroscopy: a text and atlas. Chicago: Year Book, 1989:174–178.
18. Gimpelson RJ. Hysteroscopic Nd:YAG laser ablation of the endometrium. J Reprod Med 1988;33:872–876.
19. March CM, Israel R. Hysteroscopic management of recurrent abortion caused by septate uterus. Am J Obstet Gynecol 1987;156:834–842.
20. Fedele L, Ferrazi E, Dorta M, Vercellini P, Candiani GB. Ultrasonography in the differential diagnosis of "double" uteri. Fertil Steril 1988;50:361–364.
21. Letterie GS, Wilson J, Miyazawa K. Magnetic resonance imaging of mullerian tract abnormalities. Fertil Steril 1988;50:365–366.

22. Hulka JF, Peterson HA, Phillips JM, Surrey MW. Operative hysteroscopy: American Association of Gynecologic Laparoscopists' 1993 membership survey. J Am Assoc Gynecol Lap 1995;2: 131–132.
23. Hulka JF, Peterson HA, Phillips JM, Surrey MW. Operative laparoscopy: American Association of Gynecologic Laparoscopists' 1993 membership survey. J Am Assoc Gynecol Lap 1995;2: 133–136.
24. Shirk GJ, Gimpelson RJ, Krewer K. Comparison of tissue effects with sculptured fiberoptic cables and other Nd:YAG laser and argon laser treatments. Lasers in Surg Med 1991;11:563–568.
25. Daly DC, Walters CA, Soto-Albors C, Riddick DH. Hysteroscopic metroplasty: surgical technique and obstetric outcome. Fertil Steril 1983;39:623–628.
26. Valle RF, Sciarra JJ. Hysteroscopic treatment of the septate uterus. Obstet Gynecol 1986;67: 253–257.
27. Kazer RR, Meyer K, Valle RF. Late hemorrhage after transcervical division of a uterine septum: a report of 2 cases. Fertil Steril 1992;57:930–932.
28. Valle RF, Sciarra JJ. Intrauterine adhesions: hysteroscopic diagnosis, classification, treatment and reproductive outcome. Am J Obstet Gynecol 1988;158:1459–1470.
29. Donnez J, Nisolle M. Hysteroscopic lysis of intrauterine adhesions (Asherman's syndrome). In: Donnez J, Niselle M, eds. An atlas of laser operative laparoscopy and hysteroscopy. New York: Parthenon, 1994;305–312.

ACKNOWLEDGMENT

The author acknowledges the invaluable assistance of Marsha L. Bagby, R.N., in the preparation of this manuscript for publication.

Chapter 6
Operative Hysteroscopy
Endometrial Ablation

Frank DeLeon

Excessive menstrual blood loss exceeding 80 mL per menses and lasting more than 7 days is defined as menorrhagia. This physically incapacitating condition occurs in 10% of women (1). Its etiology may be due to organic causes such as fibroids, polyps, hematologic disorders or, more commonly, due to dysfunctional uterine bleeding (DUB). Dysfunctional uterine bleeding is defined as excessive uterine bleeding due to no demonstrable organic cause and mostly due to abnormality of the hypothalamic pituitary axis, resulting in chronic anovulation. The treatment of dysfunctional uterine bleeding is medical with hormonal therapy. However, medical therapy may only be temporarily successful, and patients may require further definitive therapy in the form of hysterectomy.

Hysterectomy is the most common major gynecologic operation performed in the United States, with nearly 600,000 of these procedures reported in 1990 by the Department of Health and Human Services (2). Although there are many indications for hysterectomy, dysfunctional uterine bleeding unresponsive to medical therapy and dilatation and curettage is the indication given in as many as half of these procedures (3). Hysterectomy, however, is an expensive option in our health care system to treat patients with dysfunctional uterine bleeding, and carries a mortality rate of 0.1–0.2% (4), and a morbidity rate as high as 59% (5). An alternative to hysterectomy to treat dysfunctional uterine bleeding unresponsive to medical therapy is endometrial ablation, first reported by Goldrath et al. in 1981 (6). This chapter will describe the technique of endometrial ablation and discuss its advantages and disadvantages in the treatment of abnormal uterine bleeding, and provide recommendations to the novice for developing hands-on experience in learning this procedure.

HISTORY OF ENDOMETRIAL ABLATION

The goal of an effective endometrial ablation is to destroy the basalis layer of the endometrium to prevent its regrowth, causing amenorrhea. This technique was first described in 1981 by Goldrath et al. (6) when he used the Nd:YAG laser to destroy the endometrium of patients with menorrhagia unresponsive to medical treatment. This endometrial destruction is similar to Asherman's description in 1948 of patients with a syndrome of infertility with amenorrhea associated with a previous uterine instrumentation and infection (7). Although the clinical result of amenorrhea with endometrial ablation is similar to Asherman's syndrome, the endometrial cavity response may differ in appearance. The cavity after an ablation is usually shrunken and shows destruction and distortion, whereas with true Asherman's syndrome there is varying severity of adhesion formation ranging from minimal adhesion to completely agglutinated walls.

In 1987 DeCherney et al. (8) described the effective use of the resectoscope, using a cutting loop electrode to destroy and scarify the lining of the uterus in a group of 21 patients with intractable uterine bleeding. In this group there were 14 with blood dyscrasias, four were poor anesthetic risks, and three refused hysterectomy. Only one of the 21 patients treated required a repeat ablation treatment. In 1987 Vancaillie (9) described the rollerball technique to perform effective endometrial ablation in 15 patients with only one failure occurring, which was subsequently treated by vaginal hysterectomy.

INDICATIONS AND CONTRAINDICATIONS

Endometrial ablation is ideal in the treatment of intractable uterine bleeding in a patient who has completed childbearing, has failed medical therapy, and does not wish to have a hysterectomy. It is also the method of choice in patients who have medical contraindications to hysterectomy. This includes patients with heart disease, chronic renal failure, or hematologic disorders, where laparotomy would place the patient at very high risk. These patients should be thoroughly screened by diagnostic hysteroscopy to exclude patients with benign intrauterine tumors such as polyps, myomas, or other pathology that may explain the abnormal bleeding. Other indications, such as treatment of premenstrual syndrome (10) and to shorten the length of a normal menstrual period, are extremely controversial and should be weighed against potential hazards associated with the surgical procedure. Another potential use of endometrial ablation is in women with postmenopausal bleeding with no abnormal pelvic findings and a benign endometrium, who are unresponsive to hormonal therapy and refuse hysterectomy.

To offer the patient the best results with endometrial ablation, ideally they should be properly selected. Candidates for the procedure should have a normal uterus size without any pathology, such as submucous myomas, endometrial hyperplasia, or adenomyosis. This procedure should not be advised to the patient if the uterus is excessively large or sounds greater than 12 cm.

PATIENT PREPARATION

Preoperative preparation involves counseling regarding the realistic outcome of the surgery and explanation of the procedure, including possible complications. Since endometrial ablation causes amenorrhea in only 60 to 70% of patients, it is important that patients understand that they may experience only shorter and lighter periods. The importance of adequate sterilization needs to be emphasized in patients in the childbearing age and offered to be done at the same time as the ablation is performed, since pregnancy following endometrial ablation has been reported. Patients should be informed that pregnancy following endometrial ablation carries the risk of having a spontaneous abortion, tubal pregnancy, premature labor, or abnormal location of the placenta (11).

Prior to performing an endometrial ablation, patients should be evaluated with an endometrial biopsy and a diagnostic hysteroscopy to rule out benign and malignant conditions that may account for the abnormal uterine bleeding. Patient preparation also includes suppression of the endometrium. This allows easier destruction of the basalis layer of the endometrium in a shorter time, and also stops uterine bleeding, which is important in anemic patients so that they may have an opportunity to rebuild their blood volume prior to the procedure. Several agents have been used to suppress the endometrium prior to the ablative procedure. These agents are given for a minimum of one month prior to the procedure and include danazol (Danocrine) 400 mg twice a day, medroxyprogesterone acetate (Provera) 20 mg daily, Depo-Provera 150 mg intramuscularly weekly, and GnRH agonists, especially the depot 3.75-mg intramuscular dose of leuprolide acetate once a month. The use of the GnRH agonist seems to result in the thinnest endometrium and is the author's choice for endometrial suppression.

Danazol (Danocrine) is an orally active attenuated androgen. This agent has been used to significantly reduce menstrual bleeding in patients complaining of menorrhagia (12) and acts by causing atrophy of the endometrium. Danazol has androgenic side effects including weight gain and acne, and in some patients the endometrium may show decidual changes intermixed with atrophic changes.

Medroxyprogesterone acetate may be given either as the oral or intramuscular form to decrease or stop uterine bleeding. Progestin converts proliferative endometrium to secretory endometrium and several histological changes occur including edema, vascular proliferation, and neovascularization of the endometrium. Atrophy of the endometrium, however, is not observed during short pretreatment courses of one month's duration.

Leuprolide acetate (Lupron) has been used extensively in patients with excessive uterine bleeding associated with uterine fibroids (13). By suppressing pituitary gonadotropins and ovarian estrogen production, GnRH agonists can also effectively induce atrophic endometrial changes prior to endometrial ablation (14).

An alternative to medical suppression to thin the endometrium prior to an ablation is a mechanical preparation by means of suction curettage. Evaluation of 28 patients treated by suction curettage revealed no significant difference from 109 patients pretreated medically prior to endometrial ablation (15). Advantages of mechanical preparation include reduction in costs, absence of side effects, and allowing to have a specimen for histopathologic evaluation.

DISTENSION

Endometrial ablation is an operative hysteroscopic procedure that depends on adequate uterine distension. Although several distending media have been utilized including Hyskon, electrolyte- and nonelectrolyte-containing low viscosity solutions, it is the latter medium that is most frequently used. Low viscosity nonelectrolyte-containing solutions include glycine 1.5%, sorbitol 3%, and mannitol. In the United States, glycine 1.5% is most commonly used as the medium of choice since it is readily available in operating rooms and is found in 3-liter bags. Glycine can be delivered via a mechanical pump at preset pressures of 80 mm Hg or, alternatively, the most common technique is to use gravity with the 3-liter bag connected to urologic tubing. A urologic bag collecting system is used to monitor the fluid that is collected, and when subtracted from the fluid used, an accurate determination of the total fluid absorbed by the patient can be made. Most ablations will require 3 to 6 liters of low viscosity fluid to maintain a clear field of vision. The amount of fluid will decrease with experience and shortening the operative time.

Sorbitol 3% is also a popular nonconductive, hypoosmolar low viscosity solution, miscible with blood, used for endometrial ablations. Both sorbitol 3% and glycine 1.5% are found in 3-liter bags and can be delivered by gravity alone, by putting a large pressure cuff around the bag and raising the intravenous pole as high as possible, or electrically via a pump such as the one developed by Storz, which can regulate a constant preset pressure.

It is imperative to monitor fluid intake and output closely to avoid fluid overload, which can lead to dilutional hyponatremia and pulmonary edema. We prefer to use a urology drape with a reservoir that can be hooked up to wall suction to adequately monitor fluid output.

INSTRUMENTATION

Destruction of the endometrium using the resectoscope can be achieved by using a rollerball electrode or wire loop electrode. It is important to understand the components of the resectoscope as well as ancillary equipment required for its proper use prior to performing a procedure on patients.

A resectoscope that is modified for endometrial ablation consists of 5 distinct units (Fig. 6.1). The first unit is a 0, 12, or 30° viewing telescope with an outer diameter of 3.5 mm. Although the 30° offset hysteroscope is excellent for viewing the cornual openings, the 12° angle telescope allows the rollerball to be seen when it is fully extended into the cavity (Fig. 6.2). The hysteroscope is then

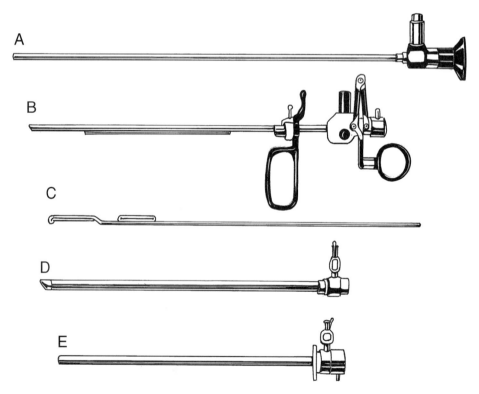

Figure 6.1. Components of 26 French continuous flow resectoscope. **A.** 3.5 mm hysteroscope. **B.** Working element. **C.** Electrode. **D.** Inner sheath. **E.** Outer sheath.

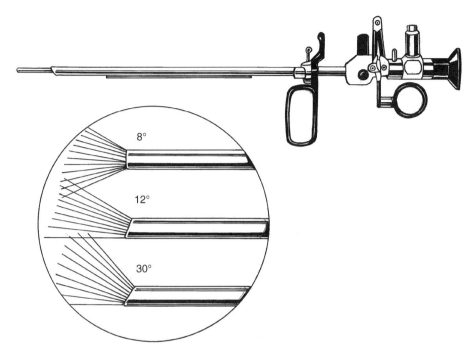

Figure 6.2. Assembled continuous flow resectoscope. Close-up of directions of view offered by straight forward (0°) and for oblique (12°) and (30°) hysteroscope.

placed within the resectoscope sheaths with the electrode in place (Figs. 6.3–6.5). There are two sheaths, inner and outer, that allow continuous inflow and outflow of irrigation, which is essential to maintain a clear field of vision during the procedure. The fourth unit is the working element. This allows the movement and control of the rollerball and cutting loop electrode in a forward and backward movement. The fifth unit is the electrode. There are several that can be used for an endometrial ablation. These electrodes include rollerball, rollerbar, and a variety of loop electrodes. The loop electrode is used primarily for shaving lesions such as myomas and polyps, but can be used for endometrial ablation as well. More popular, however, is the use of the rollerball or the slightly larger rollerbar, which has a larger surface contact area than the loop electrode, and has less risk of uterine perforation. Between the rollerball and rollerbar we prefer the latter, since more surface area can be covered, helping in finishing the procedure more efficiently. It is possible, however, that both of the loop electrodes and rollerball or rollerbar may be necessary, such as in a case where there is a small polyp or myoma that can be removed with the loop electrode prior to the ablation with the rollerbar. For this reason, one should have a variety of electrodes available at the time of the procedure. Once fully assembled, a continuous flow is established to remove debris from the front of the telescope, thus keeping the field clear (Fig. 6.6).

In addition to the resectoscope, an illumination source, an electrical surgical generator, a video camera, and video monitor are essential to perform endometrial ablations. The light source for operative hysteroscopy should be able to de-

80 GYNECOLOGIC ENDOSCOPY: Principles in Practice

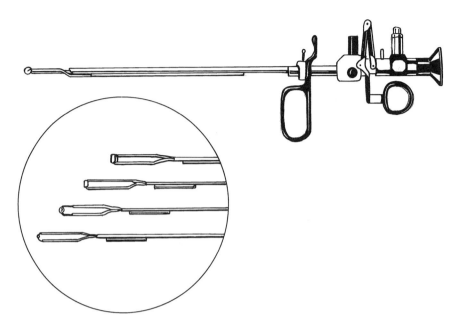

Figure 6.3. Close-up of interchangeable and disposable electrodes. These electrodes include rollerball, rollerbar, and loop.

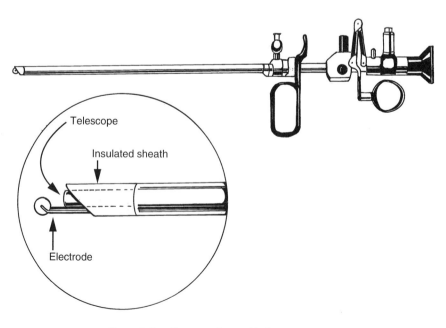

Figure 6.4. Close-up of assembled resectoscope.

Chapter 6: Endometrial Ablation 81

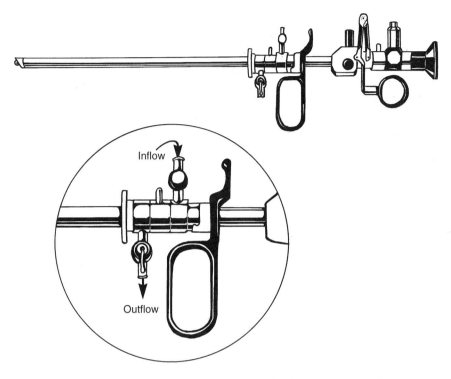

Figure 6.5. Inflow and outflow channels of inner and outer sheaths of a continuous flow resectoscope.

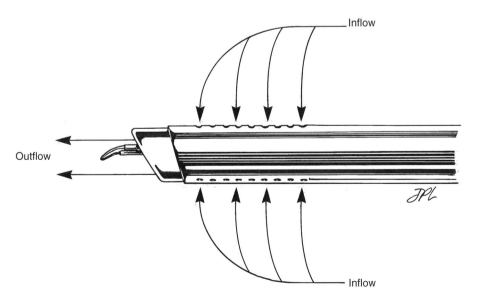

Figure 6.6. Close-up of tip of the inner and outer sheath of the resectoscope, which allows continuous outflow and inflow of liquids.

82 GYNECOLOGIC ENDOSCOPY: Principles in Practice

liver bright images when a television monitor is used. A xenon or halogen light source can be used that delivers at least 250 watts. For operative hysteroscopy it is preferred to use a video camera, since it is less tiring than direct visualization through the hysteroscope, and ancillary personnel can view the surgery as well. An electrosurgical generator is needed that can deliver a wattage range up to 120 watts to perform in cutting, coagulation, and blended modes. An example of an electrosurgical generator that is commonly used includes the Valley Lab electro-coagulation source SSE2L.

An example of the operating room setup for endometrial ablation is illustrated in Figures 6.7–6.10.

TECHNIQUE

Endometrial ablation can be performed effectively under general anesthesia or regional anesthesia. After placing a single-hinged speculum in the vagina, the cervix is grasped with a single-toothed tenaculum. The cervix is then dilated to the diameter of the outer sheath of the resectoscope, usually 8 or 9 mm. Excessive dilatation can result in fluid leakage during the procedure, while insufficient dilatation can result in cervical trauma. One should strive to obtain a watertight seal when introducing the resectoscope. The rollerball electrode is properly fastened to the working element and the resectoscope is assembled and plugged in the unipolar mode using 40–70 watts. The sheaths of the resectoscope are easier to introduce into the uterus if an obturator is initially used to the level of the en-

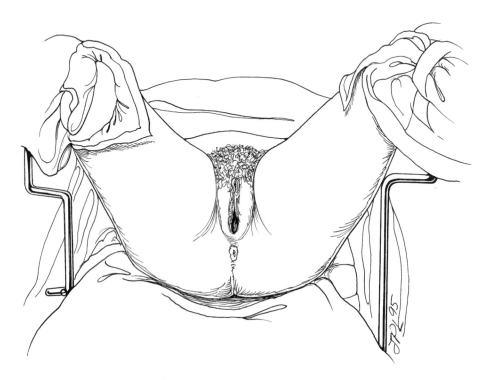

Figure 6.7. Dorsal lithotomy position.

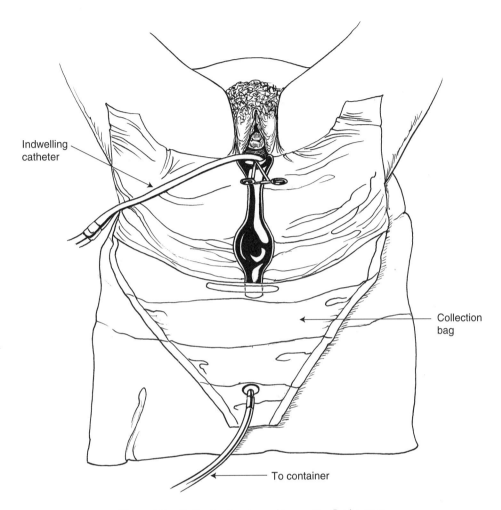

Figure 6.8. Collection bag is used to monitor fluid output.

docervix, and then removed to attach the remainder of the resectoscope. Alternatively, under direct view the resectoscope can be introduced while the irrigating solution is flowing. This latter approach, however, may result in more cervical trauma and lodging of cervical tissue into the open distal end of the resectoscope. The fluid medium is then allowed to flow as one gently inspects the endometrial cavity. The ablation is begun only after the patient has been properly grounded. The rollerball ablation of the endometrium is begun near the ostia, rolling the bar toward the internal cervical os (Fig. 6.11). The movement is always toward the operator. The endometrium is coagulated in a systematic way continuing with the posterior wall, lateral walls, and anterior wall. The endometrium that is coagulated appears brownish-white in color, in contrast to noncoagulated endometrium, which has a pinkish appearance. Coagulation of endometrial tissue results in collection of tissue on the rollerball, which may need to be cleaned intermittently. In addition, bubbles may interfere with adequate visualization.

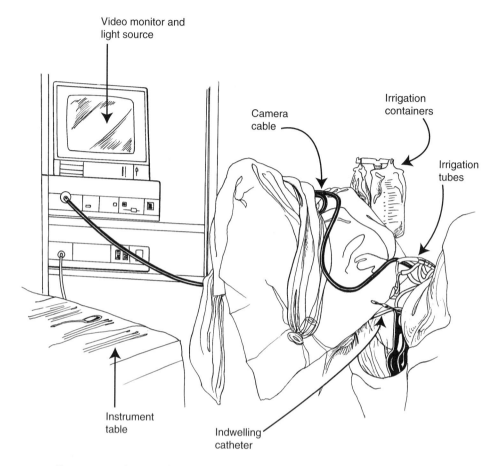

Figure 6.9. Side view of patient and instrument positioning for endometrial ablation.

Both of these problems may be remedied by removing the working element and leaving the sheaths in the uterine cavity. The continuous irrigation forces the excess tissue buildup and bubbles out of the uterine cavity. Endometrial ablation using the resectoscope rarely takes over 30 minutes to complete.

The exact power settings or waveforms that are optimal for endometrial destruction are controversial. Thermal energies between 50 and 100 watts have been reported (16, 17). Using hysterectomy samples, Onbargi et al. (18) evaluated endometrial destruction and thermal myometrial penetration using wattages ranging from 40 to 160 when using both coagulating and cutting waveforms. Higher power settings (greater than 60 watts), using both waveforms failed to demonstrate consistently greater depths of destruction than lower settings. This may be explained by an increase in resistance (impedance) of the tissue when using higher power settings, which results in depletion of electrolytes caused by quicker desiccation of the tissue. Furthermore, this study also revealed that regardless of the power setting used, the maximum amount of tissue damage caused in the myometrium was not excessive. No more than 4.2 mm were affected, which represents approximately 20% of the uterine wall thickness.

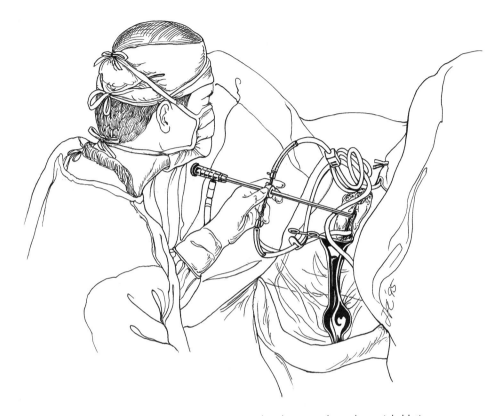

Figure 6.10. Instrument and irrigation tube placement for endometrial ablation.

This study illustrates that power settings between 60 and 120 watts may be used with equally good tissue destruction. At our institution, we rarely exceed power settings of 70 watts during an endometrial ablation and use the blended mode.

ELECTRORESECTION

Resection of the endometrium is an alternative to the rollerball method. The use of the wire loop to destroy the endometrium in patients with intractable uterine bleeding was first described by DeCherney et al. (8). With this technique, resection of the endometrium begins in the anterior fundus, is always directed toward the surgeon when the power is on, and uses 70–100 watts of pure cutting energy. The same procedure is performed in a circumferential manner until the entire surface is resected. The accumulation of endometrial chips during the procedure can obscure the view, and it is important to clear the cavity intermittently by physically removing the chips with irrigation or small forceps. Of 11 patients treated with total resection of the endometrium, Magos et al. reported 55% amenorrhea and 45% hypomenorrhea (19). Another option for endometrial ablation reported by Serden et al. is the use of the combination of the two above-mentioned techniques (20). The loop electrode is first used to remove a 3- to 4-mm section of endometrium using a cutting current of 70–120 watts, followed by rollerball abla-

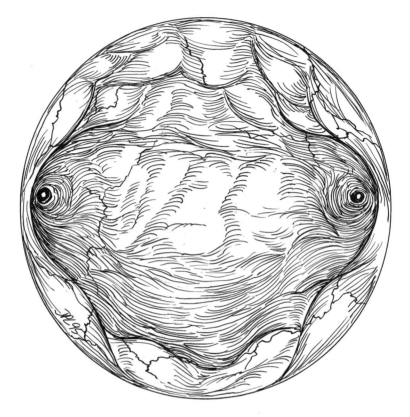

Figure 6.11. Panoramic view of uterine fundus.

tion with 65 watts of coagulation current. Of 96 patients treated in this manner, 50% were amenorrheic, 20% had hypomenorrhea, 17% had eumenorrhea, and 7% were unimproved.

Comparing these two hysteroscopic endometrial ablation techniques, it is the author's opinion that the use of the rollerball or bar with a properly prepared endometrium appears to be the safest and quickest method to learn and offers equally good results.

ND:YAG LASER

A hysteroscopic alternative to the resectoscope for endometrial ablation is the use of the Nd:YAG laser first reported by Goldrath et al. in 1981 (6) (Fig. 6.12). After adequate visualization of the entire uterine cavity, the laser fiber can be inserted through the operating channel of the hysteroscope. The Nd:YAG laser fiber can then be used either as a touch or non-touch technique (21) (Fig. 6.13). With the touch technique, the laser fiber is activated with 40–50 watts of energy and dragged on the endometrial surface beginning on the fundus, down toward the endocervix, in successive strokes. This is done in a systematic way so that the entire surface is eventually covered. With the non-touch or blanching technique, the laser fiber is placed a few mm away from the endometrial surface while the laser

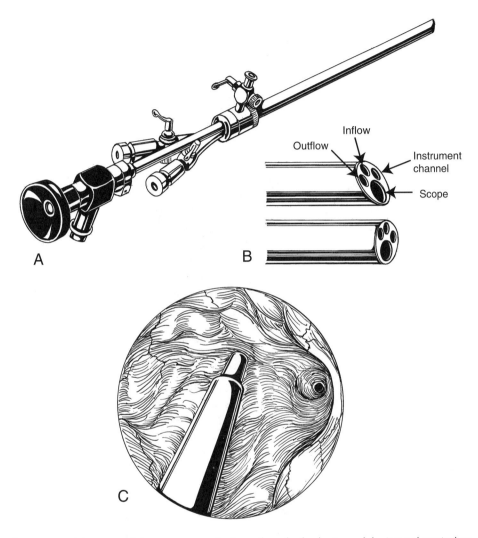

Figure 6.12. Movement of the resectoscope is always from the fundus toward the internal cervical os. **A.** Operating sheath used for Nd:YAG laser endometrial ablation. **B.** Sheath with separate channels. **C.** Laser fiber is seen protruding from the hysteroscopic sheath.

energy is activated. The non-touch technique using 50 watts of power output is usually used, since it is faster, has deeper penetration, and appears to have a better success rate in terms of amenorrhea than the touch technique; 65% versus 12% (21). Due to the thinner 600 micron Nd:YAG fiber diameter when compared to rollerball, it generally takes longer to complete an endometrial ablation with the laser method.

Sapphire tips can be used on Nd:YAG laser fibers to convert laser energy into heat. This has allowed their use intra-abdominally for ablation of endometriosis, since it diminishes the lateral thermal damage caused on normal tissue. The sapphire tips are cooled with a coaxial flow of gas or water through the fiber. When gas is used, the flow rate is 1–2 liters per minute; when used in the

88 GYNECOLOGIC ENDOSCOPY: Principles in Practice

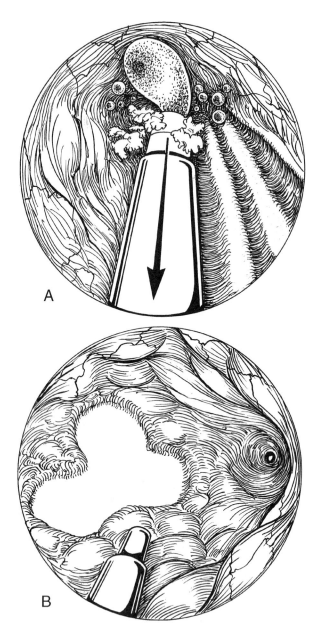

Figure 6.13. Dragging (touch) technique (**A**) and non-touch technique (**B**) performed with the Nd:YAG laser.

abdomen this is not a major problem. However, their use hysteroscopically has resulted in several deaths from gas embolism, and therefore they are now contraindicated for this use.

It is the author's opinion that although the laser ablation technique is now over 13 years old with long follow-up and a good safety record, its expense and long learning curve make it a less popular method to learn than the rollerball method. Ideally gynecologists should learn both methods and select their preference. However, it is more probable that hospitals would approve a $5000 resectoscope than a $100,000 instrument to perform the same function.

POSTOPERATIVE CARE

One of the biggest advantages of endometrial ablation is that it is an outpatient procedure. Patients are observed in the recovery room and discharged the same day when stable. Patients should expect a serosanguineous vaginal discharge for a few days, and may experience mild pain. Intercourse and vaginal tampons should be avoided until a postoperative visit two weeks after the procedure.

RESULTS OF ENDOMETRIAL ABLATION

The success rate of endometrial ablation in treating abnormal uterine bleeding by Nd:YAG laser and resectoscope techniques is reported as high as 90% (16, 17, 20, 21). More data are available using the Nd:YAG technique than the rollerball, since it has been available for more than a decade.

The definition of success rate of endometrial ablation by either electrocoagulation or laser depends on the objective of the treatment. If one examines the incidence of total amenorrhea following endometrial ablation, it varies between 40–67% (16, 17, 21, 22). However, if one includes hypomenorrhea in the group of successful outcomes, the overall effectiveness of this procedure raises to over 90%. When counseling patients it is important to emphasize that the goal of the procedure is to treat menorrhagia without necessarily causing total amenorrhea. Up to 10% of patients may not respond to this treatment and may require a second attempt at ablation. Patients that fail to respond to endometrial ablation may harbor underlying pathology such as uterine fibroids and adenomyosis.

Although the results of the Nd:YAG laser use are similar to the use of the resectoscope, there are distinct disadvantages. The Nd:YAG is an expensive modality costing between $60,000 and $100,000. It also requires special operating room cooling hookup and technical help. At the same time, using the laser method usually takes longer to complete an ablation than the resectoscope. For these reasons the resectoscope using the rollerball has become the method of choice for ablation by most gynecologists.

COMPLICATIONS

Endometrial ablation carries a complication rate similar to any other advanced operative hysteroscopy procedure. According to the 1988 survey by the American Association of Laparoscopists, where they reviewed the complication rate in 7293 consecutive operative hysteroscopies, the perforation rate was 1.3% and the major complication rate, mostly due to fluid absorption, was 0.17% (23). This is similar to the findings of a recent survey by the Royal College of Obstetricians and Gynecologists of patients who had endometrial ablation by British doctors (24). The perforation rate in this survey was 1.2% and serious complications, mostly from fluid absorption, were 0.5%. Other complications associated with endometrial ablation include major vessel hemorrhage, bowel and bladder burns, infection, and anesthetic complications.

Uterine perforation can result from a forceful introduction of the rigid resectoscope into the uterus, especially when the cervix has not been adequately dilated, but is more commonly associated with the laser fiber or loop electrode advancing through the myometrium without the surgeon's knowledge. If a perforation is suspected or confirmed, especially in the lateral sidewall, a laparoscopy should be performed to evaluate possible bowel injury. If a uterine perforation is visualized without bowel involvement, observation or bipolar coagulation to the uterus to stop any bleeding may be all that is necessary. The endometrial ablation can then be finished under direct laparoscopic observation. If a bowel injury is detected, a laparotomy is indicated to determine the extent of the injury. It is important to remember that unipolar injury is usually more extensive than one can visualize. Patients who complain postoperatively of increasing abdominal pain, and have clinical signs of peritonitis, should also be suspected of having a thermal injury to the bowel.

To explore the possibility that bowel injury can occur without a uterine perforation, Indman et al. (25) treated the cornu of six patients for five seconds with a rollerball using power settings of 50–150 watts while measuring the maximum temperature rise of the uterine serosa. The temperature rise in all of these patients did not exceed 6° C, indicating that without a true perforation, it is highly unlikely that severe thermal bowel damage can occur.

To avoid uterine perforation, the rollerball, loop electrode, or laser tip should be visualized at all times with the ablation always performed toward the surgeon. The incidence of uterine perforation with endometrial ablation is less than 1%, and patients with marked retroflexion, retroversion, a scarred uterine cavity, or an atrophic uterus are more predisposed to this complication.

Hemorrhage can result from penetration into myometrial vessels, perforation of the entire thickness of the uterine wall into uterine vessels, or even pelvic vessels. Postoperative bleeding, however, is usually related to inadequate coagulation of small endometrial vessels. These small vessels collapse due to the tamponade effect of the distending media and do not bleed during the procedure, but open up once the pressure effect of the media is removed. These bleeding points can be easily identified by slowly lowering the intrauterine pressure at the end of the procedure and individually coagulating them until the bleeding is stopped. Alternatively, the intrauterine placement of a pediatric Foley catheter for several hours can also control this type of bleeding.

The fluids most commonly used for endometrial ablation are glycine 1.5% and sorbitol 3%, which do not contain electrolytes. The use of large amounts of nonelectrolyte-containing solutions during endometrial ablation can result in severe and lethal complications of hyponatremia, pulmonary edema, water intoxication, and encephalopathy due to excessive fluid absorption. This complication is similar to the "TURP syndrome," associated with prostatectomies when there is excessive tissue resection and fluid absorption, and is well documented in the urologic literature (26). Hyponatremia leading to encephalopathy can result from the excessive absorption of hypotonic fluids (glycine 1.5% and sorbitol 3%) via opened uterine veins, as well as retention of water secondary to endogenous elevated plasma levels of arginine vasopressin (27). Hyponatremic encephalopathy should be suspected in patients having an endometrial ablation under general anesthesia who show signs of decreased body temperature, decrease in oxygen saturation, tremulousness, and dilated pupils. Postoperatively these patients may complain of headache, nausea, emesis, and continued tremulousness. Intraoperatively, if there is fluid deficit with signs of hyponatremia, a measurement of electrolytes should be ordered immediately. If severe hyponatremia is evident, termination of the case should be a priority, with simultaneous treatment with hypertonic sodium chloride. In four documented cases of endometrial ablation complicated by hyponatremic encephalopathy, Arieff et al. (28) reported one fatality. To avoid this type of complication with glycine 1.5% and sorbitol 3%, they recommend isotonic mannitol, which does not lead to hypo-osmolality.

To avoid excessive fluid absorption, careful monitoring of the volume of fluid media infused, intravenously as well as through the hysteroscope, and recovered during the procedure is therefore mandatory. It is recommended that every 15 minutes, the circulating nurse should make the operator aware of the amount infused and recovered to calculate any deficit which presumably has been absorbed by the patient. If the deficit reaches one liter, the surgeon should decide whether the procedure can be terminated soon and make the anesthesiologist aware of the estimated time of finishing. If the deficit reaches 1500 mL, the procedure should be terminated to avoid fluid overload and potential pulmonary edema. The use of diuretics and limiting intravenous fluids may also be necessary. In addition to fluid overload problems, use of glycine 1.5% has also been associated with transient blood oxygen desaturation, hypercapnea, and coagulopathy. Of 46 patients undergoing endometrial ablation, Goldenberg et al. (29) reported six patients with decreased oxygen saturation and increased PCO_2, all of which occurred within 20 to 30 minutes from the beginning of the procedure. In addition, four of the six patients had significant blood coagulopathy.

High viscosity fluids such as Dextran 70 (Hyskon, Pharmacia) have also been associated with severe complications and are not preferred media for endometrial ablation. These complications include anaphylactic reactions, pulmonary edema, and bleeding coagulopathies.

Infection from endometrial ablation is an extremely rare occurrence following hysteroscopic procedures and can be treated easily with oral antibiotics. Other potential complications include electrical and laser energy damage to the patient and surgeon, and anesthetic complications. In addition to immediate operative and postoperative complications, one should be aware of delayed complications. These include pelvic pain and possible future development of endometrial cancer.

Recently, Townsend et al. (30) reported six women over an 18-month period who had previous endometrial ablation and simultaneous tubal ligation, who presented with persistent pelvic pain that began 6–10 months following the procedure. On repeat laparoscopy, one or both of the proximal parts of the fallopian tubes were noted to be swollen, causing symptoms similar to an ectopic pregnancy. This post ablation-tubal sterilization syndrome is treated by removal of the affected tube. The proposed etiology of this syndrome is regeneration of the endometrium at the cornual area, with menstrual blood passing out into the fallopian tube.

There has also been the concern that clusters of viable endometrial cells could be hidden by scarring and could develop into endometrial cancer in the future. There are now two case reports of this delayed complication in the literature. Cooperman et al. (31) have recently reported a patient who presented with vaginal bleeding and was diagnosed with endometrial carcinoma five years after having an endometrial ablation. This previously theoretical complication has now become evident after five years of follow-up and emphasizes the importance of patient selection and close future postoperative follow-up, especially in those women at high risk of developing endometrial cancer. To further illustrate this latter point, Ramey et al. (32) have reported a 39-year-old multigravid woman with severe polycystic ovaries who was treated with endometrial ablation; within six months a repeat hysteroscopy was performed due to bleeding, and revealed grade I, well-differentiated adenocarcinoma of the endometrium. Although this patient had a normal endometrial curettage prior to the ablation, the possibility exists that a small focus of adenocarcinoma could have been initially missed.

ALTERNATIVES

Present conservative alternatives to endometrial ablation to control excessive uterine bleeding are investigational and include the use of heat by radiofrequency (33) and the use of a balloon filled with heated sterile 5% dextrose to thermally destroy the endometrium (34). Radiofrequency electromagnetic energy to heat the endometrium using a probe inserted through the cervix resulted in 80% amenorrhea or hypomenorrhea. The use of heated balloons to 170° F to destroy the endometrium resulted in 83% reduction in bleeding or amenorrhea in a recent study by Singer et al. (34).

DEVELOPING PRACTICAL EXPERIENCE IN ENDOMETRIAL ABLATION

Physicians wishing to become proficient in advanced operative hysteroscopic techniques such as endometrial ablation should be well versed in the following areas:

A. Basic diagnostic hysteroscopy skills,
B. Recognition of normal and abnormal uterine anatomy,
C. Basic understanding of electrosurgery and laser physics,
D. Knowledge of resectoscope and ancillary equipment needs.

It is highly recommended that developing technical knowledge and hands-on experience with endometrial ablation be systematic. This begins with didactic and reading material, followed by laboratory experience with inanimate and animal models, which is then followed by observation of live cases. Before proceeding on their own, physicians should perform at least five endometrial ablations under supervision, since most complications with this procedure occur within the first few.

DIDACTIC EXPERIENCE

Didactic sessions should include information on equipment, indications, alternatives, patient preparation, technique, expected results, and complications associated with this procedure. If one is not familiar with electrosurgery and laser physics, these should be reviewed prior to hands-on experience. Exposure to current literature and videos is very helpful.

LABORATORY

Laboratory experience should include review of the necessary equipment and the actual assembly and disassembly required for endometrial ablation. Specific exercises should follow that are conducted on tissue models and, if possible, animal models.

Physicians should become familiar with the following equipment and assembly:

  I. Resectoscope Instrumentation
     1. Continuous flow sheaths
     2. Obturator
     3. Compatible telescope viewing angles 0, 12, 30°
     4. Working element
     5. Electrosurgical setup
     6. Electrodes, rollerball, rollerbar, loop electrode
     7. Laser fibers
 II. Ancillary Instrumentation
     A. Light source
        1. System components
        2. Setup with hysteroscopic equipment
     B. Video system
        1. System components
        2. Setup with hysteroscopic equipment
     C. Video monitor
        1. Setup with video system
     D. Methods and instruments for media instillation
        1. System components
        2. Setup with hysteroscopic equipment
     E. Energy sources
        1. Electricity
           a. Biophysics
           b. Generator settings
           c. Setup with hysteroscopic equipment
           d. Precautions
        2. Laser Nd:YAG
           a. Biophysics
           b. Delivery systems
           c. Setup with hysteroscopic equipment
           d. Precautions
III. Distension Media
     A. Instillation methodology
        1. Mechanical pump
        2. Gravity flow
     A. Collecting System
        1. Urologic drape
        2. Wall suction

94 GYNECOLOGIC ENDOSCOPY: Principles in Practice

TISSUE MODELS

In order to gain practical experience with the technique of rollerball ablation and laser ablation, a tissue model prepared in a training box is highly recommended. Sophisticated training boxes are usually available from most instrument companies, but may also be homemade for self-training and resident teaching (see Chapter 9).

RECOMMENDED LAB EXERCISES FOR ENDOMETRIAL ABLATION WITH THE RESECTOSCOPE (35)

1. Review standard tray and equipment needed for endometrial ablation.
2. Assemble and disassemble resectoscope, including the use of 0, 12, and 30° angle telescope and connect rollerball, rollerbar, and loop electrodes.
3. Assemble intravenous tubing and electrosurgical cord.
4. Practice inserting resectoscope in sow bladder model and examine walls in a systematic fashion. Repeat with different angle scopes.
5. Practice the extension and return of the electrode with the spring mechanism. Make contact with the electrode and bladder walls in a systematic way.
6. Practice withdrawal of the electrode while maintaining the rollerball in contact with the bladder wall using only the spring return, using only the resectoscope with the electrode fully extended, and a combination of the two steps.
7. Assess tissue effects and media changes caused by using cutting, blend, and coagulation waveforms.
8. Assess tissue effects with varying wattages, 40–100 watts.
9. Assess tissue effects with varying times of contact to the bladder wall.
10. Assess tissue effect from the use of rollerball versus loop electrode on the bladder surface.

Endometrial Ablation Exercises with the Nd:YAG Laser

1. Review set-up of Nd:YAG laser unit and assembly with quartz fiber.
2. Review safety precautions.

Non-Contact Technique

3. Insert telescope with operating sheath into sow bladder or bovine uterus and initiate distension.
4. Strategically inspect bladder lumen or uterine cavity.
5. Pass quartz fiber down operating channel.
6. Observe fiber while being extended into cavity of bladder or uterus with 0, 12–15, and 25–30° angle telescopes.
7. Practice contact of cavity surfaces with tip of fiber, with and without using Albarran bridge.
8. Assess tissue and media effects at different wattages and durations of activation.

Contact Technique

Contact laser tissue effects require the thickness of a bovine uterus.

1. Follow steps 3–7 for non-contact technique.
2. Practice dragging fiber against all surfaces of the cavity, with and without Albarran bridge.
3. Practice strategic patterning of uterine cavity.
4. With laser activated, repeat dragging exercise over entire uterine cavity.
5. Practice touchup non-contact technique at cornu.
6. Observe tissue effects from varying wattage settings and duration of contact.

REFERENCES

1. Hallberg L, Hogdahl AM, Nilsson L, et al. Menstrual blood loss—a population study: variation at different ages and attempts to define abnormality. Acta Obstet Gynecol Scand 1966;45:320.
2. Health United States 1991. Hyattsville, MD: United States Department of Health and Human Services, 1992:231.
3. Goldfarb HA. A review of 35 endometrial ablations using Nd:YAG laser for recurrent menometrorrhagia. Obstet Gynecol 1990;76:833.
4. Wingo PA, Huezo CM, Rubin GL, et al. The mortality risk associated with hysterectomy. Am J Obstet Gynecol 1985;152:803.
5. Schofield MJ, Beanett AM, Redman S, et al. Self-reported long-term outcomes of hysterectomy. Br J Obstet Gynaecol 1991;98:1129.
6. Goldrath MH, Fuller TA, Segal S. Laser photovaporization of endometrium for the treatment of menorrhagia. Am J Obstet Gynecol 1981;140:14.
7. Asherman JG. Traumatic intrauterine adhesion. J Obstet Gynecol British Empire 1948;55:23–26.
8. DeCherney A, Diamond MP, Eavy G, Polan ML. Endometrial ablation for intractable uterine bleeding: Hysteroscopic resection. Am J Obstet Gynecol 1987;70:668–670.
9. Vancaillie T. Electrocoagulation of the endometrium with the ball-end resectoscope. Obstet Gynecol 1989;74:425–427.
10. Lefler HT, Lefler CF. Origins of premenstrual syndrome: Assessment by endometrial ablation. J Am Assoc Gynecol Laparoscopists 1994;1:207–212.
11. Hill DJ, Peter JM. Pregnancy following endometrial ablation. Gynaecol Endoscopy 1992;1:47–49.
12. Chimbira TH, Anderson ABM, Naish C, et al. Reduction of menstrual blood loss by danazol in unexplained menorrhagia: lack of effect of placebo. Br J Obstet Gynaecol 1980;87:1152.
13. Friedman AJ, Barbieri RL, Doubilet PM, et al. A randomized, double-blind trial of a gonadotropin-releasing hormone agonist (leuprolide) with or without medroxyprogesterone acetate in the treatment of leiomyomata uteri. Fertil Steril 1988;49:404–409.
14. Brooks PG, Serden SP. Preparation of the endometrium for ablation with a single dose of leuprolide acetate depot. J Reprod Med 1991;36:477.
15. Gimpelson RS. Mechanical preparation of the endometrium prior to endometrial ablation. J Reprod Med 1992;37:691–694.
16. McLucas B. Endometrial ablation with the rollerball electrode. J Reprod Med 1990;35:1055–1058.
17. Daniell JF, Kurtz BR, Ke RE. Hysteroscopic endometrial ablations using the rollerball electrode. Obstet Gynecol 1992;80:329–332.
18. Onbargi LC, Hayden R, Valle RF, Del Priore G. Effects of power and electrical current density variations in an in vitro endometrial ablation model. Obstet Gynecol 1993;82:912–918.
19. Magos AL, Baumann R, Turnbull AC. Transcervical resection of the endometrium in women with menorrhagia. BMJ 1989;298:1209–1212.
20. Serden SP, Brooks PG. Treatment of abnormal uterine bleeding with gynecologic resectoscope. J Reprod Med 1991;36:697.
21. Lomano JM. Dragging technique versus blanching technique for endometrial ablation with the Nd:YAG laser in the treatment of chronic menorrhagia. Am J Obstet Gynecol 1988;159:152.

22. Townsend DE, Richart RM, Paskowitz RA, Woolfork RE. Rollerball coagulation of the endometrium. Obstet Gynecol 1990;76:310–313.
23. Peterson HB, Hulka JF, Phipps JM. 1988 Membership survey on operative hysteroscopy. J Reprod Med 1990;35:590–591.
24. Macdonald R, Phipps J, Singer A. Endometrial ablation: a safe procedure. Gynaecol Endoscopy 1992;1:7–9.
25. Indman PD, Brown WW. Uterine surface temperature changes caused by electrosurgical endometrial coagulation. J Reprod Med 1992;37:667.
26. Gale DN, Notley RG. TURP without the TURP syndrome. Br J Urol 1985;57:708–710.
27. Thomas TH, Morgan DB. Post-surgical hyponatremia: the role of intravenous fluids and arginine vasopressin. Br J Surg 1979;66:540–542.
28. Arieff AI, Ayus JC. Endometrial ablation complicated by fatal hyponatremic encephalopathy. JAMA 1993;270:1230–1232.
29. Goldenberg M, Zolti M, Seidman DS, Beider D, Mashiack S, Etchin A. Transient blood oxygen desaturation, hypercapnia, and coagulopathy after operative hysteroscopy with glycine used as the distending medium. Am J Obstet Gynecol 1994;170:25–29.
30. Townsend DE, McCausland V, McCausland A, Fields G, Kauffman K. Post-ablation tubal sterilization syndrome. Obstet Gynecol 1993;82:422–424.
31. Copperman AB, DeCherney AH, Olive DL. A case of endometrial cancer following endometrial ablation for dysfunctional uterine bleeding. Obstet Gynecol 1993;82:640–642.
32. Ramey JW, Koonings PP, Given FT, Acosta AA. The process of carcinogenesis for endometrial adenocarcinoma could be short: development of a malignancy after endometrial ablation. Am J Obstet Gynecol 1994;170:1370–1371.
33. Phipps JH, Lewis VB, Prior MV, Roberts T. Experimental and clinical studies with radiofrequency induced thermal endometrial ablation for functional menorrhagia. Obstet Gynecol 1990;76:876–881.
34. Singer A, Almanza R, Gutierrez A, Huber G, Bolduc LR, Neuwirth R. Preliminary clinical experience with a thermal balloon endometrial ablation method to treat menorrhagia. Obstet Gynecol 1994;83:732–734.
35. Brill AI, Munro MG, De Leon FD, Sanfillipo JS, Vancaillie TG, Younger JB. Resident training in hysteroscopy: a suggested syllabus from CREOG. Washington, DC: CREOG Training Guidelines: Advanced Surgical Techniques for Residency Training Programs in Obstetrics and Gynecology.

Chapter 7

Laparoscopically Assisted Vaginal Hysterectomy

Robert L. Summitt, Jr.

In 1982, Dicker et al. (1) reported that 3.5 million American women underwent hysterectomy for benign conditions between 1970 and 1978. The vaginal approach was used in 28% of cases and the abdominal approach was used in 72%. In a more recent report, Wilcox and coworkers (2) reported that from 1988 to 1990, 1.7 million women in the United States had a hysterectomy performed, 75% by the abdominal approach and 25% by the vaginal approach. When complication rates for hysterectomies are compared by approach, vaginal hysterectomy is associated with much lower morbidity (23%) than abdominal hysterectomy (43%) (3). Therefore, if more of the hysterectomies that are performed could be completed by the vaginal route, improved patient outcomes and potentially greater health care savings could be achieved. However, the reports of Dicker (1) and Wilcox (2) show that while the numbers of hysterectomies performed annually have increased, the relative percentage of vaginal hysterectomies has not risen. Instead, this percentage has actually fallen.

In an effort to reduce the percentages of hysterectomies performed by the abdominal approach, with its attendant morbidity and slower recovery, the laparoscope has been introduced as a tool to assist with removal of the uterus through the vagina while maintaining the advantages of abdominal exposure. In addition, variations of the laparoscopic technique allow supracervical hysterectomy or a coning of the cervix combined with removal of the fundus, thereby avoiding entry of the vagina or removal of the cervix (4, 5). With the recent introduction of this new technology has come a burgeoning demand by less experienced surgeons for training in the technique, and a definite familiarity on the operating schedules of many hospitals with the procedure referred to as laparoscopically assisted vaginal hysterectomy (LAVH). However, no clear indications for LAVH exist. Variations in technique are controversial with regard to expense, equipment, potential complications, and sheer necessity of the benefits that their surgical steps can lend. In an effort to consolidate the surgical techniques of assisting a hysterectomy with the laparoscope, classification criteria have been derived in order to allow communication among surgeons and institutions, and to critically analyze the benefits and risks of the technical alternatives. With new surgical technology has also come a new set of complications. Suggestions for credentialing practices at national and institutional levels have been discussed but are difficult to agree upon.

This chapter will review the subject of laparoscopically assisted vaginal hysterectomy. Particular emphasis will be placed on its background and potential indications. Our own technique will be presented along with the variations by others. The reader should be able to develop a critical assessment of this technique and subsequently use it prudently and safely.

BACKGROUND

Early Experience

The technical feasibility of a laparoscopically assisted vaginal hysterectomy was first reported by Reich in 1989. Using laparoscopic electrosurgical instrumentation and aquadissection, the uterus and left ovary of a 38-year-old woman were removed through the vagina. Indications for removal of the uterus were pelvic pain and hypermenorrhea unresponsive to medical therapy and prior conservative surgery. Laparoscopic surgical assistance was selected because of the history of endometriosis and severe pelvic adhesions, documented and treated by three prior laparoscopic surgeries. The patient was able to go home on the fourth postoperative day and resumed full activity within three weeks. With the successful assistance of laparoscopy to aid in performing a vaginal hysterectomy, it was concluded that the laparoscopic approach to hysterectomy could provide patients a chance to avoid abdominal surgery and its long recovery period. No guidelines were provided to select these patients.

Shortly after the initial report by Reich (6), Kovac et al. (7) published a study describing the use of laparoscopy to intraoperatively determine whether women who were initially felt to be candidates only for abdominal hysterectomy, could successfully undergo a vaginal hysterectomy. Using a laparoscopic scoring system, the investigators found that 42 of 46 women (91%), could successfully undergo an uncomplicated vaginal hysterectomy. In 17 women preoperatively suspected of having ovarian pathology, eight were found to have none. The remaining nine women with ovarian masses successfully underwent vaginal hysterectomy and oophorectomy by standard vaginal techniques. Several patients with Stages III and IV endometriosis were able to undergo vaginal surgery after the disease was destroyed laparoscopically. Laparoscopy confirmed that only three of 24 women who had prior pelvic surgery would require an abdominal route for hysterectomy. While the benefit of laparoscopy to assist in determining the route of hysterectomy was suggested by this study, no portion of the hysterectomy was performed with pelviscopic techniques. However, the ground was laid for the progress in developing laparoscopically assisted vaginal hysterectomy.

A second case report of laparoscopic hysterectomy was published by Nezhat et al. (8) in 1990. In this particular case, a multifire endoscopic stapler was used to ligate and divide uterine pedicles, allowing a shorter operating time than the initial case report (6) in which bipolar cautery and scissors were used.

Following these initial case reports (6, 8), several case series were published, demonstrating the feasibility and potential safety of the operation in experienced hands (9–13). In one of the larger pure series, Liu (10) reported data from 72 cases performed between June 1990 and January 1991. Bipolar cautery and scissors were used to ligate and divide round ligaments, infundibulopelvic or mesosalpinx/utero-ovarian ligaments, and uterine arteries. The procedures were completed through the vagina. Of the 72 cases, there were no intraoperative complications. Mean operating time was 120 minutes and the mean hospital stay was 1.18 days. Only two postoperative complications were noted: one umbilical wound infection and one patient with a fever of unknown source. In 1992, Padial and coworkers (12) also published a large review of LAVH procedures ($n = 75$). Again, no intraoperative complications occurred except blood loss <1000 mL on two cases, in both instances primarily during the vaginal phase of the operation. Mean hospital stay was 2.73 days, and 8 patients (10.8%) had postoperative fevers. In addition to collecting data from LAVH procedures, Padial compared this information to that obtained from a review of 100 unmatched consecutive vaginal and abdominal hysterectomies. As a group, LAVH was associated with less pain, fewer analgesic requirements, and earlier ambulation than both vaginal and abdominal hysterectomies. Hospital stays were shorter for the LAVH patients, and the incidence of postoperative fever was lower. However, it must be kept in mind that abdominal and vaginal hysterectomies were performed by other physicians with different practice patterns, and that data collection was retrospective.

With the results of early success in both small and large case series, and the results of unmatched retrospective comparisons, LAVH was felt to be a promising addition to the techniques of hysterectomy, being superior not only to abdominal hysterectomy, but also vaginal hysterectomy in many respects. Claims of reduced morbidity, less postoperative pain, and shorter hospital stay compared to abdominal and vaginal hysterectomies were made (10, 12). Although not a substitute for simple vaginal hysterectomy, claims of easier adnexectomy and better inspection of the pelvis (9, 10, 12) have resulted in greater utilization of LAVH, substituting for an otherwise standard vaginal hysterectomy by many surgeons.

Comparative Studies

When evaluating new surgical technology, comparative studies with standard techniques provide the most valuable information in understanding the usefulness of the new procedure, especially when these studies are randomized and prospective. To date, there have only been two randomized controlled prospective comparative trials between LAVH and abdominal (TAH) or vaginal (TVH) hysterectomy (14, 15). Other comparative studies exist, both retrospective and prospective, but control within these studies is lacking. In spite of this, some generalizations can be made.

LAVH and TAH

Most comparisons between LAVH and TAH have not addressed preoperative selection criteria stringently. When studies are retrospective, postoperative management is difficult to correlate because of intrinsic, perceived biases affecting postoperative care. However, most intraoperative findings in this research are consistent, and some postoperative data can be extrapolated to make broad conclusions.

Intraoperatively, LAVH is associated with longer operating times than TAH, with mean times ranging from 35 to 50 minutes longer (14, 16, 17). Blood loss during surgery has been found to be either less (14, 17) with LAVH or, in two studies (18, 19), not statistically different from, TAH. With little effect on the need for transfusion, these few statistical differences in blood loss are not clinically important. Because of longer operating times and the use of disposable and/or highly technical laparoscopy equipment, hospital costs and patient charges are more with LAVH (16–18). No differences have been found between the two operations with regard to the incidence of intraoperative complications.

The postoperative parameter of hospital stay has been shorter for LAVH than TAH. Mean LAVH hospital stays are approximately 2.4 days, and stays after TAH range from 4.4 to 6 days (14, 16, 17). The differences in hospitalization days have been correlated with health care savings for LAVH. However, these correlations must be viewed in light of uncontrolled physician biases in postoperative management and, in some cases, retrospective abstraction of data.

Other immediate postoperative advantages have been associated with LAVH when compared to TAH. Pain scores and pain medication use are significantly less following LAVH (16, 19). In general, the incidence of postoperative complications is lower after LAVH (16, 17). The most commonly reviewed complication is febrile morbidity, being more frequent following TAH. In addition, wound complications are more common in women undergoing TAH. No statistical differences in the incidence of postoperative transfusions have been noted (17).

While many propose LAVH provides a reduction in health care costs when compared to TAH, few objective data exist to support these claims. In fact, studies that have attempted to analyze and compare total hospital costs and charges between LAVH and TAH have shown that LAVH is either no different, or is associated with higher costs (17, 18). Boike et al. (17) reported that although the mean hospital stay for LAVH was 2.5 days compared to 4.5 days for TAH, the mean hospital costs were $12,814 versus $10,511, respectively. The higher costs for LAVH were primarily related to charges for disposable laparoscopic equipment and secondarily related to anesthesia charges. In a comparative study of LAVH and TAH in which no disposable laparoscopic surgical instruments and no disposable staplers were used, Howard and Sanchez (18) showed no statistical differences in total hospital costs. Interestingly, they emphasized if an individual patient in the TAH group, who developed adult respiratory distress syndrome postoperatively, was excluded from analysis, the mean cost for TAH would have been less than LAVH (but not significantly different). Some suggest that more rapid convalescence and return to work can offset the hospital costs and provide more global health care savings. While this conceptual result is a desirable one, it is difficult to calculate because of varied patient backgrounds and their monetary value to the work force.

The subject of patient selection for the procedures of LAVH or TAH has been controversial. Few studies have addressed the question of who is the appropriate candidate for LAVH and who should still have a TAH. Most prospective comparative studies have selected patient groups who have a common indication for hysterectomy. While this is desirable for control, these indications have often been ones in which a standard vaginal hysterectomy could potentially have been performed (16, 18, 19). In addition, the results simply show technical and postoperative differences between procedures, lending only minimal information to the decision making process needed for selection. Retrospective analyses review broad categories of indications, but are also hindered by uncontrolled selection biases prior to surgery. However, these studies provide information with regard to the current patient selection practices of physicians. Nezhat et al. (14) prospectively compared LAVH and TAH in women with preoperative diagnoses of either endometriosis or leiomyomata; both indications selected as appropriate for the abdominal route only. While endometriosis is not questioned as a directive for the abdominal route, the uterine size in the women with fibroids would have potentially been amenable to the vaginal route. Phipps et al. (16) prospectively compared LAVH and TAH among women with menorrhagia and fibroids (less than eight gestational weeks in size), pelvic pain, or Stage I endometrial cancer. Again, women with menorrhagia and small fibroids, and some with pelvic pain, could potentially have had a simple TVH. Boike et al. (17) retrospectively reviewed hospital records at Northwestern Memorial Hospital from September 1, 1991 to August 31, 1992 to determine the number and route of hysterectomies performed during that 1-year period. They found that surgical indications for LAVH more closely resembled those for TAH than TVH, with uterine leiomyomas being the most common indication. However, uterine weights were significantly greater in the TAH group, and similar between the LAVH and TVH groups.

LAVH and TVH

As noted earlier, some surgeons have suggested significant intraoperative and postoperative advantages for LAVH over TVH. Padial et al. (12) reviewed 75 consecutive LAVH procedures, and then retrospectively compared the outcomes to the first 100 consecutive TVH and TAH procedures performed over the same time period. When compared to vaginal hysterectomy, LAVH patients reported less pain, required less postoperative analgesia, and were able to ambulate earlier. There was also a lower incidence of postoperative fever associated with LAVH. Interestingly, the operating times were similar between the two operations. There was one case of visceral trauma and one case of re-exploration in the TVH group, but neither of these operative complications occurred with LAVH. Similar findings were noted by Bronitsky et al. (20) who retrospectively compared 25 LAVH procedures to 25 TVH and 25 TAH procedures selected at random. LAVH had a shorter hospital stay than TVH. LAVH patients also required less injectable and oral pain medication. LAVH was associated with longer operating times, and overall was a more expensive procedure. With these findings, and case series by others, some have begun to favor LAVH over TVH, not only claiming less pain, shorter hospital stay, and fewer complications, but also easier adnexectomies, a better view of the pelvis, and superior flexibility in the patient who has had prior surgery or limited access in the vagina.

In 1992, Summitt et al. (15) published the only randomized, prospective, controlled trial comparing LAVH and TVH. Candidates for the study were women who were judged eligible for the vaginal route, including uterine fibroids up to 16 gestational weeks in size. Women were not excluded based upon prior surgeries. A total of 56 women was enrolled in the study and randomly assigned to a procedure (27 to TVH, 29 to LAVH). All procedures were to be performed on an outpatient basis, with discharge occurring on the afternoon of surgery. Both groups were comparable demographically. When assessing intraoperative parameters, mean surgical and anesthesia times were significantly longer for LAVH. Estimated blood loss was greater for vaginal hysterectomy (376.1 mL versus 203.8 mL). There was no difference between groups with regard to final uterine weights. All 27 patients undergoing TVH were discharged on the day of surgery, whereas 3 of the 29 women undergoing LAVH stayed in the hospital. One LAVH was converted to TAH because of exploration necessary to control bleeding from the inferior epigastric artery. Another incurred a cystotomy, which was repaired laparoscopically, and a third developed a fever immediately after surgery secondary to a herniation of a cecal epiploica through a lower trocar site. No differences were noted between groups with regard to the incidence of postoperative fever. There was no difference in the use of intramuscular narcotics immediately after surgery. Women undergoing LAVH required statistically more oral pain medication on postoperative day 2. Women in the LAVH group also had lower hematocrit values on postoperative days 1 and 2. In the TVH group, one woman was admitted 9 days after surgery with an infected vaginal cuff hematoma, and another was found to have a vesicovaginal fistula at 2 postoperative weeks. Mean hospital charges between TVH and LAVH groups were examined. Charges for LAVH were significantly higher ($7905 versus $4891) than TVH. This was primarily the result of disposable laparoscopy equipment and longer operating/anesthesia times.

In summary, this prospective study showed no advantage of LAVH over TVH in women who could undergo a vaginal hysterectomy, even a difficult one. LAVH was not associated with less pain, or earlier ambulation and discharge. Adnexectomies were completed in all patients when indicated, regardless of the group. And last, LAVH was much more expensive, even when performed on an outpatient basis.

INDICATIONS

When considering the appropriate indications for LAVH, the concept of indications for hysterectomy must be distinguished from indications for the route of hysterectomy. For it is the route of hysterectomy that should be considered when discussing indications for LAVH. Based upon current sound information available, indications for LAVH are listed in Table 7.1.

Gynecologic conditions that require the abdominal route and preclude a vaginal approach are appropriate for LAVH. In general, these are conditions that affect adnexal structures and require extensive dissection or evaluation to remove the adnexae and complete the procedure. Endometriosis is a typical example of one of these disease processes. In cases where pain persists in spite of conservative therapy, adnexal structures are often fixed by dense adhesions, or the cul-de-sac may be obliterated. The laparoscopic approach to dissection can avoid an abdominal incision and its attendant morbidity, while maintaining visualization needed to free structures that are to be removed. This obviously could not be achieved by a vaginal approach. Davis and coworkers (21) have reported one of the largest series of LAVH cases for endometriosis, being able to successfully perform the procedure in 40 of 46 women with Stages III and IV endometriosis. Six

Table 7.1. Indications for Laparoscopically Assisted Vaginal Hysterectomy

1. Documented endometriosis
2. Known pelvic adhesions
3. Adnexal mass with an indicated hysterectomy
4. Prior major pelvic surgery in two or more cases
5. Inadequate pelvis or no mobility of the uterus
6. Stage I endometrial cancer

women required conversion to a laparotomy because of bowel involvement or dense adhesions. In many cases the presence of an adnexal mass noted in a pre or postmenopausal woman who is undergoing a hysterectomy will direct a surgeon to the abdominal route. The laparoscope can be used as both a diagnostic and surgical tool, to evaluate the mass for the possibility of malignancy and then assist in adnexectomy and hysterectomy. Boike et al. (17) showed significant association in this indication between LAVH and TAH. Strict criteria have been identified to assess the adnexal mass intraoperatively (22). The surgeon must be prepared to proceed to a laparotomy and staging procedure if the frozen section diagnosis reveals a malignant tumor. Mild pelvic adhesions do not necessarily contraindicate a vaginal approach to hysterectomy, but known dense adhesions may prevent removal of the uterus or access to the adnexae without a transabdominal approach. Many surgeons will utilize the abdominal route for hysterectomy when the patient has had one or more pelvic operations. However, Coulam and Pratt (23) demonstrated that previous pelvic and abdominal surgery does not preclude vaginal hysterectomy, even after procedures such as a uterine suspension and cesarean section. In some cases, their approach required detachment from the abdominal wall. The laparoscopic approach may have been a better alternative in these difficult cases. However, predicting severe adhesions secondary to prior surgeries is not always possible. Being selective in choosing candidates for LAVH who have had prior surgeries is necessary; in particular, selecting those with two or more major surgeries that have directly involved the uterus, such as a uterine suspension or myomectomy. An inadequate pelvic or vaginal outlet, or a lack of uterine mobility, is still a controversial indication for LAVH. The laparoscopic approach most commonly detaches the adnexal structures, broad ligaments, round ligaments, and possibly the upper cardinal ligament complex. From experience, this dissection does not usually improve uterine mobility, nor avoid a contracted vagina. The classic studies of Mengert (24) must still be considered, as he showed that the major supports of the uterus are the uterosacral ligaments and lower cardinal ligament complex, structures most accessible through the vagina. Until these supports are severed, descent of the uterus will not improve. Alternative laparoscopic techniques for hysterectomy such as supracervical hysterectomy, the CASH procedure, or total laparoscopic hysterectomy, may overcome the problems of limited vaginal access or mobility, but the frequency of their use would be rare, and their utility for this particular indication has yet to be tested.

One of the most promising indications for LAVH is Stage I endometrial cancer (25, 26). The advantage offered by laparoscopy is the ability to perform lymph node sampling and avoid laparotomy, which has been required in the past. Successful procedures have been reported, with excellent yields of lymph node material (26). Hospital stays are shorter and morbidity is less when compared to the standard transabdominal approach. Before the full role of LAVH can be defined for gynecologic cancers, long-term prospective series will be necessary to demonstrate satisfactory survival rates.

The presence of leiomyomata uteri is not listed among the indications for LAVH. Laparoscopy adds little benefit to a hysterectomy procedure for fibroids when the uterine size is 16 gestational weeks or less (15). Morcellation techniques have been described and are quite capable of removing large uteri through the vagina (27, 28). The attempted placement of a laparoscope in the patient with a larger uterine fundus may prove injurious to the patient. In addition, visualization in the pelvis may be limited. Because uterine weights have not differed between groups undergoing LAVH and TVH in retrospective reviews, it does not appear that surgeons have yet begun to convert the transabdominal route to the vaginal route with the laparoscope for large leiomyomata uteri (17).

The laparoscopic route for hysterectomy should also not be indicated when oophorectomy is desired in what would otherwise be a simple vaginal hysterectomy. Sheth (29) has clearly shown that planned oophorectomy is possible in as many as 94% of vaginal hysterectomies. While it is not always possible to predict potential difficulty in a vaginal oophorectomy, it is not yet reasonable to begin with laparoscopy.

SURGICAL TECHNIQUES

Because LAVH is an alternative technique for hysterectomy in cases that would typically be performed using a standard abdominal approach, the basic principles of abdominal surgery should be maintained using many of the procedural steps of abdominal hysterectomy, and making few changes to allow laparoscopic assistance. Significant changes in hysterectomy technique should not occur in order to use the laparoscope, as this could lead to unexpected complications. The procedural steps described in this section for standard LAVH technique represent a combination of routine abdominal hysterectomy steps performed with laparoscopic scissors and graspers, and modified, but safe, steps to ligate pedicles with bipolar cautery or stapling devices, which facilitate the more advanced laparoscopic techniques. Alternative surgical techniques for hysterectomy assisted by the laparoscope are described later, and their utility discussed.

Standard LAVH Technique

LAVH, like other advanced laparoscopic operations, is a highly technical procedure, making the surgeon extremely dependent upon his/her equipment. In addition to a standard vaginal hysterectomy tray of instruments, current laparoscopy equipment in good working order should be available, including an extra laparoscope, both bipolar and unipolar instrumentation, a suction/irrigation unit, and a state-of-the-art video monitor unit with at least two screens. If additional equipment is desired, such as multifire stapling devices, the surgeon must be familiar with their use. A laser is not necessary for LAVH.

Prior to beginning the actual operation, attention must be directed to patient positioning and preparation. After the induction of general anesthesia, the patient is placed in the lithotomy position using candy cane-type suspension stirrups. By placing the stirrups at a low adjustment point, the thighs are kept out of the laparoscopic operative field while the patient's entire lower extremity is abducted enough to allow the assistants to properly position themselves for the vaginal portion of the case. A standard povidone-iodine preparation of the abdomen and vagina is used. A Hulka tenaculum is inserted into the uterus and attached to the cervix to manipulate the uterus. A Foley catheter is then inserted and the patient is draped. All patients should receive preoperative antibiotic prophylaxis with a first-generation cephalosporin or doxycycline if she is allergic to penicillin.

Chapter 7: Laparoscopically Assisted Vaginal Hysterectomy   105

Three trocars are initially placed into the abdomen. As we usually use a multifire linear stapling device for part of the operation, trocars consist of three 12-mm ports to allow insertion of the instrument. If a stapling device is not anticipated, we use one 12-mm and two 5-mm trocars. The primary trocar is inserted at the umbilicus, and the other two are inserted in both lower quadrants, approximately 10 mm above the pubic rami, and lateral to the inferior epigastric arteries (Fig. 7.1). If needed, an additional 5-mm trocar may be placed suprapubically for a suction/irrigation unit.

With all trocars in place, the abdomen and pelvis are inspected in order to assess the anatomy and note any pathology such as adhesions or pelvic masses. The anatomy must be normalized as much as possible prior to beginning the hysterectomy. The first true step of the operation is identical to that performed with a transabdominal approach: development of the bladder flap. The round ligament on one side is elevated, cauterized approximately 5 cm below the uterine origin, and then cut. The vesicouterine space beneath the peritoneum is developed bluntly with scissors across the lower uterine segment, and the peritoneum is cut as progress is made (Fig. 7.2). When the contralateral round ligament is finally transected, the bladder is dissected sharply off the lower uterine segment and cervix. Careful use of cautery will maintain hemostasis. Injury to the bladder is avoided by incising areolar tissue and fibrous attachments as close to the uterus and cervix as possible.

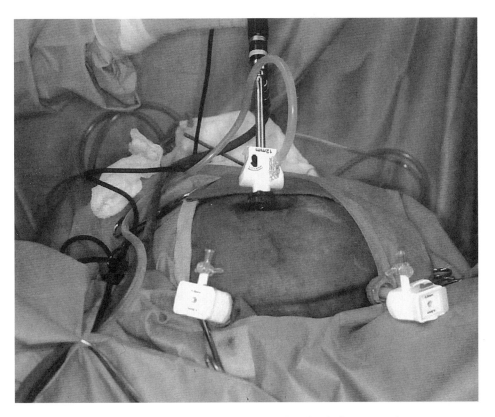

Figure 7.1.   Three 12-mm trocars appropriately placed at the beginning of surgery.

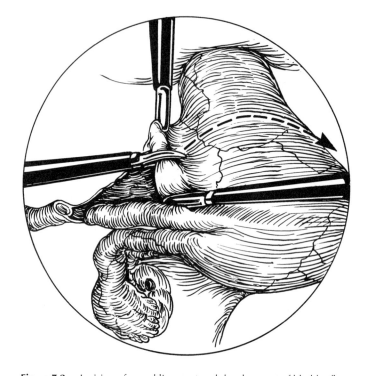

Figure 7.2. Incision of round ligament and development of bladder flap.

With the bladder flap developed, the next step of the procedure is to open the lateral retroperitoneal spaces and identify the ureters. This step is of paramount importance in order to avoid intraoperative occlusion or transection of the ureters. The dissection may be performed in one of two ways, depending upon whether oophorectomy is to be performed. If the ovaries are to be removed, the peritoneal incision for entering the retroperitoneal space is identical to an open procedure. The incision in the peritoneum is begun at the lateral aspect of the previously developed bladder flap. The incision is directed cephalad, lateral to the infundibulopelvic vessels. After an incision of approximately 10 cm is created, the lateral retroperitoneum is opened inferiorly, using blunt dissection with a probe or rounded grasping instrument. The ureter will be located deep in the space on the medial leaf of the broad ligament. If the ovaries are to remain, an alternative approach to ureteral exposure is used, beginning the dissection in the cul-de-sac, opening the medial leaf of the respective broad ligament. This is achieved by identifying the ureter through the peritoneum, and then lifting and incising the peritoneum halfway between the ureter and the infundibulopelvic vessels (Fig. 7.3). This incision is directed to the cervicouterine junction, parallel to the ureter. The lower edge of the incised peritoneum is then lifted medially and the ureter again exposed using blunt dissection. This maneuver aids in pushing the ureter downward. The lower cut edge of peritoneum is also a point of identification for the ureter, allowing stapling or cautery of structures above while avoiding injury to the ureter.

With the ureters exposed and the bladder flap developed, ligation and divi-

Chapter 7: Laparoscopically Assisted Vaginal Hysterectomy

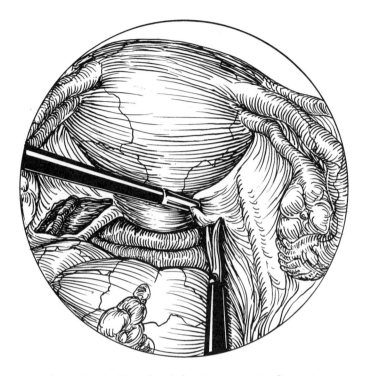

Figure 7.3. Incision of medial peritoneum to visualize ureter.

sion of uterine pedicles may now be performed. If removing the ovaries, a perforation in the already open medial peritoneum of the broad ligament is made, just below the infundibulopelvic vessels. The opening should extend 2–3 cm. The vascular bundle may be ligated with a vascular linear stapling device by passing the anvil through the peritoneal perforation and incorporating the entire structure. Alternatively, bipolar cautery may be used to desiccate the infundibulopelvic ligament. A 2–3-cm segment must be desiccated prior to cutting in order to maintain hemostasis. Prior to division of the infundibulopelvic vessels by either method, the ureter must be identified.

When leaving the ovaries, the first pedicle is developed adjacent to the uterus, dividing the fallopian tube and utero-ovarian ligament. We prefer using a linear stapler for this step because of its speed. In most cases, the stapler is inserted through the ipsilateral lower quadrant trocar. However, when the uterus is small, it is inserted through the umbilical port. The stapling device encloses the tube and utero-ovarian ligament, placing it as close to the uterus as possible (Figs. 7.4 and 7.5). Prior to firing the stapler, the tip must be observed above the lower cut edge of medial peritoneum, again avoiding the ureter. Bipolar cautery and dissecting instruments may certainly be used for this step, but do take longer in the presence of large tissue pedicles.

When the uterus is not exceptionally enlarged, the next step consists of ligation of uterine arteries. To avoid mass tissue bunching, and potential injury to the ureter, we prefer to dissect the uterine artery free of its fibrous attachments and then desiccate the vessel with bipolar cautery prior to division. A linear stapling

108 GYNECOLOGIC ENDOSCOPY: Principles in Practice

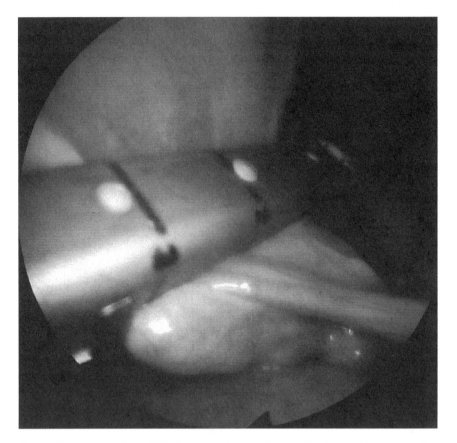

Figure 7.4. Incorporation of right fallopian tube and utero-ovarian ligament in linear stapler.

device may also be used for this step, but only when the uterine artery is easily visible and the ureter has been pushed inferiorly and out of danger (Fig. 7.6). It is not absolutely necessary to ligate the uterine arteries via the laparoscopic approach as they are most often easily reached through the vagina. However, laparoscopic ligation may reduce blood loss slightly.

After occlusion and division of the uterine arteries, an anterior colpotomy incision is made. This is performed by distending the anterior fornix of the vagina with a moist sponge and then incising the anterior vaginal wall, close to the cervix, with unipolar cutting current.

With the colpotomy completed, the operating team then moves to the vaginal operating field, leaving the trocars in place and turning off the gas to the abdomen. If adjustments in leg position are needed, they are made now. Typically, the vaginal portion of the operation is begun by entering the posterior cul-de-sac sharply and then clamping and suture-ligating the uterosacral ligaments bilaterally. The remaining vaginal mucosa is incised until it communicates with the anterior colpotomy incision. A retractor can easily be placed anteriorly, elevating the bladder. At this point, only one more bite is usually needed on each side of the uterus to facilitate removal. Care must be taken to correctly place the clamps in order that communication with the superior dissection is achieved. If clamps are

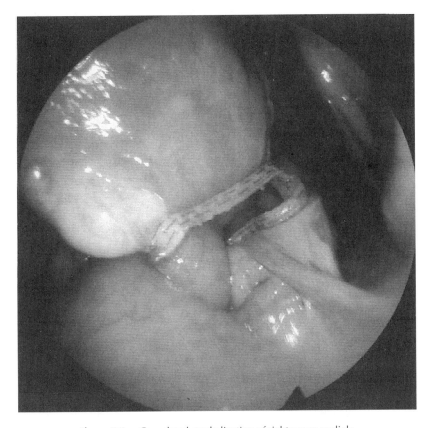

Figure 7.5. Completed staple ligation of right upper pedicle.

placed too close to the uterus, dissection may be directed medial to the superior dissection planes.

Once the uterus is removed and the vagina closed, the abdomen is reinsufflated and the pelvis is inspected. Irrigation of the pelvis removes any clots and allows inspection of all pedicles and the cuff for hemostasis. The procedure is completed by closing the fascia and skin of all incisions. No catheter is placed as our patients are typically discharged on the afternoon of surgery. However, typical hospital stays of 1–3 days are enjoyed at other institutions.

Alternative Laparoscopic Techniques for Hysterectomy

Laparoscopic Supracervical Hysterectomy

A resurgence of the supracervical hysterectomy technique has occurred as a method to simplify the laparoscopic approach to hysterectomy. Additional claims of shorter operating times, lower morbidity, and shorter convalescence have been made (30). To offset the argument of a persistent risk of cervical cancer, researchers note the current low incidence, and typically perform some form of destructive procedure to eliminate the endocervical canal (30, 31). Surgeons also claim that the supracervical technique eliminates lower urinary tract dysfunction, reduces the risk of prolapse, and preserves unaltered sexual function.

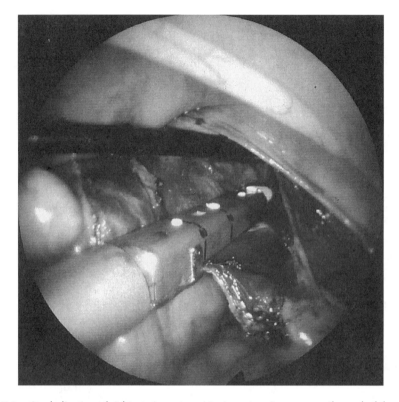

Figure 7.6. Staple ligation of right uterine artery. Uterine artery is seen near the end of the stapling device.

In general, laparoscopic supracervical hysterectomy begins in the same manner as LAVH. However, after the uterine arteries have been ligated, the fundus is separated from the cervix, usually with either unipolar cautery or a neodymium:YAG (Nd:YAG) laser. The superior aspect of the cervical stump is then either oversewn or simply cauterized to obtain hemostasis. The fundus is typically removed through an enlarged umbilical incision. However, Donnez and Nisolle (5) described removal of the fundus through a posterior colpotomy incision. To reduce the likelihood of cervical cancer, some have described removal of the transition zone with loop electrocautery, or thermally destroying the transition zone (5, 31). In the absence of dysplasia, this should have little effect on reducing cancer incidence, as a new transition zone can readily form.

Controversy still surrounds the use of supracervical hysterectomy, whether it is used transabdominally or laparoscopically. Most of the proposed advantages of laparoscopic supracervical hysterectomy have yet to be proven objectively. Lyons (30) showed shorter operating times and less blood loss when using the supracervical technique, comparing it in a nonrandomized fashion to LAVH. Fewer complications, less pain, and shorter convalescence have not been satisfactorily demonstrated. With regard to prolapse or sexual function after laparoscopic supracervical hysterectomy, no data currently exist. Past information from transabdominal studies is inconclusive. Prior studies of urinary function show that total and supracervical hysterectomies are no different when postoperative function is compared (32). The role of supracervical laparoscopic hysterectomy is therefore unclear. Future randomized comparative studies analyzing postoperative outcomes objectively may be helpful.

The CASH Procedure

In 1991, Semm (4) described the CASH procedure as a new method for laparoscopic hysterectomy. CASH is an eponym for: Classic Abdominal S.E.M.M. (Serrated Edged Macro-Morcellated) Hysterectomy. This procedure is similar to the supracervical laparoscopic hysterectomy in that the fundus is removed and the cervix left intact. However, it differs by using a calibrated uterine manipulator, inserted through the cervix and fundus, that allows a serrated resection device to pass along the guide and "core-out" the cervical canal. Theoretically, this effectively removes the endocervical glands, thereby reducing the risk of cervical cancer. In addition, by leaving the cervix intact with its ligamentous and neural attachments, the risk of prolapse is reduced and sexual sensation is undisturbed. The CASH technique requires additional skill training beyond laparoscopy in order to use the morcellating tools. However, proponents claim that the learning curve is easily climbed and that eventually operating times are no different than LAVH. Claims regarding cervical cancer, risk of prolapse, and sexual function, like supracervical hysterectomy, have yet to be fully answered.

Laparoscopic Doderlein Hysterectomy

A variation on the vaginal portion of LAVH has used the Doderlein technique (33). As with the traditional description for the vaginal hysterectomy, the laparoscopic Doderlein hysterectomy uses an anterior colpotomy to draw the uterine fundus into the vagina. This is performed after the adnexae have been detached laparoscopically. In most cases, the uterine arteries are ligated during the vaginal portion of the procedure. Proponents of this technique relate that the laparoscopic dissection facilitates delivery of the fundus through the anterior colpotomy, eventually leading to an easier vaginal position than the standard Heaney technique. Any differences between techniques have not been proven.

CLASSIFICATION SYSTEMS

Because of variations in operative technique among gynecologic surgeons who perform LAVH, supracervical laparoscopic hysterectomy, or CASH, it is difficult to assimilate intraoperative and postoperative data in order to analyze outcomes. To this end, classification systems are being proposed in order that quantifiable comparisons can be made among institutions and practitioners. A comprehensive system could allow analysis of suitable technical steps, incidence of complications, and cost. It could provide a basis for meaningful research to be conducted between multiple sites. Lastly, it might facilitate education of surgeons, provide a stepwise progressive method for learning, and potentially assist with credentialing by hospitals and institutions.

To date, no consensus has been reached with regard to an accepted classification system for laparoscopic hysterectomy. However, one of the most thoughtful formats for classification has been proposed by Munro and Parker (34). This system (Tables 7.2 and 7.3) classifies laparoscopic assisted hysterectomy into four types based upon levels of dissection and increasing surgical complexity, extending from the ovarian vessels to the cardinal-uterosacral ligament complex. Type I hysterectomy is characterized by ligation and division of at least one of the ovarian artery pedicles; Type II includes the addition of either unilateral or bilateral occlusion and division of the uterine arteries. Type III hysterectomy includes dissection of part but not all of the uterosacral-cardinal ligament complex, and Type IV consists of dissection and detachment of the entire complex on at least one side. Each type of hysterectomy is further classified into subgroups based upon dissection and/or division of surrounding anatomic structures. A similar system classifies subtotal laparoscopic hysterectomy.

The use of a classification system such as the one described has yet to be tested for its utility. However, the value is promising. A consensus as to an ultimate classification system will be difficult to reach, but remains an important goal.

COMPLICATIONS

Laparoscopically assisted vaginal hysterectomy shares a number of potential known complications with the more standard abdominal and vaginal ap-

Table 7.2. Classification System for Laparoscopically Directed and Assisted Total Hysterectomy[a]

Type 0	Laparoscopically directed preparation for vaginal hysterectomy	
Type I[b]	Dissection up to but not including uterine arteries	
	Type IA	Ovarian artery pedicle(s) only
	Type IB[c]	A + anterior structures
	Type IC	A + posterior culdotomy
	Type IDC	A + anterior structures and posterior culdotomy
Type II[b]	Type I + uterine and vein occlusion, unilateral or bilateral	
	Type IIA	Ovarian artery pedicle(s) plus unilateral or bilateral uterine artery and vein occlusion only
	Type IIB[c]	A + anterior structures
	Type IIC	A + posterior culdotomy
	Type IID[c]	A + anterior structures and posterior culdotomy
Type III[b]	Type II + portion of cardinal-uterosacral ligament complex; unilateral or bilateral, plus:	
	Type IIIA	Uterine and ovarian artery pedicles with unilateral or bilateral portion of the cardinal-uterosacral complex only
	Type IIIB[c]	A + anterior structures
	Type IIIC	A + posterior culdotomy
	Type IIID[c]	A + anterior structures and posterior culdotomy
Type IV[b]	Type II + total cardinal-uterosacral ligament complex; unilateral or bilateral, plus:	
	Type IVA	Uterine and ovarian artery pedicles with unilateral or bilateral detachment of the total cardinal-uterosacral ligament complex only
	Type IVB[c]	A + anterior structures
	Type IVC	A + posterior culdotomy
	Type IVD[c]	A + anterior structures and posterior culdotomy
	Type IVE	Laparoscopically directed removal of the entire uterus

From Munro MG, Parker WH. A classification system for laparoscopic hysterectomy. Obstet Gynecol 1993;82: 624–629. With permission.
[a]The system describes the portion of the procedure completed laparoscopically.
[b]A suffix "o" may be added if unilateral or bilateral oophorectomy is performed concomitantly (e.g., Type IoA).
[c]The B and D subgroups may be further subclassified according to the degree of dissection involving the bladder, and whether an anterior culdotomy is creased: 1 = incision of vesicouterine peritoneum only, 2 = dissection of any portion of the bladder from the cervix, 3 = creation of an anterior culdotomy.

Table 7.3. Classification System for Laparoscopically Directed Subtotal (Supracervical) Hysterectomy

Type ST I	Up to but not including uterine arteries
	A, Without cervical epithelial excision or ablation
	B, With cervical canal ablation
	C, With cervical canal excision
Type ST II[a,b]	Including occlusion of uterine arteries (unilateral or bilateral)
Type ST III[a,b]	Including occlusion and division of uterine arteries (unilateral or bilateral)

From Munro MG, Parker WH. A classification system for laparoscopic hysterectomy. Obstet Gynecol 1993;82:624–629. With permission.
[a]A suffix "o" may be added if unilateral or bilateral oophorectomy is performed concomitantly (eg, Type ST IoA).
[b]Types ST II and ST III are subgrouped (A, B, and C) in a fashion identical to that for ST I procedures.

proaches. However, the addition of laparoscopy using large trocars, and the introduction of new manipulations to facilitate hysterectomy via endoscopy have led to two additional categories of complications.

Shared complications with standard hysterectomy techniques can occur intraoperatively or postoperatively. In most cases, the vaginal portion of LAVH is performed using a Heaney technique. Intraoperative complications, although rare, can include hemorrhage from the vaginal cuff or lower uterine pedicles. They can also include incidental cystotomy if an anterior colpotomy was not created laparoscopically. The most common complication after standard hysterectomy is febrile morbidity. In general, the incidence of febrile morbidity is lower for LAVH than TAH (19), but Carter et al. (19) found no differences when comparing outcomes of 38 patients. There appears to be no difference in the incidence of fever between LAVH and TVH (15). Causes of fever most commonly include vaginal cuff cellulitis, infected vaginal cuff hematoma, and atelectasis.

Although the use of large diameter (10–12-mm) trocars is not unique to LAVH, the high frequency with which this procedure is being performed is resulting in an association with trocar complications. The two most noted complications are abdominal wall vascular injury and intestinal herniation through the trocar sites. Several reports of LAVH have documented injury to the inferior epigastric artery upon insertion of a large trocar into the lower quadrant of the abdominal wall (15, 19, 35). These injuries have typically resulted in significant bleeding and difficulty controlling hemorrhage. They appear to occur more often in obese patients where the abdominal wall cannot be transilluminated or the vessels cannot be visualized through the peritoneum. Trocar site herniations have recently become associated with the use of large caliber trocar sheaths. Boike et al. (36) presented 19 cases of bowel herniation following laparoscopy. Eleven of these cases were LAVHs. Herniations most commonly occur in the lower quadrants, but have been reported at the umbilicus (19, 35, 36). Early diagnosis is mandatory as this complication could lead to bowel necrosis and resection. Fascial closure of all trocar sites is recommended following LAVH. However, in Boike's (36) study, a significant number of herniations occurred through sites in which closure had been documented in the operative report.

The second additional category of complications unique to LAVH includes those that result from manipulations necessary to perform hysterectomy steps endoscopically. In some cases the complications are a result of new and unfamiliar steps, whereas others are secondary to the use of new equipment or technology. Complications in this category consist of injuries to the urinary tract or gastrointestinal tract. Bladder perforation is a commonly reported injury. This may result during bladder flap dissection in a patient with prior surgery in this area, such as a cesarean section (15). If recognized, the cystotomy can usually be repaired with endoscopic suturing. Ureteral injuries are being reported more often. Most of these injuries are associated with the use of endoscopic stapling devices (35, 37). The staplers are placed too low, in many cases attempting to ligate uterine arteries, without adequate identification of the ureter. This is why it is imperative to dissect and identify the location of the ureter. Bowel injuries are less common than urinary tract injuries. However, injuries to the rectum during posterior colpotomy have been noted.

The incidence of specific complications with LAVH is unknown. This is because of limited general experience and some degree of underreporting. In spite of the complications noted above, LAVH can be a safe procedure. The surgeon must dictate extreme care with each step, especially involving the urinary tract, and avoid overextending his level of skill.

TRAINING AND CREDENTIALING

Laparoscopically assisted vaginal hysterectomy is a technically advanced operation demanding a great deal of operative skill from the surgeon. Unfortunately, no consensus has identified the best method for teaching this procedure, and there exists great controversy and variation in regard to credentialing a surgeon for the technique.

Approximately 20–25 cases are needed to complete the learning curve for LAVH. Initiating this learning process integrates several processes. First, a didactic course of basic and advanced laparoscopy is necessary. In addition, integral review of LAVH technique, indications, and complications is needed. Secondly, laboratory training in laparoscopy, specifically the steps for LAVH, is needed. Familiarity with stapling devices, cautery instruments, and cutting tools must be obtained on foam or inanimate training models. Simulation of stapling upper pedicles or performing adenexectomies can be achieved on the inanimate models. Next, animal models provide living tissue specimens that closely reproduce the steps for LAVH. Goat or sheep models are preferred, as the pelvis and uterus are large enough in these animals to practice most steps. Steps to practice in the animal models include development of the bladder flap, dissection of ureters, stapling of upper pedicles, ligation of uterine arteries, and severing of the fundus. In smaller animals such as the pig, the bladder flap may need to be simulated by undermining and cutting the peritoneum superior to the bladder and over the pubis, as adequate space may be limited between the bladder and uterus.

Training beyond the laboratory requires supervision from a skilled endoscopic surgeon. Training now blends with credentialing. The trainee should scrub during 3–5 LAVH procedures prior to serving as the primary surgeon. Then, 5–10 procedures should be performed as primary surgeon with a credentialing physician as the assistant. Hospitals or institutions *must establish minimum requirements for new surgeons* performing LAVH. They are presently the controlling factors for the new LAVH surgeon. Until a more global governing body is formed, patients and their doctors are dependent upon this institutional control.

Laparoscopically assisted vaginal hysterectomy, like any other procedure, must be used prudently and for the proper indications. It must remain an alternative for abdominal hysterectomy and avoid being a substitute for an otherwise possible vaginal hysterectomy. Proper skill and care must be used during the operations to prevent complications and maximize the intraoperative and postoperative benefits.

REFERENCES

1. Dicker RC, Scally MJ, Greenspan JR, et al. Hysterectomy among women of reproductive age: trends in the United States. JAMA 1982;248:323.
2. Wilcox LS, Koonin LM, Pokras R, et al. Hysterectomy in the United States, 1988–1990. Obstet Gynecol 1994;83:549–555.
3. Dicker RC, Greenspan JR, Straus LT, et al. Complications of abdominal and vaginal hysterectomy among women of reproductive age in the United States. Am J Obstet Gynecol 1982;144:841–848.
4. Semm K. Hysterektomie per laparotomiam oder per pelviskopiam. Geburtsh u Frauenheilk 1991;51:996–1003.
5. Donnez J, Nisolle M. Laparoscopic supracervical (subtotal) hysterectomy (LASH). J Gynecol Surg 1993;9:91–94.
6. Reich H, DeCaprio J, McGlynn F. Laparoscopic hysterectomy. J Gynecol Surg 1989;5:213–216.
7. Kovac RS, Cruikshank SH, Retto HF. Laparoscopy-assisted vaginal hysterectomy. J Gynecol Surg 1990;6:185–193.
8. Nezhat C, Nezhat F, Silfen SL. Laparoscopic hysterectomy and bilateral salpingo-oophorectomy using multifire GIA surgical stapler. J Gynecol Surg 1990;6:287–288.
9. Minelli L, Angiolillo M, Caione C, Palmara V. Laparoscopically-assisted vaginal hysterectomy. Endoscopy 1991;23:64–66.
10. Liu CY. Laparoscopic hysterectomy: a review of 72 cases. J Reprod Med 1992;37:351–354.
11. Langebrekke A, Skar OJ, Urnes A. Laparoscopic hysterectomy: initial experience. Acta Obstet Gynecol Scand 1992;71:226–229.
12. Padial JR, Sotolongo J, Casey MJ, Johnson C, Osborne NG. Laparoscopy-assisted vaginal hysterectomy: report of seventy-five consecutive cases. J Gynecol Surg 1992;8:81–85.
13. Maher PJ, Wood EC, Hill DJ, Lolatgis NA, Laparoscopically assisted hysterectomy. Med J Aust 1992;156:316–318.
14. Nezhat F, Nezhat C, Gordon S, Wilkins E. Laparoscopic versus abdominal hysterectomy. J Reprod Med 1992;37:247–250.
15. Summitt RL, Stovall TG, Lipscomb GH, Ling FW. Randomized comparison of laparoscopy-assisted vaginal hysterectomy with standard vaginal hysterectomy in an outpatient setting. Obstet Gynecol 1992;80:895–901.
16. Phipps JH, John M, Nayak S. Comparison of laparoscopically assisted vaginal hysterectomy and bilateral salpingo-oophorectomy with conventional abdominal hysterectomy and bilateral salpingo-oophorectomy. Br J Obstet Gynaecol 1993;100:698–700.
17. Boike GM, Elfstrand EP, DelPriore G, et al. Laparoscopically assisted vaginal hysterectomy in a university hospital: report of 82 cases and comparison with abdominal and vaginal hysterectomy. Am J Obstet Gynecol 1993;168:1690–1701.
18. Howard FM, Sanchez R. A comparison of laparoscopically assisted vaginal hysterectomy and abdominal hysterectomy. J Gynecol Surg 1993;9:83–90.
19. Carter JE, Ryoo J, Katz A. Laparoscopic-assisted vaginal hysterectomy: a case control comparative study with total abdominal hysterectomy. J Am Assoc Gynecol Laparosc 1994;1:116–121.
20. Bronitsky C, Payne RJ, Stucky S, Wilkins D. A comparison of laparoscopically assisted vaginal hysterectomy vs traditional total abdominal and vaginal hysterectomies. J Gynecol Surg 1993;9:219–225.
21. Davis GD, Wolgamott G, Moon J. Laparoscopically assisted vaginal hysterectomy as definitive therapy for stage III and IV endometriosis. J Reprod Med 1993;38:577–581.
22. Parker WH, Berek JS. Management of selected cystic adnexal masses in postmenopausal women by operative laparoscopy: A pilot study. Am J Obstet Gynecol 1990;163:1574–1577.

23. Coulam CB, Pratt JH. Vaginal hysterectomy: Is previous pelvic operation a contraindication? Am J Obstet Gynecol 1973;116:252–260.
24. Mengert WF. Mechanisms of uterine support and position. I. Factors influencing uterine support (an experimental study). Am J Obstet Gynecol 1936;31:775–781.
25. Photopulos GJ, Stovall TG, Summitt RL. Laparoscopic-assisted vaginal hysterectomy, bilateral salpingo-oophorectomy, and pelvic lymph node sampling for endometrial cancer. J Gynecol Surg 1992;8:91–94.
26. Childers JM, Surwit EA. Case report: Combined laparoscopic and vaginal surgery for the management of two cases of stage I endometrial cancer. Gynecol Oncol 1992;45:46–51.
27. Grody MHT. Vaginal hysterectomy: the large uterus. J Gynecol Surg 1989;5:301–312.
28. Kovac SR. Intramyometral coring as an adjunct to vaginal hysterectomy. Obstet Gynecol 1986;67:131–136.
29. Sheth SS. The place of oophorectomy at vaginal hysterectomy. Br J Obstet Gynaecol 1991;98:662–666.
30. Lyons TL. Laparoscopic supracervical hysterectomy: A comparison of morbidity and mortality results with laparoscopically assisted vaginal hysterectomy. J Reprod Med 1993;38:763–767.
31. Pelosi MA, Pelosi MA, III. Laparoscopic supracervical hysterectomy using a single-umbilical puncture (mini-laparoscopy). J Reprod Med 1992;37:777–784.
32. Stanton SL, Cardozo LD. Results of colposuspension operation for incontinence and prolapse. Br J Obstet Gynaecol 1979;86:693–697.
33. Saye WB, Espy GB, Bishop MR, Slinkard P, Miller W, Hertzmann P. Laparoscopic Doderlein hysterectomy: a rational alternative to traditional abdominal hysterectomy. Surg Laparosc Endos 1993;3:88–94.
34. Munro MG, Parker WH. A classification system for laparoscopic hysterectomy. Obstet Gynecol 1993;82:624–629.
35. Nezhat C, Nezhat F, Bess O, Nezhat CH. Injuries associated with the use of a linear stapler during operative laparoscopy: review of diagnosis, management and prevention. J Gynecol Surg 1993;9:145–150.
36. Boike GM, Miller CE, Spirtos NM, et al. Incisional bowel herniations following operative laparoscopy: a series of nineteen cases and review of the literature. Am J Obstet Gynecol 1995;172:1726–1733.
37. Woodland MB. Ureter injury during laparoscopy-assisted vaginal hysterectomy with the endoscopic linear stapler. Am J Obstet Gynecol 1992;167:756–777.

Chapter 8
Laparoscopic Sterilization
Gary H. Lipscomb

Laparoscopic tubal occlusion as a method for human sterilization was first performed by Bösch in Switzerland (1). Independently, two American gynecologists, Powers and Barnes, developed a similar procedure in the United States (2). During the 1940s, female sterilization in the United States was generally performed only for medical indications. Elective sterilizations were subjected to a formula where age times parity had to be greater than or equal to 120 before the procedure could be considered. This general lack of demand for sterilization coupled with technical difficulties with the early laparoscopic equipment resulted in few American physicians attempting the new procedure. American interest remained dormant until the changing cultural climate of the late 1960s resulted in a demand for a safe, minimally invasive female sterilization procedure.

During this interim period, technical advances in optics and instrumentation pioneered by the Germans, Italians, and French made laparoscopy a much easier and safer procedure. Raoul Palmer of Paris adopted the use of the Trendelenburg position and uterine manipulator to give better access to the fallopian tubes and ovaries (3). He also popularized the use of biopsy forceps and unipolar current for tubal sterilization. Following the publication of the first textbook in English on laparoscopy (4), a resurgence of interest in laparoscopy occurred in the United States. Propelled by the increasing demand for elective sterilization, laparoscopy became the most common method of interval sterilization in the United States by the mid-1970s. Conversely, sterilization became the most common indication for laparoscopy (5).

Many methods of laparoscopic tubal sterilization have been described. The most commonly used methods today include the use of electrocoagulation, Silastic bands, or mechanical clips to achieve occlusion of the fallopian tubes. Other potentially useful but uncommon techniques include endocoagulation and the laparoscopic Pomeroy procedure.

ELECTROCOAGULATION

Laparoscopic electrocoagulation is the oldest technique of laparoscopic sterilization. Electrocoagulation utilizing unipolar current gained widespread popularity during the early years of laparoscopic sterilization, but fell into disfavor following reports of increasing numbers of bowel burns resulting from the procedure. Although most bowel injuries were subsequently shown to be trocar injuries and not electrical burns, the majority of laparoscopists abandoned the use of unipolar electric current for sterilization (6). Today, the inherently safer bipolar electric current has essentially replaced unipolar current for tubal sterilization. Because of the widespread tubal destruction associated with electrocoagulation, this method is less affected by tubal thickness and mobility than many other methods. Thus, electrocoagulation may be preferable when the tube is edematous and thickened, or cannot be easily mobilized for mechanical device placement. Conversely, the greater tubal damage associated with electrocoagulation makes tubal reversal more difficult should the patient regret her decision. Regardless of the method chosen for tubal occlusion, electrocoagulation should always be readily available during laparoscopic tubal sterilization, both as a backup method of sterilization and for control of unexpected bleeding.

During sterilization with bipolar electrocoagulation, the fallopian tube is identified and grasped at the midisthmus region, approximately 2.5–3.0 cm from the uterotubal junction, with the bipolar forceps. The tube is tented up to ensure the forceps are not in contact with any other structure, and the current applied until coagulation is complete. Unlike the widespread coagulation seen during unipolar electrocoagulation, tissue destruction with bipolar current is confined to the area between and immediately adjacent to the bipolar paddles (7). Therefore, it is generally necessary to repeat the electrocoagulation an additional two times at immediately adjacent sites to duplicate the same amount of coagulation seen with unipolar current. Destruction of a minimum of 2 cm of tube has been suggested as adequate by some authorities (8), although others, including Kleppinger, advocate coagulation of at least 3 cm to ensure sterilization (Fig. 8.1) (9).

If unipolar electrocoagulation is used, the initial site of coagulation should

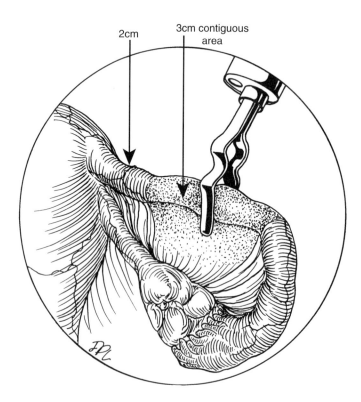

Figure 8.1. Laparoscopic bipolar electrocoagulation. Three-cm contiguous area of tube desiccated (note 2 cm proximal stump uncoagulated).

be chosen to allow any subsequent application to be closer to the uterus. Unipolar current returns to the ground through the path of least resistance. After the initial coagulation of the tube, the desiccated area has increased resistance, thus unipolar current applied distal to this site may flow to the end of tube instead of through the uterus. If the distal end of the tube should touch bowel, a bowel burn could theoretically occur.

Classically, the fallopian tube was cut and divided following coagulation. A segment of tube can also be removed for histologic evaluation as part of this procedure. Some authorities now believe that division of the tube significantly increases the chance of tuboperitoneal fistula and subsequent ectopic pregnancy (10, 11). The risk of a tear in the mesosalpinx with subsequent hemorrhage is also increased with this technique. Furthermore, any tissue submitted to pathology is often so distorted that an accurate tissue diagnosis cannot be made. As a result, most laparoscopists today do not divide the tube after electrocoagulation.

Although gynecologists use electrosurgery on an almost daily basis, many are unfamiliar with the physics involved. The unfortunate designation of current as "cut" and "coag" is especially confusing, as "cut" current can coagulate and "coag" current can cut depending on the manner in which it is used. A more appropriate scientific designation is nonmodulated current for "cut," and modulated current for "coag." When used in a contact mode, nonmodulated (cut) current is a far more efficient desiccator of tissue than modulated (coag) current. In a similar situation, modulated current produces a rapid carbonization of the tubal surface, which impedes deeper electrocoagulation. Thus, nonmodulated current is the most appropriate current to use for tubal sterilization.

Electrosurgical units designed solely for tubal electrocoagulation generate only nonmodulated (cut) bipolar current, while "Bovie" type electrosurgical generators permit the selection of either modulated (coag) or nonmodulated (cut) current in the bipolar mode. Unfortunately, many surgeons and operating room nurses automatically select the less powerful "coag" mode for tubal sterilization. The result may be a tubal lumen that remains viable despite the visual appearance of complete tubal coagulation (12).

Many gynecologists also use a "blanch, swell, and collapse" visual endpoint to determine complete tubal coagulation. However, it is uncertain whether this method is completely reliable (12). Consistent adequate coagulation is best achieved by using an ammeter to document cessation of current flow rather than depending on a visual endpoint. Alternatively, a timed coagulation period of at least 10 seconds at 25 watts of nonmodulated current will usually assure complete tubal occlusion (12, 13).

The use of electrosurgical generators with bipolar forceps produced by different manufacturers has been suggested as a cause of insufficient tubal coagulation (8). However, subsequent research would seem to indicate that complete coagulation is more dependent on selection of the proper waveform and power setting rather than generator-forceps mismatch (12–14).

The most serious and feared complication occurring with the use of electrocoagulation is thermal injury to the bowel. The use of bipolar current eliminates the majority of risk of this complication. Care to ensure that only the fallopian tube is grasped with the forceps and that the tube is not touching other intraabdominal structures should further reduce the risk of this complication.

SILASTIC RINGS

Efforts to replace electric current with a safer means of laparoscopic sterilization led to the development of Silastic rings for tubal occlusion (15). The Silastic ring (Fig. 8.2) is a nonreactive silicone rubber ring with an inner diameter of 1 mm. To permit radiographic identification, 5% barium sulfate is incorporated into the ring. The rings are applied with a specialized applicator device consisting of two concentric cylinders, the inner one of which contains grasping prongs at its distal end (Fig. 8.2). The movement of these cylinders is controlled by a single ring grip (Fig. 8.2). The Silastic band is stretched over the inner ring using a cone-shaped applicator. Bands should not be loaded on the applicator until ready for use to prevent possible loss of elastic memory. Applicators are also available that accommodate two rings so that removal for reloading between banding is not required.

The preloaded Silastic ring applicator may be introduced either through a second suprapubic puncture or through the operating channel of an operative laparoscope. The grasping forceps are extended and the fallopian tube is grasped approximately 2.5–3.0 cm distal to the uterotubal junction. The tube is drawn into the inner sleeve by retracting the tongs until resistance is felt. The ring is then

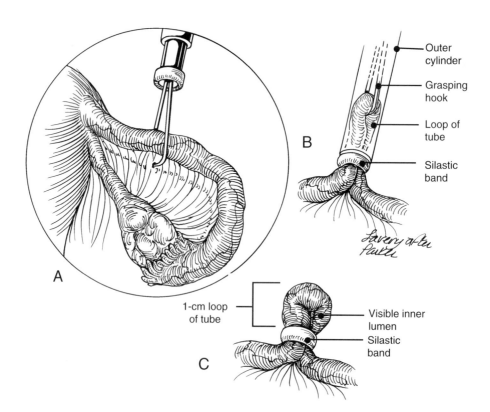

Figure 8.2. Silastic band placement. **A.** Forceps grasp tube 2.5–3.0 cm from cornu. **B.** Loop of tube pulled into outer cylinder and ring pushed off. **C.** Adequate 1-cm knuckle of tube with inner lumen (butt sign).

pushed off the applicator and onto the tube using the sliding mechanism on the applicator. An adequate knuckle of tube should be approximately one centimeter long with an obvious inner loop (Fig. 8.2).

This knuckle of tube then undergoes necrosis from interruption of its blood supply. Complete absorption of the knuckle occurs in 3–6 months, at which time the proximal and distal stump usually separate completely. The ring itself usually becomes covered with peritoneum and remains near the original occlusion site, but may fall free into the abdominal cavity (Fig. 8.3). Occasionally this characteristic has resulted in lawsuits when uninformed surgeons, operating for an ectopic pregnancy, have assumed that the absence of a ring on the tube indicated incorrect initial ring placement.

Difficulties with Silastic ring placement can occur with thickened or adhesed fallopian tubes. These conditions often hinder complete retraction of the tube into the applicator. The end result is often application of the ring to a knuckle containing only serosa, or complete transection of the tube. This complication can generally be prevented by: (a) slow withdrawal of the tube into the sleeve, thus allowing time for the tube to conform to the sleeve diameter, and (b) slightly advancing the entire applicator as the tube is drawn up to avoid countertraction from the fixed uterine end of the tube. In the case of edematous or thickened tubes, using a "milking" action with the tongs will often allow edematous tubes to be drawn into the sleeve. Alternatively, the "Yoon three-grasp technique" may be used to allow ring placement on edematous tubes (Fig. 8.4) (16). With excessively thick, edematous tubes or scarred tubes, the use of an another method such as cautery should be considered as an alternative to attempted mechanical occlusion.

If the tube is transected, Silastic rings may be placed proximal and distal to the transection, interrupting blood supply to the rent. Alternatively, electrocoagu-

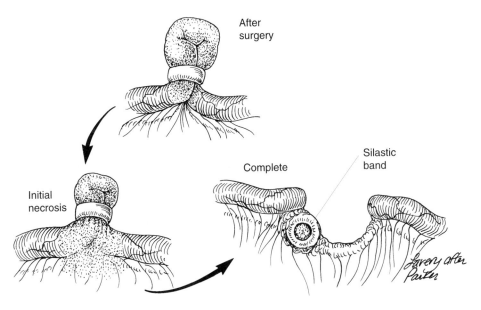

Figure 8.3. Knuckle absorption after band placement.

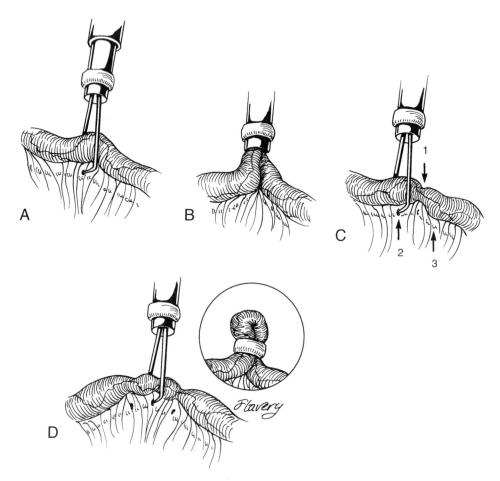

Figure 8.4. Yoon three-grasp technique. **A.** Thickened tube grasped at normal position. **B.** Tube partially retracted into applicator to squeeze edema fluid from tube, then dropped. **C.** Procedure repeated on either side of initial site. **D.** Tube regrasped at initial site and band placed.

lation of the free ends also may be used to achieve both hemostasis and tubal occlusion.

MECHANICAL CLIPS

Sterilization by mechanical clip is potentially the most reversible of all the laparoscopic methods. Originally, mechanical clips for tubal occlusion were essentially identical to the hemostatic clips used to occlude small bleeding vessels during surgery. These original clips had an unacceptably high failure rate. Such failures occurred when necrosis of the tubal muscularis beneath the clip eliminated the pressure on the deeper endosalpinx and allowed the tubal lumen to reopen. To prevent this complication, modern clips are designed to maintain a constant pressure as the tube undergoes necrosis. When properly placed, only 4 mm of tube and virtually none of the tubal blood supply is destroyed. Thus, elective tubal reanastomosis is more easily accomplished after mechanical clip tubal occlusion (17). The disadvantage of this limited destruction is that precise and accurate placement is required to achieve acceptable failure rates.

Today, there are primarily two mechanical clips in widespread use, the Hulka-Clemens clip and the Filshie clip (18, 19). The Filshie clip, widely used outside the United States, is currently unavailable in this country, but is expected to be available shortly, pending FDA approval. The Hulka-Clemens clip consists of two toothed jaws of Lexan plastic joined by a metal hinge pin. The lower jaw possesses a distal hook. The stainless steel pin (gold plated to reduce peritoneal irritation) maintains the clip in an open position. When completely advanced, the spring closes and locks the jaws. The Hulka applicator is 7 mm in diameter with a three ring configuration at the handle. A fixed distal lower jaw cradles the clip while the mobile upper jaw opens and closes the clip. A center piston, when advanced, locks the clip closed (Fig. 8.5). The Filshie clip is made of titanium and silicone. It is technically a simpler device than the Hulka-Clemens clip. A thick silicone coating instead of a metal spring is used to provide constant pressure on the tube.

Application of the Hulka-Clemens clip is described here, but the Filshie clip is applied in a similar manner. The loaded Hulka clip applicator is introduced with the clip in the closed position and the clip opened after the applicator is intraabdominal. The clip is placed perpendicular to the tube at a site 2.5–3.0 cm from the uterotubal junction. The clip may be repeatedly opened and repositioned until ideal position is achieved. The center piston is then advanced to permanently lock the clip and unseat it from the applicator. The applicator is withdrawn, leaving the clip in place on the tube (Fig. 8.6).

ENDOCOAGULATION

A technique of laparoscopic sterilization using true cautery to coagulate the fallopian tubes has been developed by Semm (20). This system uses direct electric current to heat grasping forceps to 100–120° C. Coagulation occurs as a result of

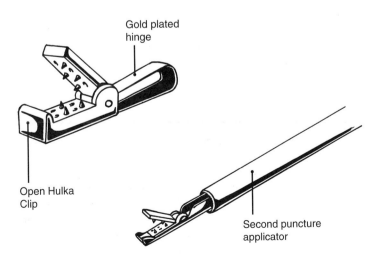

Figure 8.5. Hulka clip and applicator.

124 GYNECOLOGIC ENDOSCOPY: Principles in Practice

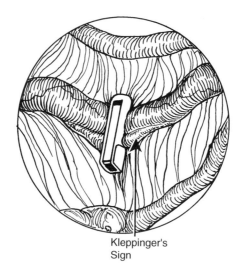

Kleppinger's Sign

Figure 8.6. Properly positioned Hulka clip. Note perpendicular placement with entire tube within clip.

heat transfer from the forceps and not by heat generated from the effect of current passing through the tissue. This method, although rarely used in the United States, is popular in many parts of Europe. Proponents believe that endocoagulation is less likely than high frequency electrocoagulation to stimulate tubal recanalization.

During endocoagulation as described by Semm, the tube is grasped 1–3 cm from the uterotubal junction. The tube is then coagulated in two adjacent areas. Semm continues to recommend transection of the tube following endocoagulation.

LAPAROSCOPIC POMEROY

One of the disadvantages of most laparoscopic sterilization techniques is the lack of a tissue specimen to document sterilization. Methods such as the Soderstrom snare technique (21), which can provide such a specimen, have not gained widespread acceptance. Recently, a laparoscopic version of the Pomeroy tubal ligation has been advocated (20, 22). The laparoscopic Pomeroy may be performed using either two lower abdominal operating ports, or one midline suprapubic port and an umbilical operating laparoscope.

After the fallopian tube has been identified a ligature of #0 plain gut with a pretied Roeder knot is inserted through one of the lower abdominal ports. The laparoscopic forceps are inserted through the opposite lower abdominal port or alternatively through the operating channel of an operating laparoscope. The forceps are passed through the endoloop, and the isthmic portion of tube is grasped and elevated through the loop. The loop is secured around the knuckle of tube and the suture tail cut with scissors and removed (Fig. 8.7). A second loop may be placed to double ligate the knuckle as described in the initial report of the Pomeroy procedure (23). Alternatively, sutures may be placed and secured using extracorporeal knot tying techniques. The ligated segment is excised with scissors

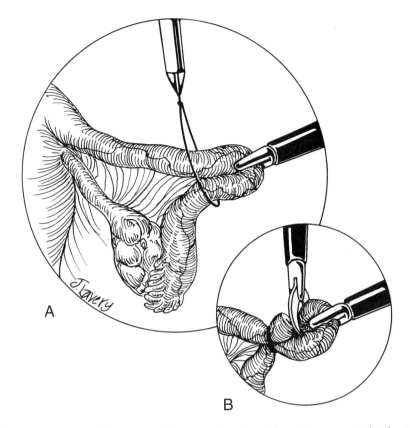

Figure 8.7. Laparoscopic Pomeroy. **A.** Tube drawn though endoloop. **B.** Loop excised with scissors.

and submitted for pathological examination. This method of sterilization is more complicated than other methods of laparoscopic sterilization and requires more operative laparoscopic skill. However, because this technique uses many of the basic skills required for more complex operative laparoscopy, it has been advocated as a training step in preparation for these more complicated procedures (24).

APPLICATION OF LOCAL ANESTHESIA

The use of mechanical devices for tubal occlusion is often associated with more postoperative discomfort than with electrocoagulation (25, 26). Electrocoagulation destroys the neural innervation, thus rendering the tube anesthetic. On the other hand, mechanical occlusion of the tube may be considered occlusion of a small hollow viscus and produces a similar crampy abdominal pain. Postoperative nausea and vomiting also are reported to be increased with these methods. These side effects can be minimized or eliminated, however, if the fallopian tubes are first anesthetized with a local anesthetic (25–27).

Because of its high protein binding and long duration of action, 0.5% bupivacaine is an excellent choice as the local anesthetic. For best results, the local anesthetic should be applied to each tube prior to and not after occlusion. Five milliliters of 0.5% bupivacaine per tube will provide prolonged tubal anesthesia.

An aspiration cannula can be used to flow the bupivacaine over all surfaces of the tube. Topical application of bupivacaine has been shown to be equal to tubal injection and is technically much simpler (26).

STERILIZATION FAILURES

Luteal Phase Pregnancy

Luteal phase pregnancy is defined as a pregnancy diagnosed after an interval tubal sterilization, but in which contraception occurred before the sterilization procedure. Luteal phase pregnancy has been reported to occur at a rate of one to fifteen per 1000 interval sterilizations (28, 29). Technically speaking, a luteal phase pregnancy is not a true sterilization failure since, by definition, the pregnancy preceded the sterilization. Nevertheless, the result is an undesired pregnancy. A variety of strategies has been suggested to reduce the incidence of luteal phase pregnancies. These include performing sterilization procedures before the date of estimated ovulation, concurrent D & C, use of effective contraception and/or sexual abstinence before sterilization, and preoperative pregnancy testing. At our institution, we have found that the use of same-day urine pregnancy testing using an enzyme-linked immunosorbent assay has virtually eliminated luteal phase pregnancies (29).

Failed Tubal Occlusion

Sterilization failures from failed tubal occlusion fall into three categories: (*a*) misidentification of the fallopian tube, (*b*) incomplete occlusion of a properly identified tube, and (*c*) selection of an incorrect portion of the fallopian tube for occlusion. On occasion, pelvic structures such as the round ligament, ovarian ligament, and infundibulopelvic ligament may be mistaken for a fallopian tube and mistakenly ligated. This mistake is primarily caused by inadequate visualization of the pelvic structures. Factors that may contribute to poor visualization include poor optics, inadequate light, failure to adequately elevate the uterus, inadequate pneumoperitoneum, and pelvic adhesions. With the exception of pelvic adhesions, these factors are easily avoided with the use of proper equipment and technique, and should be a rare cause of sterilization failure.

A more common cause of true sterilization failure is failure to completely occlude the fallopian tube. This is frequently encountered with the use of mechanical occlusive devices. The mechanical clips are particularly vulnerable to poor placement. Great care must be taken to fully include the tube within the clip. With correct application, the mesosalpinx on the surface of the tube is pulled upward to resemble the flat triangle shape of an envelope flap (Kleppinger's "envelope" sign). A grasper inserted through another abdominal port or the operating laparoscope can be used to place the tube on tension prior to clip application. This decreases the likelihood that the lumen will roll out of the clip during application. The use of mechanical devices on edematous or dilated tubes frequently results in only partial tubal occlusion. When Silastic rings are used, the tubal serosa, but not tubal lumen, may be pulled into the ring. This knuckle of serosa can closely resemble a truly adequate "knuckle." However, close observation will reveal the absence of the vertical crease formed when an entire loop of tube is included in the ring. Some have compared the appearance of an adequate knuckle to that of a baby's bottom, with accompanying gluteal crease (butt sign; Fig. 8.2).

Incomplete tubal occlusion with electrocoagulation is generally associated with either application of current for too short a time interval or use of modulated (coag) current as discussed previously in this chapter. The use of timed electrocoagulation or ammeter and nonmodulated current should eliminate this cause of tubal sterilization failure.

The isthmic portion of the fallopian tube is the proper site of tubal occlusion regardless of the occlusion method chosen. The isthmus of the tube has a thick muscularis with a narrow lumen. In contrast, the ampulla has a thin muscularis, wide lumen, and voluminous rugae. Attempted occlusion with mechanical devices may not incorporate all of the tubal lumen resulting in sterilization failure (30). Electrocoagulation of the tubal ampulla is more likely to produce complete occlusion, but will not achieve the same failure rate as coagulation of the isthmic portion of the tube (31).

On the other hand, coagulation of the tube too close to the cornu may lead to uteroperitoneal fistula formation. In 1930, Sampson described sprouts of endosalpinx growing out of the traumatized mucosa of the tubal stump (32). McCausland suggested that coagulation of the proximal isthmic fallopian tube tends to activate this process, which can then invade the tubal muscularis, penetrate the serosa, and result in a fistula (33). He named this endosalpingoblastosis. Recanalization frequently results in a fistula sufficient to allow passage of sperm, but usually not the ovum (34, 35). This may be one explanation of the high ratio of ectopic to intrauterine pregnancies following failure of sterilization by electrocoagulation.

Technical Failures

Technical failures result when a sterilization procedure is performed correctly but a pregnancy still occurs. Historically, failure rates for all laparoscopic sterilization methods have been reported to be one to four per 1000 procedures with no difference between clips, rings, or electrocoagulation. However, much of these data are based on relatively small groups without reliable long-term follow-up. Preliminary unpublished data from the Collaborative Review of Sterilization (CREST) have indicated higher failure rates for all methods than previously reported. In particular, electrocoagulation may have a cumulative failure rate of 1–3% at 10 years after surgery.

Chromopertubation

The transcervical injection of dye to assess tubal patency (chromopertubation) at laparoscopic sterilization has been advocated as a method to reduce failures to incomplete tubal occlusion (16, 36). Unfortunately, lack of dye spill is not an absolute indicator of tubal occlusion, since tubal spasm during dye injection may produce temporary blockage of patent tubes. Moreover, dye spillage does not necessarily indicate sterilization failure. Older studies involving hysterosalpingography after laparoscopic sterilization have shown the risk of subsequent pregnancy appears to be very low despite "patent tubes" (37–39). In one study, immediate resterilization of tubes "patent" by chromopertubation did not reduce the true failure rate. This suggests that anatomic distortion and tubal dysfunction, as well as delayed tubal fibrosis, may be partially responsible for the action of tubal sterilization (37).

Chromopertubation is also not without potential risks. Fistula formation, infection, displacement of devices used for tubal occlusion, and increased sterilization failures have all been suggested as potential side effects. Although studies suggest these risks are minimal, there appears to be no evidence to support the routine use of chromopertubation at laparoscopic sterilization (40).

Sterilization Under Local Anesthesia

Various investigators have reported their experiences with the use of local anesthesia as an alternative to general anesthesia for laparoscopic sterilization (27, 41–43). While this technique appears safe, effective, and is used widely in many countries, only a small proportion of laparoscopic sterilization in this country utilize this technique. This could potentially be secondary to a lack of residency training or because the operator is not experienced with the technique involved.

Local anesthesia is associated with advantages as well as disadvantages (Table 8.1). While local anesthesia is essential for patients with a contraindication to general anesthesia, almost all patients are candidates. Relative contraindications involve the extremely obese patient, or those who have had multiple abdominal procedures, making the need for laparotomy more likely.

When local anesthesia is used, the patient is managed preoperatively and postoperatively a bit differently (Table 8.2). Initially, the patient is given ibuprofen (800 mg), 30 minutes prior to surgery to decrease uterine contractility when the Hulka tenaculum is placed into the uterus, and when the uterus is manipulated during the procedure. Just prior to beginning the procedure the patient is asked to void, thereby eliminating the need to place a catheter in the bladder. Again, this step is used to minimize any discomfort caused by bladder catheterization. The patient is given atropine, 0.4 mg, and midazolam, 1 mg, intravenously just prior to beginning the pelvic examination and vaginal/abdominal prep. The patient's mental status is assessed after 4 to 5 minutes, and if she is not

Table 8.1. Advantages and Disadvantages of Laparoscopic Tubal Sterilization Under Local Anesthesia

Advantages	Disadvantages
• Avoidance of potential respiratory/cardiac complication	• Additional physician training
• Decreased anesthesia time	• Gentle tissue manipulation
• Decreased recovery time	• Patient may be more anxious
• Shorter operative time	• Patient may move if she experiences pain
• Decreased patient cost	
• Decreased nausea/vomiting	
• Patient may observe the procedure (enhanced understanding)	
• Avoidance of potential air embolism	
• Decreased postoperative pain medication requirement	

Table 8.2. Medications for Sterilization Using Local Anesthesia

Drug	Dose	Purpose	Timing
Ibuprofen	800 mg p.o.	Decrease uterine cramping	30 min. preop.
Atropine	0.4–0.6 mg i.v.	Vaginal blockage	O.R. arrival
Midazolam	2.5 mg i.v.	Sedation/amnesia	Abdominal prep
Alfentanil	0.5–1.0 mg i.v.	Narcosis	After Midazolam
Bupivacaine	25 cc (0.5%)	Local anesthetic	Variable

sufficiently sedated, an additional 0.5 to 1.0 mg of alfentanil is given to provide sufficient patient comfort.

Like tubal occlusion with general anesthesia, the pneumoperitoneum can be created using carbon dioxide or nitrous oxide. Some investigators feel that nitrous oxide pneumoperitoneum produces less abdominal discomfort than does carbon dioxide. Once the uterine manipulator is inserted, an umbilical field block is created with 5 mL of a 0.5% solution of bupivacaine. This is followed by the creation of a diamond-shaped fascial block using 10 mL of the 0.5% bupivacaine solution. Each point of the "diamond," as well as the center, is injected with 1 mL below the fascia and 1 mL above the fascia as the needle is withdrawn along the tract. The center of the diamond corresponds to the planned entry site of the trocar (Fig. 8.8). A direct trocar insertion technique is utilized, gas instilled into the abdomen, and the operating laparoscope is inserted. A cannula is passed through the operating port of the laparoscope, and approximately 10 mL of 0.5% bupivacaine solution is dripped over all surfaces of the fallopian tubes, the broad ligaments to the round ligaments, and on the ovaries and uterine fundus. Thus, the total bupivacaine dose for laparoscopic sterilization done in this manner is 125 mg (25 mL of 0.5% solution). The recommended is 2.5 mg/kg, or 175 mg for a 70 kg patient.

While the tubal occlusive method used in the past has been electrocoagulation, Lipscomb et al. have shown that the use of Silastic rings is associated with less intraoperative discomfort and a shorter operative time than is electrocoagulation (27). Unlike when general anesthesia is used, when local anesthesia is used, the electrical current is applied in an incremental manner to prevent heat buildup and discomfort. The remainder of the surgical procedure is performed as usual. Postoperatively, the patient spends only a short time in the recovery room and then is discharged home. A nonsteroidal antiinflammatory is used for pain control, and the patient is allowed to return to her normal activities when she becomes completely alert.

Cost containment is yet another issue when sterilization is being considered. Handa et al. (44) reviewed all laparoscopic sterilizations at San Francisco General Hospital performed over a 2-year period. Patients receiving local anesthesia were compared to patients receiving general anesthesia. In their study, general anesthesia was used in 81 (39%) cases. The average cost of each procedure was $1200 for local anesthesia and $3971 for general anesthesia. These authors estimated that more than $277 million dollars per year could be saved if local anesthesia were used in 50% of the laparoscopic tubal ligations performed in the United States.

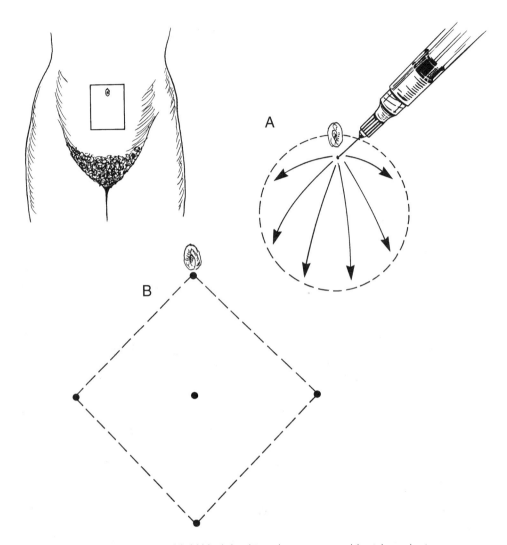

Figure 8.8. Diamond field block for skin, subcutaneous, and fascial anesthesia.

TEACHING MODULE FOR LAPAROSCOPIC STERILIZATION

The teaching of laparoscopic sterilization is generally taught/learned by operating room observation and supervision by either a senior resident or faculty.

It has been demonstrated that residents given a pretest just several days prior to performing their first laparoscopic sterilization procedure lacked basic knowledge and principles required to perform the procedure. It was further demonstrated that these same residents could be taught the required principles following completion of a teaching module. It was further shown in this study that the failure rates following laparoscopic sterilization were significantly reduced following completion of this teaching module (45).

The teaching module consisted of a 40-minute videotape accompanied by a monograph of the videotape script. The videotape demonstrated basic laparoscopic techniques and laparoscopic sterilization techniques for the tubal ring (Falope Ring Band, Cabot Medical, Langhorne, PA), electrocautery, and the spring-loaded clip (Hulka-Clemen, Richard Wolf, Rosemont, IL). In addition, these videotapes included a discussion of laparoscopic complications and their management. Following completion of the teaching module, the resident was given a test, which consisted of 23 single-answer multiple-choice (A-type) questions and eight multiple-multiple (K-type) questions. Residents were required to have a score of at least 83% before being allowed to perform laparoscopic sterilizations.

Initially, the resident's performance is monitored through the entire laparoscopic procedure. Gradually, this monitoring is reduced until the resident is able and comfortable with the performance of the procedure on his/her own.

A teaching module like this one could be used for many gynecologic and surgical procedures, and could also be used for testing nonsurgical treatment alternatives. It seems reasonable that the approach could be used by anyone wishing to learn or review the technique of laparoscopic sterilization.

CONCLUSION

Laparoscopic sterilization remains the most common means of interval sterilization in the United States. Multiple ways are available to achieve tubal occlusion with each method having both advantages and disadvantages. The correct methods for any particular patient should be based on that patient's anatomy, as well as the physician's comfort and experience with the methods available. It also appears that laparoscopic sterilization using local anesthesia should be offered to all patients considering laparoscopic tubal occlusion.

REFERENCES

1. Bösch PF. Laparoskopie. Scheiz. Z. Krankenhaus-u. Anstaltsw 1936;6:62.
2. Powers FH, Barnes AC. Sterilization by means of peritoneoscopic tubal fulguration: preliminary report. Am J Obstet Gynecol 1941;41:1038–1043.
3. Palmer R. Essai de sterilization tubaire celioscopique par electrocoagulation isthique. Bull Fed Soc Gynecol Obstet Lang Fr 1962;14:298.
4. Steptoe PC. Laparoscopy in gynaecology. Edinburgh: E & S Livingstone, 1967.
5. Philips J, Hulka J, Keith C, Hulka B, Keith L. Laparoscopic procedures: a national survey for 1975. J Reprod Med 1977;18:219.
6. Levi BS, Soderstrom RM, Dali DS. Bowel injuries during laparoscopy—gross anatomy and histology. J Reprod Med 1985;30:168.
7. Ryder RM, Hulka JF. Bladder and bowel injury after electrodesiccation with Kleppinger bipolar forceps. J Reprod Med 1993;38:595–598.
8. Soderstrom RM, Levy BS. Bipolar systems—do they perform? Obstet Gynecol 1987;69:425–427.
9. Kleppinger RK. Laparoscopic tubal sterilization. In: Garcia CR, Mikuta JJ, Rosenblum NJ, eds. Current therapy in surgical gynecology. 1st ed. Philadelphia: BC Decker, 1987:80–86.
10. Cunanan R, Courey N, Lippes J. Complications of laparoscopic tubal sterilization. Obstet Gynecol 1980:55:501–506.
11. Shah A, Courey N, Cunanan R. Pregnancy following laparoscopic tubal electrocoagulation and division. Am J Obstet Gynecol 1977;129:459–460.

12. Soderstrom RM, Levy BS, Engel T. Reducing bipolar failures. Obstet Gynecol 1989;74:60–63.
13. Tucker D, Brenda JA, Mardan A, Engel T. The interaction of electrosurgical bipolar forceps and generators on an animal model of fallopian tube sterilization. Am J Obstet Gynecol 1991;165: 443–447.
14. Tucker D, Brenda JA, Sievert CE, Engel T. The effect of electrosurgical coagulation waveform on a rat uterine model of fallopian tube sterilization. J Gynecol Surg 1992;8:235–241.
15. Yoon IB, Wheeless CR, King TM. A preliminary report on the new laparoscopic sterilization approach: the silicone rubber band technique. Am J Obstet Gynecol 1974;120:132–136.
16. Yoon IB, King TM. A preliminary and immediate report on a new laparoscopic tubal ring procedure. J Reprod Med 1975;15:54–56.
17. Hulka JF, Nolble AD, Letchworth AT, et al. Reversibility of clip sterilization. Lancet 1982;2:927.
18. Hulka JA, Fishburne JI, Mercer JP, et al. Laparoscopic sterilization with a spring clip: a report of the first fifty cases. Am J Obstet Gynecol 1973;116:715.
19. Filshie GM, Casey D, Pogmere JR, et al. The titanium/silicone clip for female sterilization. Br J Obstet Gynaecol 1981;88:655–662.
20. Semm K. Course of endoscopic abdominal surgery. In: Freidrich ER, trans. Operative manual for endoscopic abdominal surgery. Chicago: Year Book, 1987:130–213.
21. Soderstrom RM, Smith MR. Tubal sterilization: a new laparoscopic method. Obstet Gynecol 1971;38:152–154.
22. Murray JE, Hibbert ML, Heth SR, Letterie GS. A technique for laparoscopic tubal ligation with endoloop sutures. Obstet Gynecol 1992;80:1053–1055.
23. Bishop E, Nelms WF. A simple method of tubal sterilization. NY State J Med 1930;30:214–216.
24. Parson MT, Hill DA. The benefits of the loop ligature (endoloop) laparoscopic sterilization procedure in a residency program. J Gynecol Surg 1994;10:15–20.
25. Koetsawang S, Srisupandit S, Apimas Champion CB. A comparison study of laparoscopic sterilization with the use of the tubal ring. Am J Obstet Gynecol 1984;150:931–933.
26. Borgatta L, Gruss L, Barad D, Ong C, et al. Randomized trial of local anesthetic application for the relief of postoperative pain after tubal sterilization with Falope rings. Am J Gynecol Health 1991;5:11–15.
27. Lipscomb GH, Stovall TG, Ramanathan JA, Ling FW. Comparison of Silastic rings and electrocoagulation on operative and postoperative pain during laparoscopic sterilization using local anesthesia. Obstet Gynecol 1992;80:645–649.
28. Chi I, Siemens AJ, Champion CB, Gates D, Cilienti D. Pregnancy following minilaparotomy tubal sterilization: an update of an international data set. Contraception 1987;35:171–179.
29. Lipscomb GH, Spellman JR, Ling FW. The effect of same-day pregnancy testing on the incidence of luteal phase pregnancy. Obstet Gynecol 1993;82:411–413.
30. Soderstrom RM. Sterilization failures and their causes. Am J Obstet Gynecol 1985;152:395–403.
31. Cheng MC, Wong YM, Rochat RW, Ratnam SS. Sterilization failures in Singapore: an examination of ligation techniques and failure rates. Stud Fam Plann 1977;8:109–115.
32. Sampson JA. Postsalpingectomy endometriosis (endosalpingiosis). Am J Obstet Gynecol 1930;20:443–480.
33. McCausland A. Endosalpingosis (endosalpingoblastosis) following laparoscopic tubal coagulation as an etiologic factor of ectopic pregnancy. Am J Obstet Gynecol 1982;143:12–24.
34. Makar A, Vanderheyden JS, Schatteman EA, Albert YN, Vanderkideren JJ, Van Marck EA. Female sterilization failure after bipolar electrocoagulation: a 6 year retrospective study. Euro J Obstet Gynecol Reprod Biol 1990;37:237–246.
35. Metz KG, Mastroianni L. Tubal pregnancy subsequent to transperitoneal migration of spermatozoa. Obstet Gynecol Surv 1979;34:554–560.
36. Aubert JM, Garcia A. Improving Falope-ring application in laparoscopic training. J Reprod Med 1987;32:340–341.
37. Ayers JW, Johnson RS, Ansbacher R, Menon M, LaFerla JJ, Roberts JA. Sterilization failures with bipolar cautery. Fertil Steril 1984;42:526–530.
38. Cook CL. Evaluation of ring sterilization by hysterosalpingogram. J Reprod Med 1982;27: 243–245.
39. Grunert GM. Late tubal patency following tubal ligation. Fertil Steril 1981;35:406–408.
40. Lipscomb GH, Stovall TG, Summitt RL, Ling FW. Chromopertubation at the time of laparoscopic tubal occlusion. Obstet Gynecol 1994;83:725–728.

41. Peterson HB, Hulka JF, Spielman FJ, et al. Local versus general anesthesia for laparoscopic sterilization: a randomized study. Obstet Gynecol 1987;70:903–908.
42. Fishburne JL Jr, Orman KF, Hulka JF, et al. Laparoscopic tubal clip sterilization under local anesthesia. Fertil Steril 1974;25:762–766.
43. Børdahl PE, Ræder JC, Nordentoft J, Kirste U, Refsdal A. Laparoscopic sterilization under local or general anesthesia? A randomized study. Obstet Gynecol 1993;81:137–141.
44. Handa VL, Berlin M, Washington AE. A comparison of local and general anesthesia for laparoscopic tubal sterilization. J Women's Health 1994;3:135–141.
45. Stovall TG, Ling FW, Lipscomb GH, Summitt RL Jr, Beckmann CRB. A model for resident surgical training in laparoscopic sterilization. Obstet Gynecol 1994;83:470–472.

Chapter 9

Learning Operative Endoscopy

*Michael J. Sammarco and
Thomas G. Stovall*

The manner in which new surgical techniques are learned or acquired has traditionally been taught in the clinical setting. Knowledge of the anatomy and techniques followed by observation of the procedure have been the cornerstones of surgical teaching. With the introduction of endoscopic techniques, this traditional approach has met with some problems (1). Criticisms of the manner that endoscopic skills are taught, acquired, and subsequently applied, can be found in the public press as well as specialty journals references (2, 3). There is little question that operative endoscopic skills are not easily acquired through the "see one, do one, teach one," method (4). Although there is a learning curve that is associated with all surgical procedures, this curve seems to be longer with the advanced operative endoscopic procedures. There is also a threshold that once reached, further experience will not reduce the complication rate or improve the outcome. The learning curve and thresholds for operative endoscopic procedures appear to be more individualized and less defined than in other gynecological surgical procedures. This may be secondary to the associated technical component that is necessary to perform endoscopy, or to the increased eye-hand coordination needed with these procedures. No longer are knowledge of the anatomy and knowledge of the procedure the only prerequisites to attempting the surgery; a thorough understanding of the equipment and ability to perform surgery utilizing a two-dimensional image are also required.

What is "the best" approach to learning operative endoscopy? The answer to the question is not the same for every individual. Guidelines have been proposed but there is no uniformity among institutions (5). The purpose of this chapter is to review the currently available teaching models that have been found to be effective. In addition, exercises will be presented that will help develop endoscopic skills. Finally, a section is included to review the instrumentation equipment necessary for basic operative endoscopic surgical setup.

GENERAL CONSIDERATIONS

Whether the intention is to improve existing skills or to develop new skills, exercises should be conducted under similar conditions as would be expected in the operating room. This is of particular importance for the novice. To learn a new technique with instrumentation or equipment that is not available in one's own operating room makes little sense. The importance of developing basic skills that can be applied to more complex techniques cannot be emphasized enough. New devices and instrumentation may be very effective in simplifying procedures, but these devices may not always be available. The majority of procedures can be completed using basic instrumentation. A thorough knowledge of basic operative techniques should not be taken for granted.

Keep the group small—no greater than three if possible. When initially learning endoscopy, a knowledgeable assistant is invaluable. One should feel comfortable working with both hands. This includes being equally adept at holding the camera while working, as well as working with both hands while the assistant holds the camera. Learning basic techniques on pelvic trainers equipped with stationary camera systems do not offer this aspect of training.

In keeping groups small, it allows more participation of each member. Despite the level of expertise, every effort should be made to maintain an "OR attitude." Participants should not use instruments or equipment in a manner that would be inappropriate in an OR setting. Bad habits are easily learned and difficult to alter. This is of particular importance when using reducing sleeves and ports. Acquiring good habits that eventually become second nature are of immeasurable value in allowing an actual case to proceed smoothly and efficiently.

Considering the number of different camera, video, monitor, and light source systems currently on the market, it is impossible to be familiar with every available system. What is important is to be familiar with the general principles of assembly and care for video systems. This can easily be incorporated into each training system by requiring the participants to assemble and disassemble the equipment at the beginning and the end of each session. Becoming adept at "trouble shooting" for problems is an invaluable lesson and should be emphasized continuously. These same general principles apply to instrumentation. There should be a good understanding of each type of instrument available in that particular OR. This applies to both reusable and disposable instrumentation. Although it is more cost effective to use discarded disposable reusable instruments for training, it is advantageous to train with similar instruments as those used in the OR.

Whether the purpose of the workshop is to improve individual skills or to learn basic techniques, there should be well defined goals. Training sessions should be planned to reasonably allow enough time for the completion of the exercises and not overwhelm the participants. The objective should not be to simply complete one exercise, but to apply the same basic techniques previously learned to the next exercise at hand. In this manner, basic skills are constantly being reinforced. Exercises should be challenging and applicable, but not too complex. There is no reason to waste time and effort in learning a technique that is not applicable to actual surgery. This also applies to learning a technique with instrumentation or equipment that is not generally available or that is not commonly used.

HOW TO BEGIN

The following is a minimal list of basic equipment and instruments needed for an endoscopy training workshop. It closely parallels the basic equipment list needed for most operative and diagnostic procedures (Table 9.1).

PELVIC TRAINERS

There are several types of pelvic trainers available. The most commonly used are those with a hard plastic top (opaque or transparent) with circular cutouts that have rubber inserts (Fig. 9.1). These are very durable and easy to

Table 9.1. Basic Equipment for Endoscopy Training Workshop

Video monitor, preferably 19-inch, with the necessary cables
Camera
Light source—150 watt halogen or metal halide
10-mm 0° laparoscope
Necessary light cables
Electrical generator and grounding pads
Pelvic trainer
Laparoscopic sleeves of various sizes and with reducing sleeves or caps
(There should be both disposable and reusable systems available.)
Two 5-mm graspers
Two 5-mm spring-handled atraumatic graspers
One 10-mm spoon forceps
One 5-mm scissors
Unipolar needle electrode
5-mm laparoscopic needle holder
5-mm laparoscopic knot pusher
Bipolar coagulating forceps
One 5-mm self-retaining traumatic grasping forceps

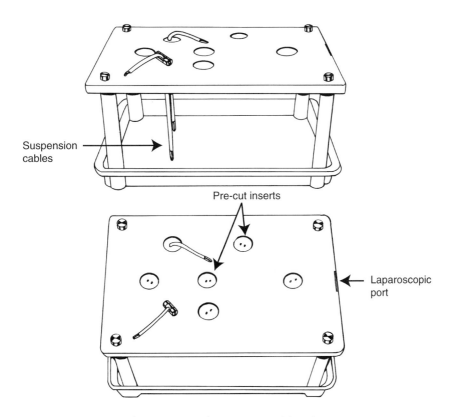

Figure 9.1. Hard top, opaque pelvic trainer.

keep clean and sanitary. They can be disassembled for cleaning and storage. The major disadvantage of these trainers is the precut holes used to place the ports. These may not be at the most advantageous position for all of the exercises. In addition, the angle that the laparoscope is placed in the trainer is not anatomical. There is often a temptation to not use laparoscopic sleeves during the exercises since the rubber inserts fit tightly around the instruments. This practice should be dissuaded. Injection techniques are more difficult to learn on these types of trainers since a needle can only be placed through a pre-selected site. The depth of the trainers is deeper than is encountered during most actual cases, but this does not usually present a problem. The use of transparent tops often decreases the frustration that often accompanies initial attempts at performing surgical techniques using a video system, but is not recommended. Learning to perform endoscopic surgery on a two-dimensional screen should be taught on a two-dimensional screen.

This second type of trainer has a soft top (Fig. 9.2). These trainers tend to be less durable and not as deep as the solid-topped trainers. The major advantage to this model is the type of top. This top "gives" and does not allow the participants to be overly rough. It also allows the ports to be positioned anywhere. This trainer can also be equipped with a transparent or opaque top. After a period of use, the tops need to be replaced for a minimal cost.

There are several other types of trainers on the market. They range from the very basic to the very complex. Any trainer can be used, but the choice should be based on one's need. Always keep in mind that the trainer's purpose is to hold models and provide a surface to position the laparoscope ports into. The more complex types, i.e., those that are entirely enclosed with the ability to insufflate, only add to the complexity of the setting up of the assembly and disassembly of the workshop (Fig. 9.3). On the other hand, the overly simplified trainers, i.e., those with a fixed camera and a transparent container, may be too unlike the actual surgical setup and would be inadequate for training the novice (Fig. 9.4).

Regardless of which trainer is chosen, the participant should always attempt to position themselves around the trainer as they would during surgery

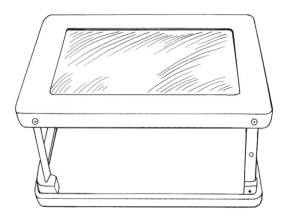

Figure 9.2.   Soft top, opaque pelvic trainer.

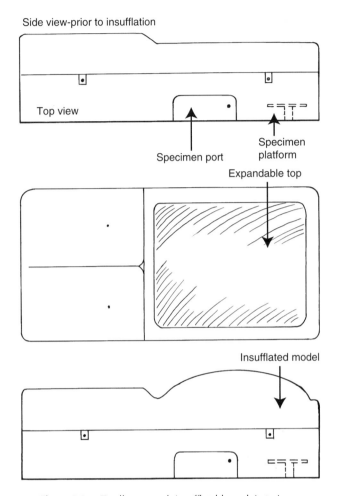

Figure 9.3. Totally encased, insufflatable, pelvic trainer.

(Fig. 9.5). This particularly applies to those manipulating the camera. It is often easier to stand directly behind the camera port. This positioning is not ordinarily possible during actual surgical cases. Neither is standing directly behind two instruments ports. If the participant is taught in these positions, it is one further adjustment that must be made when moving to the OR suite.

If using a trainer that is open on the side, wrapping a sheet around the sides will improve lighting and provide a nondistracting background to work against. It will prevent inadvertent scattering of laser energy, but may serve as a fire hazard if not moistened. If using electrosurgical or laser energy, a smoke evacuator will be needed to be placed at the edge of the trainer.

LAPAROSCOPIC MODELS

There are basically two types of models that are used for training purposes: those made from extirpated organs or tissues, and those made from plastic or other inanimate materials. Which model to use depends on the objective of the

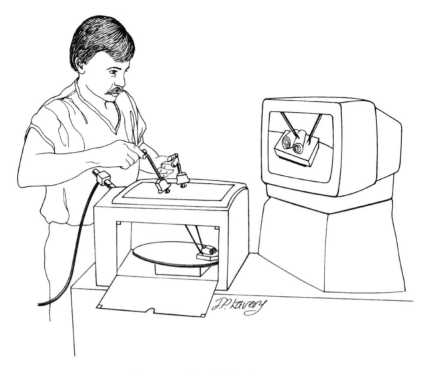

Figure 9.4. Simplified pelvic trainer.

workshop. Nontissue models have the advantage of ease of setup and cleanup, whereas the tissue models offer a better "feel." It is best to have a combination of both. This allows for more variety and keeps the workshops interesting.

Live Animal Models. When learning any surgical technique, using a live animal subject is desirable for most participants. Although used in many commercial training centers, it is impractical in smaller centers or for individual use. Their use should be reserved for the more advanced surgeon. Live animal models are relatively expensive, more time intensive, and offer no advantage for the novice. Once basic skills have been mastered, they are a useful extension to emphasize certain techniques, i.e., maintenance of adequate pneumoperitoneum, hemostasis, tissue dissection, and tissue effects of various energy modalities. Even when live animal models are used, the objective should be oriented toward the learning of a specific technique, and not in the performance of a specific surgical procedure later to be adapted to human patients. Also, when using live animal models, careful attention must be paid to fulfilling various institutional specific and State/Federal requirements (Table 9.2). Finally, the participants must be familiar with the various anatomical differences between the animal model and human subjects.

Nontissue Models. These models can be purchased or constructed. Those that are purchased are usually composed of foam or rubber. Again, the objective of the exercise should always be kept in mind when considering which type of

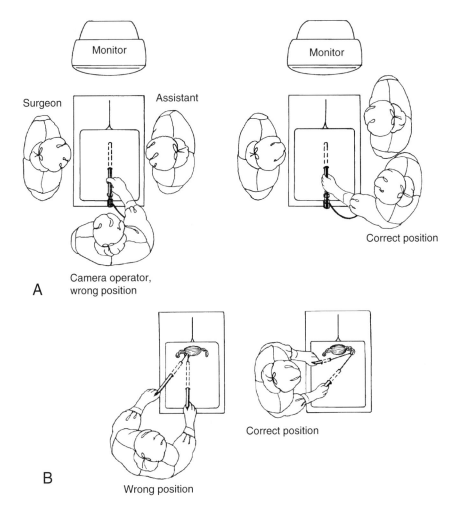

Figure 9.5. Incorrect and correct positioning during a training session. **A.** Multiple participants. **B.** Single participant.

model to use. The primary concern should be to choose a model that offers the proper spatial orientation. The following are examples of practical and easy-to-assemble models.

Uterine Models

The uterus can be composed of several different materials and subsequently mounted to a board for stabilization. The board should be at least 1 inch × 6 inches × 6 inches in size to prevent it from being easily dislodged during the exercises. The most important aspect of the uterine model, regardless of the material it is composed of, is the maintenance of its spatial orientation. The model is more beneficial if it is versatile. The ability to easily change adnexal structures is particularly important when working in groups. This will greatly improve the time efficiency of the workshop.

Table 9.2. Investigative Surgery in Non-Survival Procedures Only, Performed by Surgeons

The IACUC (institutional Animal Care and Use Committee) acknowledges the need for creativity during investigation of new procedures and devices. These activities, outside the manipulations described in the IACUC procedures, must be permitted during advancement of new surgical technologies. The limits or extent of variation from Approved Procedures shall be left to the discretion of the Veterinary Study Director or designee. Whenever significant variation is contemplated, approval of the activity should be obtained from another IACUC Veterinary Member. Any significant variation shall be documented by detailed description on the Completed Study Sheet. Documented variations shall be entered in an IACUC database for review.

Harvested Tissue
The IACUC acknowledges and promotes the use of tissues and animal cadavers resulting from nonsurvival studies. Such activities allow for more complete utilization of each individual animal and reduce overall animal usage. Specific IACUC review of such utilization is unnecessary; however, an IACUC number may be assigned to allow for documentation and product traceability.

Respect for Life
The IACUC acknowledges the need to perform multiple procedures within the same non-survival animal as part of efforts to reduce overall animal usage. The committee is concerned, however, that such multiple use always show adequate respect and concern for the life of the individual animal. Procedures or utilization which appear to disregard the intrinsic value of life should be avoided. It is incumbent upon each member of the Endosurgery Institute staff to report real or perceived unsuitable activities to the IACUC.

Humane Care and Use of Animals
The IACUC upholds the standards for Humane Care and Use of Animals used in research, testing, or educational activities as set forth by the Animal Welfare Act. Any deviations, either real or perceived, must be reported to the IACUC.

Good Science
Researchers practicing good science must be concerned with the well-being of their laboratory animals; health problems, pain, and stress may introduce unwanted variables that can invalidate study results. Concern for laboratory animals also reflects a fundamental principle of ethical animal research: experimental animals, regardless of species, should not undergo unnecessary distress or discomfort.

Attention to the animal's well-being begins with research planning. Studies should be designed to use the minimum number of animals exposed to the least amount of noxious stimulation for the shortest time.

IACUC POLICIES

Pain Category
The IACUC adopts the following categories for classification of animal discomfort. Any procedures submitted for review in category IV will receive full committee review. All animals post-operatively will be given analgesics for 24 hours unless exempted by the Study Director and approved by the Attending veterinarian.

I Includes the use of animals in procedures that involve no pain or distress. Examples: non-invasive physical monitoring, palpation, urine, and fecal sample collection.
II Includes the use of animals in procedures that involve momentary or slight pain or distress. Examples: injections, blood sample collection, anesthesia, non-survival procedures performed on properly anesthetized animals, euthanized in accordance with AVMA guidelines.
III Includes the use of animals in survival surgery procedures where appropriate anesthetics, analgesics, or tranquilizers are administered to avoid pain and distress.
IV Includes the use of animals in procedures involving pain or distress without administration of anesthetics, analgesics, or tranquilizers.

Good Surgery
Good surgery on research animals does not differ from that on human patients. In both instances, successful surgery requires good pre-operative and post-operative care; aseptic surgical procedures and facilities, appropriate equipment; and surgical competence of the persons performing the operation. Failure to fulfill these requirements can endanger not only the research animal, but also the research.

Euthanasia
Termination of experimental animals, when necessary, must be accomplished in a humane manner and in keeping with the recommendations of the American Veterinary Medical Association Panel on Euthanasia, Journal of the American Veterinary Medical Association, Vol. 188, 1986, p. 252–68.

Chapter 9: Learning Operative Endoscopy   143

Sock Uterus (Fig. 9.6).   This is easy to assemble and inexpensive. This model performs well as a suturing model. Adnexal structures can be attached to the model. This model is more difficult to use with electrosurgical techniques. Since the model is absorbent, it is usually discarded after use with extirpated tissues.

Pear Uterus (Fig. 9.7).   This model is constructed using a piece of decorative silk fruit, i.e., such as those found in floral shops or craft stores. The pear is inverted and attached to a piece of wood of the same size as previously noted. This is a more durable model than the sock uterus. Other models or tissues can be sutured to its surface or it can be used as a suturing model by itself. To help keep the model clean and reusable, a piece of cast stocking or a small sock can be used as a cover prior to attaching any additional models.

Placental Uterus (Fig. 9.8).   This model is more of a potential biohazard than the other models but offers certain advantages. Once the model is constructed, adnexal structures can be attached with suture or staples. As a model for suturing, it better demonstrates knot integrity, since placental vessels can be used for ligation. It also better demonstrates tissue effects of laser and electrosurgical energy. It requires more preparation than the other models and is usually used only once.

Grounding the Model. Since many of the exercises require the use of electrosurgical energy, the models will need to be grounded. In the case of the placental model, the grounding clip can be attached directly to the model. The other

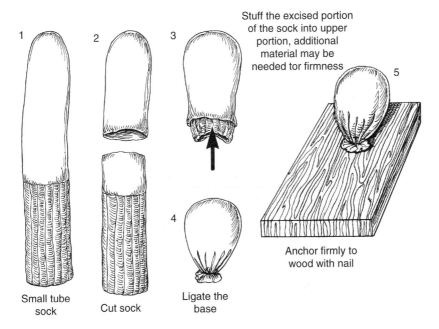

Figure 9.6.   Creating a uterine model from a sock.

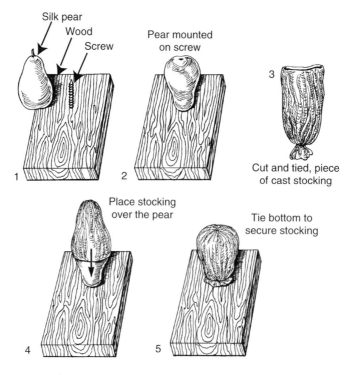

Figure 9.7. Creating a uterine model from a silk pear.

models require some modification. Placing a sheet of aluminum foil over the model, covering this with a thin layer of conducting gel, covered with a stocking, then coated with a thin layer of gel prior to attaching the adnexal structure, works well. Alternatively, the grounding clip can be attached directly to the adnexal portion of the model (Fig. 9.9).

Adnexal Structures

The choice of which material to use to construct the model for the tube, mesosalpinx, or ovary depends on the objective of the exercise. It is often beneficial to have ovarian models in place even when the primary exercise is intended for the tube, to make the exercise more practical and to maintain spatial orientations.

Tubal Models

The most versatile material to use to construct a variety of models to simulate normal tubes, mesosalpinx, and tubal pathology is the porcine uterine horn with the attached broad ligament. The first step is to obtain the specimen. The uterus should be harvested from a nulliparous feeder pig, preferably 150 to 200 lb in size. The uterine specimen can be obtained from local slaughter houses or ordered from larger companies. Usually two tubal models can be made from one uterine horn (Fig. 9.10). Portions of an umbilical cord can also be used for a tubal model with a piece of amnion for the mesosalpinx (Fig. 9.11). Other nontissue

Chapter 9: Learning Operative Endoscopy 145

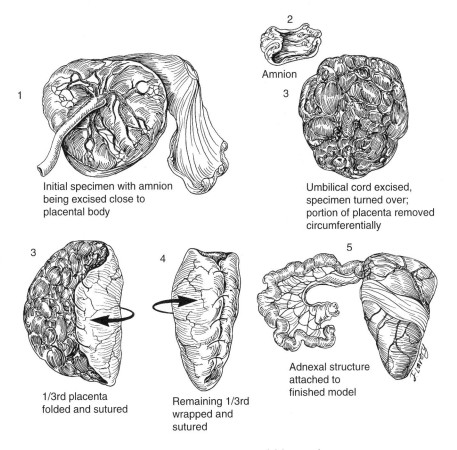

Figure 9.8. Creating a uterine model from a placenta.

models that can be used for tubal models are small rubber tubes, small Penrose drains, and fishing lure worms. These materials tend not to perform as well as the tissue models do, since they lack a mesosalpinx and are unable to conduct electricity.

Normal Tubes. These models are generally used for the demonstration of tubal ligation techniques. Tissue models perform the best. These models can demonstrate banding, clip, and electrosurgical techniques.

Tubal Ectopic Pregnancy (Fig. 9.12). This model is constructed from extirpated porcine uterine horns with the attached broad ligament to serve as the mesosalpinx. The simulated ectopic pregnancy can be made from several materials. Small pieces of fresh liver and pieces of placenta work extremely well. Ideally, at least two simulated ectopic pregnancies can be placed in each uterine horn, depending on the length of the uterine horn chosen. It is often advantageous to place a suture immediately proximal and distal to the ectopic pregnancy to stabilize its location. Nontissue materials, i.e., pieces of scrub sponge or cotton balls, can also be used to simulate the ectopic tissue.

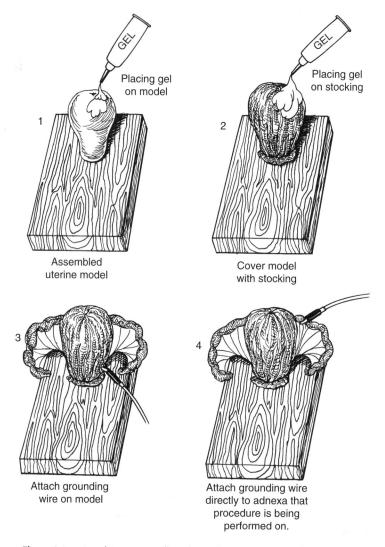

Figure 9.9. Attaching a grounding electrode to a uterine model.

Hydrosalpinx Model (Fig. 9.13). This model is constructed using the normal or ectopic tube model and attaching an extirpated gallbladder. The harvested gallbladder should be kept small. Alternatively, a previously opened hydrosalpinx can be simulated with a larger uterine horn. These models can be used to demonstrate suturing, laser, electrosurgical, or thermal techniques. (See Additional Exercises.)

Ovarian Models (Fig. 9.14)

Usually, the ovarian model will be added to the uterine model for structural relationship. This is easily accomplished by placing a small balloon within a balloon, and filling the inner balloon with water. The outer balloon can then be used for suturing the model to the surrounding structures.

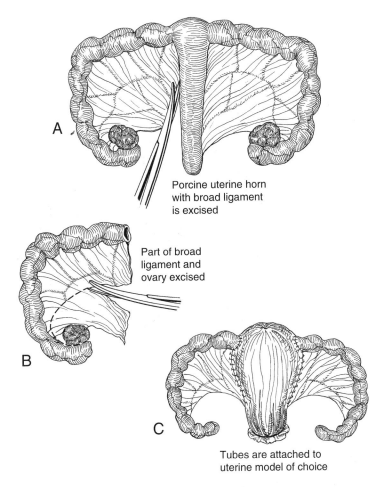

Figure 9.10. Creating a tubal model from a porcine uterus.

Extirpated gallbladders and small urinary bladders can also be used. These are useful in demonstrating vaporization or fulguration techniques, or when a cystic mass needs to be simulated for removal techniques (Fig. 9.15). (See Additional Exercises.)

Ovarian Cyst Model (Fig. 9.16). This model is constructed from an extirpated porcine gallbladder. When preparing this model, some of the liver should be left attached to the gallbladder. The gallbladder should be drained and irrigated, and then ligated prior to use. The model is then anchored to a towel with sutures or staples. The model is then placed in the pelvic trainer. Ground and clip can be attached directly to the model if necessary. This model can be used to demonstrate aspiration and dissection techniques. (See Additional Exercises.)

Adhesion Model (Fig. 9.17). Adhesions can be simulated by draping a piece of porcine or canine omentum over any of the prepared models. Chorion or amnion can also be used, but requires more preparation time.

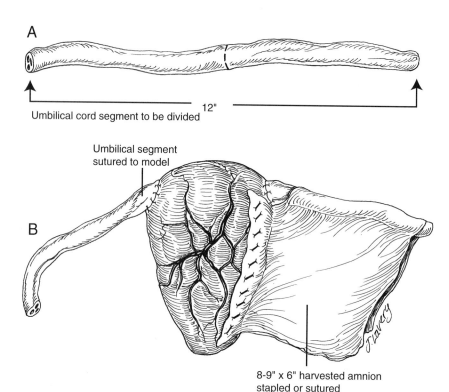

Figure 9.11. Creating a tubal model from an umbilical cord and amnion.

Suturing Models

Any of the previously described models can be used for a suturing model. These models offer the advantage of having a similar spatial relationship to the uterus as encountered during actual cases. To further develop the suturing skills, it is advantageous to be able to suture objects at different angles within the pelvic trainer. After developing these skills, it is easier to apply these techniques to structures other than the uterus if suturing is required.

Bladder Models (Fig. 9.18). An extirpated sow uterine bladder is an excellent model. The fat and surrounding connective tissue should be removed prior to using the model. The bladder is then placed on a towel or small platform to simulate its proximity to the anterior abdominal wall, and anchored loosely in place with sutures. An incision can be placed anywhere on the model. Single and two-layer closures can be demonstrated. After completion of the repair, water can be instilled through the urethra to check the integrity of the repair.

Bowel Model (Fig. 9.19). A small piece of extirpated porcine or canine small bowel can be used, but has a smaller diameter lumen and thinner wall than the human small bowel. An excellent model is a portion of a parous sow uterine horn. The midportion of the horn is loosely attached to a towel to simulate the

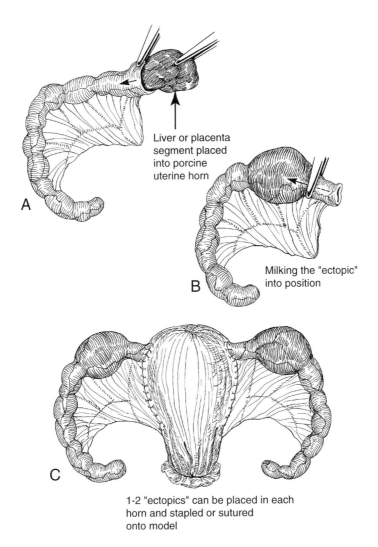

Figure 9.12. Creating an ectopic pregnancy model.

mesenteric attachment. The wall of the uterine horn is much thicker than that of the porcine or canine bowel, and is easier to grasp.

Ligature Models

Although knot tying can be demonstrated using the suture models, these models may be inadequate to demonstrate tying techniques under tension. Slippage of the endoscopic knots is always a concern during actual cases. To gain confidence of both knot security and knot tying ability, endoscopic knot tying should be practiced in the pelvic trainer while wearing surgical gloves.

Vessel Ligation Model (Fig. 9.20). Materials such as a Penrose drain, small caliber rubber tubing and umbilical cords can be used, but lack the characteristics

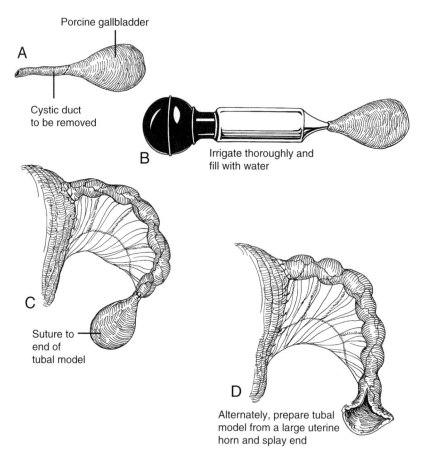

Figure 9.13. Creating a hydrosalpinx model.

of arterial venous bundles that are encountered during actual surgery. The best model is made from a small porcine uterine horn. Trimming the broad ligament from the surrounding specimen will prevent the uterine horn from coiling up when filled with water. Once filled, the model is loosely anchored to a towel or prepared uterine model. Knot security can easily be tested by cutting between two ligatures and observing for leakage.

Knot Tying Board (Fig. 9.21). To better demonstrate knot security under tension, the knot tying board is superior to the other models. As a model, it poorly simulates any direct surgical application, but can be used to practice both intra and extracorporeal knot tying techniques.

HYSTEROSCOPIC MODELS

There are basically two types of models needed to demonstrate hysteroscopic techniques: those for diagnostic hysteroscopy and those for operative hysteroscopy. The simplest models available to help familiarize and orient participants to basic hysteroscopy are fresh green peppers, melons, and other relatively

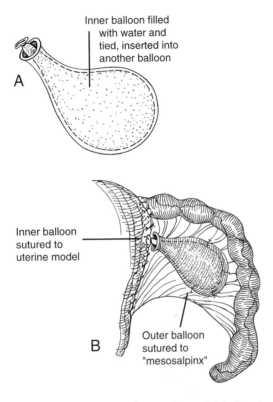

Figure 9.14. Formation of an ovarian model (balloon).

hollow vegetables. These models do not require any distension media. They help to demonstrate biopsy and cutting techniques using the operating channel. These are adequate to familiarize participants with basic instrumentation equipment assembly, but serve poorly as models to simulate an actual surgery.

Intrauterine Models

There are several models available that may be used to demonstrate intrauterine hysteroscopic techniques. It is advantageous to be familiar with all the models since none of them, by themselves, can optimally demonstrate all hysteroscopic techniques.

Sow Urinary Bladder (Fig. 9.22). Urinary bladders obtained from sows that are 300 to 350 lb perform the best. After removing all the surrounding connective tissue, the ureter should be identified and ligated. Urinary bladders are remarkably distensible. The bladder needs to be wrapped in an occlusive material. Aluminum foil works well and can easily be grounded to demonstrate electrosurgical techniques. The urethra should be left approximately six inches long. It is usually necessary to clamp the urethral opening to obtain a watertight seal. This model performs well with continuous flow systems and should be used with a nonelectrolytic solution. Ordinary tap water can be used but if the mineral con-

152 GYNECOLOGIC ENDOSCOPY: Principles in Practice

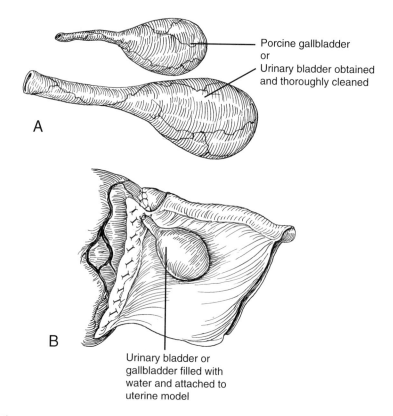

Figure 9.15. Formation of an ovarian model (porcine urinary bladder or gallbladder).

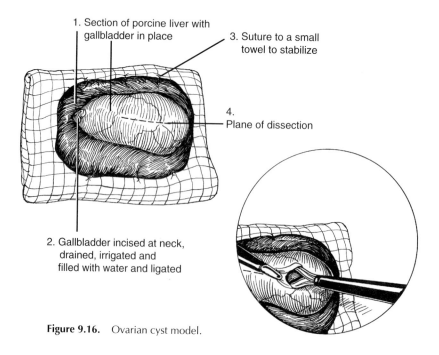

Figure 9.16. Ovarian cyst model.

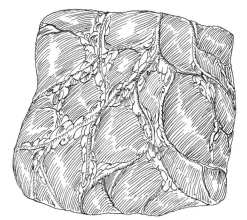

1. Obtain piece of omentum, either porcine or canine.

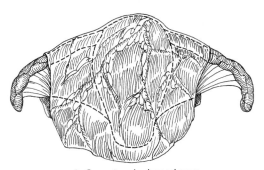

2. Omentum is draped over uterine model

Figure 9.17. Adhesion model.

tent is high, power settings of 150 to 200 watts may be required in order to demonstrate a tissue effect. Diagnostic, biopsy, and sharp dissection techniques can be easily demonstrated. Small intrauterine lesions can be simulated by placing sutures through the wall of the bladder and removing them hysteroscopically.

An intrauterine myoma can be constructed by placing a piece of smoked beef tongue, raw beef or porcine tongue, or piece of boiled beef testicle inside the urinary bladder (Fig. 9.23). Since resectoscopic techniques often generate a noticeable amount of heat within the tissue, the myoma should be anchored in place with a silk or nylon suture. Care should be taken to keep the model a reasonable size to allow enough room to manipulate the hysteroscope within the cavity.

The major drawback of the sow bladder as an endometrial model is that it perforates easily and does not demonstrate the tissue effects of the various energy sources well. In this aspect, this model is less desirable for demonstrating the Nd:YAG laser. An extirpated bovine uterus has a thick wall and can be used to demonstrate these laser techniques. To a degree, this is also true in demonstrating endometrial ablation with this model. It offers the advantage of simulating the necessary equipment instrument assembly, and spatial orientation as re-

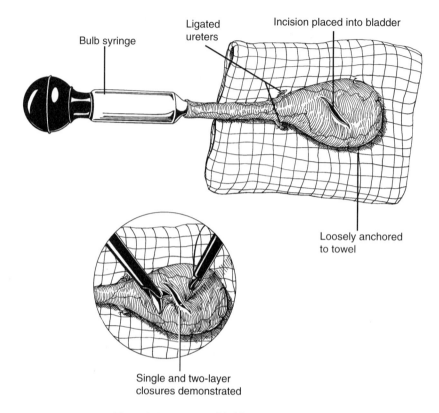

Figure 9.18. Urinary bladder suturing model.

quired to perform an actual endometrial ablation with resectoscope but does not demonstrate the relative tissue effects of the various power settings. This is better demonstrated using fresh meat or fresh liver in a resectoscope box.

Resectoscope Box (Fig. 9.24). This model is easily assembled. A nonelectrolytic solution should be used. As noted previously, tap water can also be used, but markedly higher than expected energy settings may be required, depending on the mineral content of the water. Nonelectrolytic solutions, i.e., glycine, sorbitol, or mannitol, can be used. These will add a considerable expense to the workshop. Even if these solutions are used, higher energy settings are usually required depending on the conductivity of the tissue chosen.

The advantages of this model are ease in assembly and cleanup. The tissue can be easily changed. This is an excellent tool to demonstrate the different tissue effects that are produced with various energy and waveform settings. It simulates the actual surgical procedure poorly since the surface area is fixed and a continuous flow system is not required. Resection techniques can also be demonstrated. Materials such as raw potatoes and flat squash are a better choice for demonstrating these techniques, since their consistency is more similar to myomata than are materials such as fresh liver or red meat (Fig. 9.25).

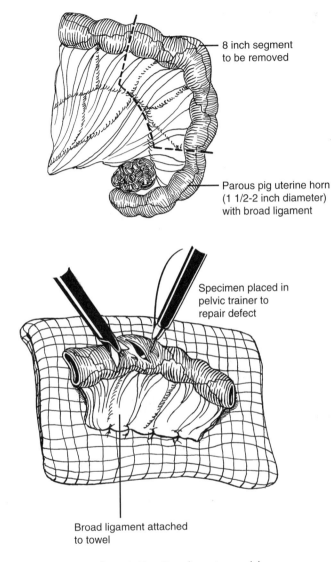

Figure 9.19. Bowel suturing model.

LIVE ANIMAL MODELS

The female pig is the most commonly used animal model since it is readily available and relatively inexpensive. Other animal models can be used (Table 9.3).

The female pig should weigh 60 to 80 pounds. It is preferable to wash the animal prior to the workshop to reduce the odor and risk of disease transmission. If possible, feeding the animal a clear liquid diet for the day prior to surgery is also useful. Other animal models have been used, i.e., goat, dog, and sheep, but the most familiarity is with the porcine model. Intravenous sedation with intubation is usually sufficient.

Table 9.3. Approved Anesthetic Options

Species	Anesthetic Option 1	Anesthetic Option 2	Anesthetic Option 3	Anesthetic Option 4
DOG	Acepromazine (0.05 mg/kg IM) Glycopyrrolate (0.01 mg/kg IM) Thiamylal sodium 2.0% IV slowly to effect	Acepromazine (0.05 mg/kg IM) Butorphanol (0.4 mg/kg IM) Glycopyrrolate (0.01 mg/kg IM) Thiamylal sodium 2.0% IV slowly to effect		
PIG	Telazol (5 mg/kg IM) Xylazine (2 mg/kg IM)	Telazol (5 mg/kg IM) Xylazine (2 mg/kg IM) and Atropine (0.05 mg/kg IM)	Acepromazine (1.1 mg/kg IM) Atropine (0.05 mg/kg IM) Ketamine (20 mg/kg IM) Xylazine (2 mg/kg IM)	Telazol (4 mg/kg IM) Xylazine (4 mg/kg IM) and Glycopyrrolate (0.01 mg/kg IM)
SHEEP, GOAT	Atropine (.02 mg/kg IM) Ketamine (11 mg/kg IM) and Xylazine (.022 mg/kg IM)	Mix 500 ml of 5% guaifenesin with 500 mg ketamine. Give 1.1–2.2 mg/kg IV of this mixture		

APPROVED ANALGESICS

Species	Analgesic	Analgesic	Analgesic
DOG	Butorphanol (0.1–0.2 mg/kg, SQ or IM)	Demerol (10 mg/kg IM q 8 h)	Buprenex (0.01–0.02 mg/kg IM, SQ or IV q 12 h)
PIGS, SHEEP, GOATS	Buprenex (0.005–.01 mg/kg IM q 12 h)		

Live animal models should be used to demonstrate different laparoscopic techniques rather than teaching a particular procedure. The animal model is extremely useful in the demonstration of hemostatic techniques with both electrosurgical instruments and the automatic stapling devices. The live animal is also useful in servicing participants in the use of new instrumentation or new energy modalities. These labs usually are very time-consuming, and generally it is more productive to introduce a live animal lab session after several sessions on the pelvic trainer. The number of participants per animal should be kept small, three or four at the most, with two being ideal. The beginner should set up all the video equipment and instrumentation to increase their familiarity and confidence with the equipment. Consolidation of the endoscopic instrumentation and equipment will reduce the time required to set up and disassemble the workshop. A checklist of the basic equipment and instruments that are required for live animal laboratories is shown in Table 9.4.

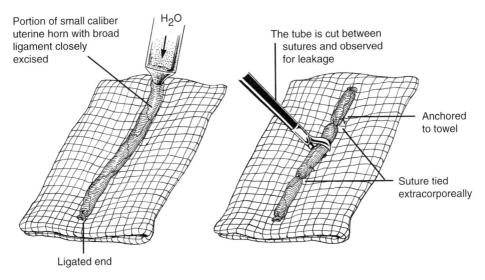

Figure 9.20. Vessel ligature model.

Potential Problems. Often the electrical plugs on the video and electrical generators, if the same as used in the OR, have different configurations than what is available in some animal labs; converters may be required. Once the laparoscopic ports have been placed, it is helpful to suture them in place. The pig abdominal wall is very thin and the ports dislodge easily. Care should be taken not to overinsufflate; the development of subcutaneous emphysema can become a problem, and interfere with completion of the necessary learning exercise.

Emphasis should be placed on both performance of the exercises in an efficient manner but also in troubleshooting equipment problems (Table 9.5). Special modalities, i.e., laser, endocoagulator or argon beam coagulator, may also be used but tend to greatly increase lab time.

ADDITIONAL EXERCISES

In addition to the exercises described within each of the applicable chapters, the following are examples of exercises that utilize the previously described models.

Hydrosalpinx Model (Fig. 9.26). There are several techniques available to perform a neosalpingostomy that can be demonstrated on this model. The prepared model can be attached to a uterus or loosely anchored to a towel. The most important aspect of this exercise is to have the model mobile. The ease in performing a neosalpingostomy depends largely on the positioning of the tube in reference to the placement of the ports. Any of the described techniques, suture, laser, or endothermal, can be shown on this model. Suturing techniques are more easily demonstrated on the "splayed tube" model than the gallbladder model.

Ovarian Cyst Model. (Reduction of cyst spillage.) Several techniques are available to reduce the spillage at the time of cyst rupture. Intraperitoneal tech-

Table 9.4. Basic Equipment for Live Animal Laboratory

Video monitoring camera.
10-mm straight laparoscope.
Light source.
Rapid insufflator, at least 6 liters per minute.
Suction/irrigator system and tubing.
Irrigation and fluid (usually tap water in refillable 3-liter bags).
Electrical generator and grounding pad.
Disposable trocars and sleeves with reducers—usually reuse these for several labs.
Scalpel, hemostats, forceps, scissors, heavy suture material, sponges, towels.

Laparoscopic Instrumentation:
(2) 5-mm graspers.
(1) 5-mm scissors.
(1) 5-mm traumatic grasper for tissue removal.
(1) 5-mm atraumatic grasper.
(2) 5-mm self-retaining spring-handled graspers.
(2) 5-mm dissectors.
(1) 10-mm spoon forceps.
(1) 1-mm–5-mm reducing sleeve.
(1) 5–4-mm reducing sleeve.
(1) 5-mm needle driver.
(1) Unipolar needle or knife and cord.
(1) Unipolar ball tip probe.
Endoscopic stapler or other available automatic devices.
Suture and needles suitable for laparoscopic suturing.
Pretied endoloop systems.

Table 9.5. Suggested Exercises for the Live Pig Model

Review of pig anatomy.
Partial salpingectomy.
Dissection and ligation of ureters.
Removal of urinary bladder using linear stapler/cutter.
Mock "appendectomy" utilizing small bowel.
Ligation of external iliac artery and/or vein with extracorporeal ligature techniques.
Simulated abdominal wall injury and repair.

niques basically utilize aspirating devices, while extraperitoneal techniques generally utilize endoscopic pouches or bags.

Aspirating Devices and Techniques (Fig. 9.27)

1. Choose a large gallbladder or thin-walled urinary bladder for the ovarian cyst model and assemble it onto the uterine model. It can be anchored only at the ovarian ligament, or an infundibulopelvic ligament can also be fashioned.

Chapter 9: Learning Operative Endoscopy 159

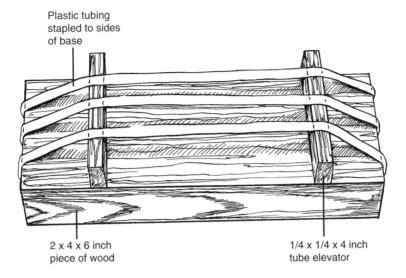

Figure 9.21. Knot tying board assembly.

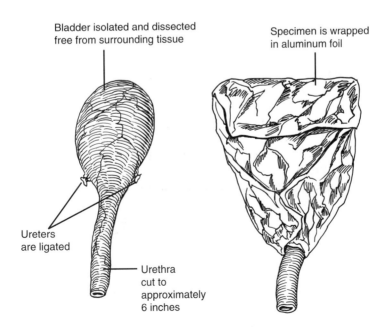

Figure 9.22. Intrauterine model (sow urinary bladder).

160 GYNECOLOGIC ENDOSCOPY: Principles in Practice

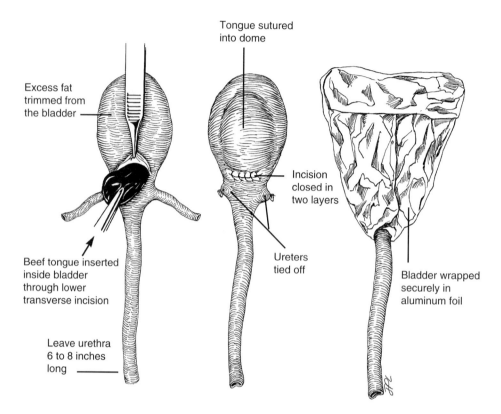

Figure 9.23. Intrauterine myoma model (sow urinary bladder).

2. The exercises can be performed before or after freeing the cyst from its attachments.
3. Place a pretied loop on the surface of the cyst.
4. Position a grasper within the loop on the surface of the cyst to stabilize the cyst wall.
5. Introduce an aspirating needle and puncture the cyst wall.
6. As the fluid is being aspirated and the cyst is collapsing, grasp the wall in close proximity to the puncture and elevate it slightly, to help reduce the amount of spillage.
7. After all the material is aspirated, remove the needle while elevating the cyst wall and puncture site.
8. Close the pretied suture, thus sealing the puncture site.
9. Sever the attachment if not previously done, and proceed to the morcellation exercises.

NOTE: The same exercise can be done utilizing a Topel aspirating needle (Cook). Omit the grasper portion of the exercise in this case.

Endoscopic pouches or bags (Figs. 9.28, 9.29). There are several products on the market that are packaged preloaded in an introducing sleeve. This exercise

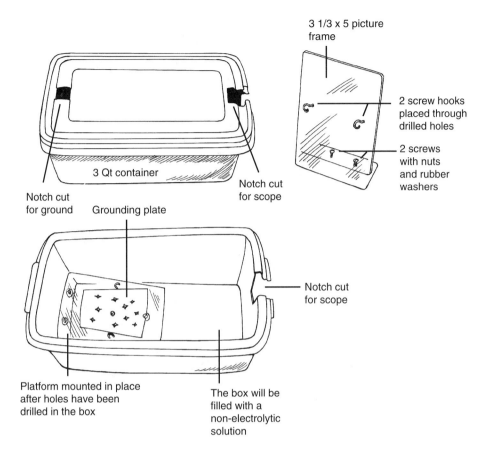

Figure 9.24. Resectoscope box.

will describe the use of a bag made from a surgical glove. For this exercise the cyst must be totally free from its attachments.

1. Take a size 5 or 6 surgical glove and cut off the upper portion.
2. Doubly ligate the distal portion with silk or other braided suture.
3. Backload the "bag" into 10- or 11-mm sleeve, leaving a small portion exposed.
4. Introduce the sleeve into the trainer.
5. Remove the bag from the sleeve by pulling it with a second grasper, not pushing it through the sleeve.
6. Position the bag beneath the center port.
7. Place a grasper through the center of the port and grasp the cyst.
8. Elevate the cyst.
9. Place the cyst within the bag, using the grasper through the lateral ports.
10. Once the cyst is within the bag, draw the bag opening into the sleeve with a twisting motion.
11. Exteriorize the bag opening by withdrawing the sleeve while grasping the bag opening with the grasper.

162 GYNECOLOGIC ENDOSCOPY: Principles in Practice

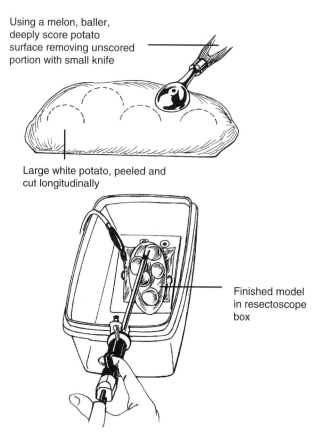

Figure 9.25. Myoma model (raw potato).

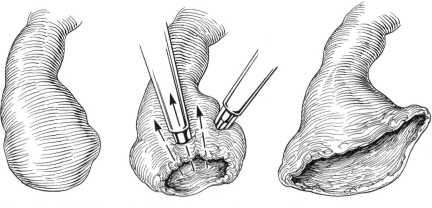

Neosalpingostomy by Bruhat technique is best demonstrated with a large uterine horn that has been splayed open. This can be done with an endothermal probe or CO_2 laser.

As the heat is applied to the area just proximal to the end of the tube, the probe is swept proximally to cause the open end to "Flower" out.

Only enough heat is applied to dehydrate and shrink the tissue, this should be done without caronixation of the tissue.

Figure 9.26. Cuff salpingostomy (Bruhat technique).

Chapter 9: Learning Operative Endoscopy   163

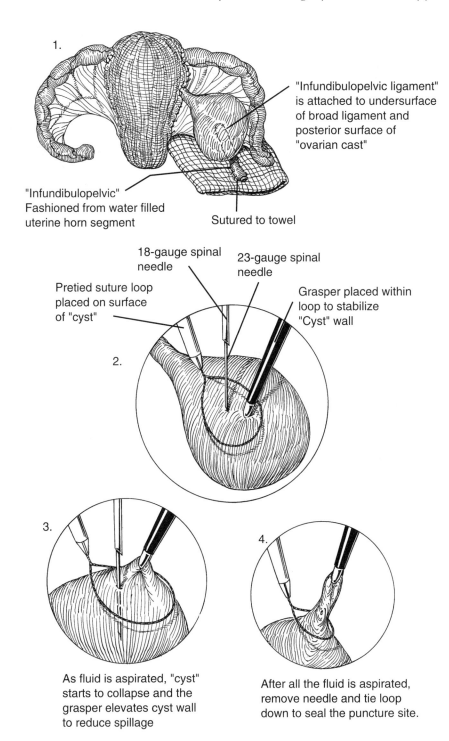

Figure 9.27.   Technique to reduce spill during an aspiration of an ovarian cyst.

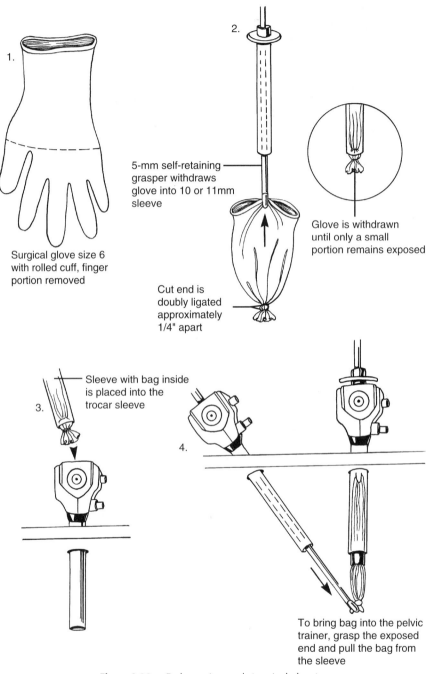

Figure 9.28. Endoscopic pouch (surgical glove).

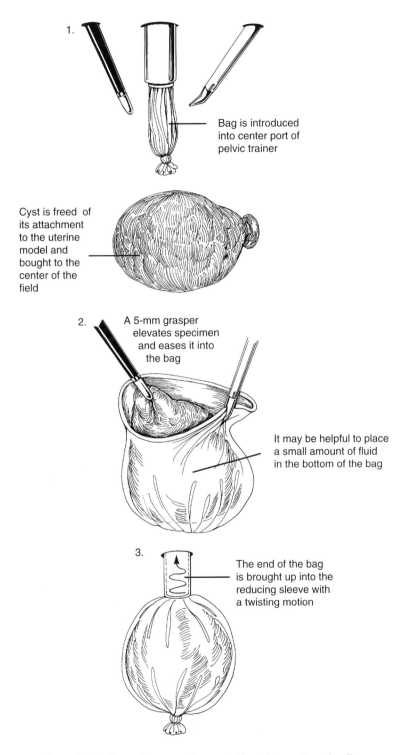

Figure 9.29. Removing an ovarian cyst without intraperitoneal spillage.

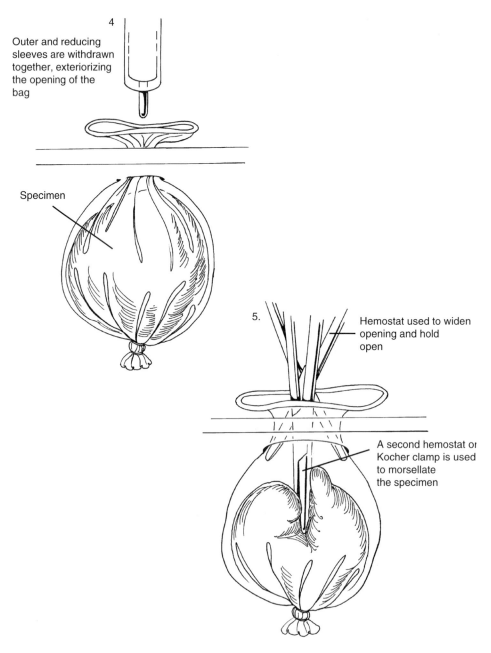

Figure 9.29. (continued)

12. Hold the bag open with a hemostat and aspirate the cyst contents while viewing the portion of the bag that remains within the trainer, to detect any spillage. Alternatively, the cyst can be ruptured with a scissors and the contents subsequently suctioned from the field.
13. After the cyst is emptied of its contents, the contents can be morcellated.

Morcellation of Tissue

These techniques can be applied as an extension of the previous exercise or designed as a separate exercise. If applied to an ovarian cyst, the morcellation exercise is generally carried out within the endoscopic bag after the opening has been exteriorized. The tissue is grasped and cut into pieces that can be removed with the hemostat or a Kocher clamp. This is a tedious technique, but closely simulates what occurs during an actual case.

Intraperitoneal Morcellation. These techniques apply to a more solid structure. Removal of large amounts of solid tissue through a 10- to 12-mm port is often time-consuming and frustrating. The exercise is designed to simulate morcellation only.

Choose a piece of tissue that is at least 3 cm × 3 cm × 3 cm in dimensions. Fibrous, dense tissue such as an empty sow urinary bladder demonstrates the "orange peel" technique, whereas a raw beef or porcine tongue is best used to demonstrate the use of a morcellator.

Orange Peel Technique (Fig. 9.30)

1. Place a 10- to 11-mm port centrally and a 5-mm port laterally.
2. Grasp the tissue with a 10-mm spoon forceps and pull it firmly against the sleeve.
3. Using a 5-mm hook scissors, start cutting the tissue proximal to the sleeve.
4. Rotate the specimen as it is being cut and continue to draw the specimen through the sleeve until it is completely removed.

Morcellator (Fig. 9.31)

1. Place a 10-mm port centrally and two 5-mm ports laterally.
2. Using self-retaining, traumatic grasper, grasp the tissue at its distal ends.
3. Morcellate the tissue until it is completely removed.

Knot Tying

These exercises are designed to improve the participant's confidence in tying sutures under tension and intracorporeal knot tying techniques.

Extracorporeal Knot Tying (Fig. 9.32)

This exercise should be done with a braided and a monofilament suture, using a slip knot and an overhand knot.

1. Place the knot tying board at the bottom of the pelvic trainer.
2. Place two 5-mm ports in each of the lateral sites.
3. Introduce the suture and pass it under all three of the bands, and back out of the pelvic trainer.
4. Tie the knot extracorporeally and observe for slippage.

168 GYNECOLOGIC ENDOSCOPY: Principles in Practice

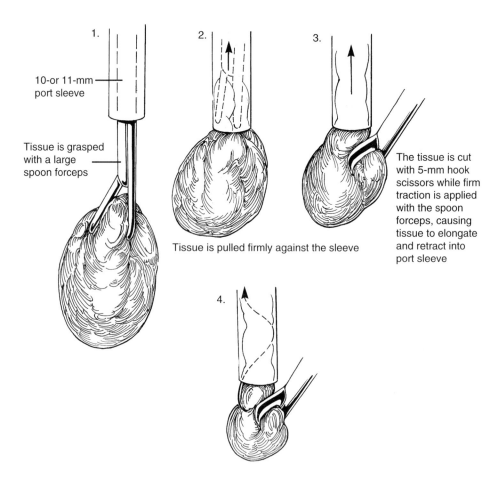

Figure 9.30. Morcellation of tissue (orange peel technique).

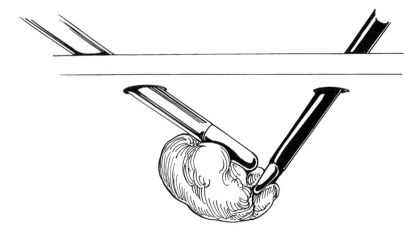

Figure 9.31. Morcellation of tissue (morcellator).

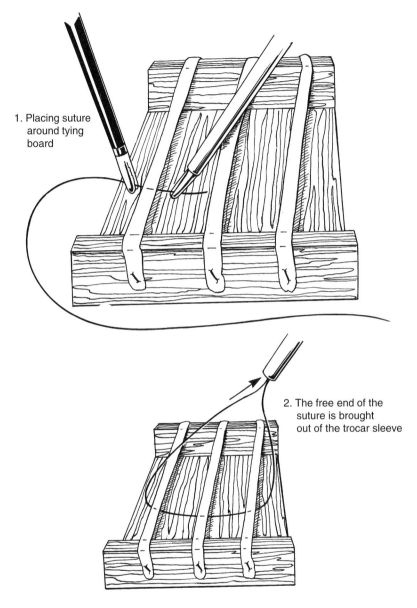

Figure 9.32. Extracorporeal knot tying—overhand knot.

Intracorporeal Knot Tying (Fig. 9.33)

Twist Technique. This exercise will emphasize accuracy and gentle tissue handling. It requires a hydrosalpinx model, one 3-mm needle driver, one 5-mm grasper, and 5-0 monofilament suture with a small, curved cutting needle cut to approximately 7-inch length.

170 GYNECOLOGIC ENDOSCOPY: Principles in Practice

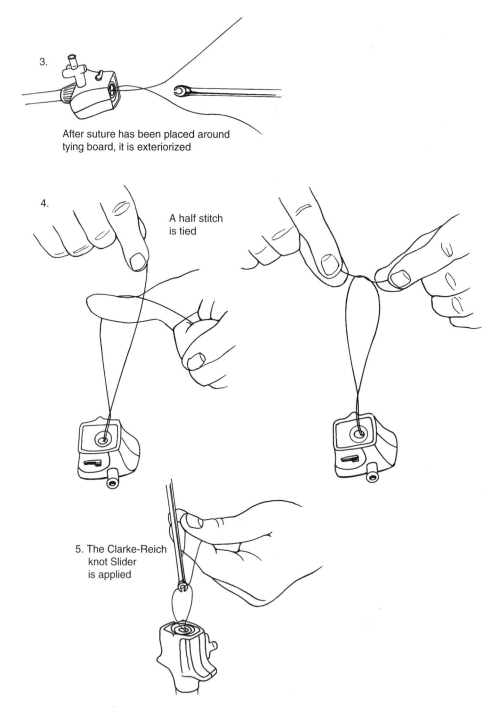

3. After suture has been placed around tying board, it is exteriorized

4. A half stitch is tied

5. The Clarke-Reich knot Slider is applied

Figure 9.32. (continued)

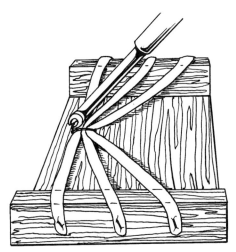

6. Using a knot, the knot is tied into place

Figure 9.32. (continued)

1. Place the assembled hydrosalpinx model in the bottom of the pelvic trainer.
2. Open the end of the hydrosalpinx by using any modality.
3. Stabilize the tissue with the grasper and place the initial stitch.
4. Gently pull the suture through the tissue.
5. Place the second stitch.
6. Grasp the suture proximal to the needle, cut the suture, and remove the needle.
7. Grasp the end of the suture with the 3-mm driver.
8. Place the 5-mm grasper against the 3-mm needle holder while placing tension on the suture.
9. Rotate the needle driver clockwise three times causing the suture to wrap around the shaft.
10. Grasp the end of the suture with the grasper and remove it from the tip of the needle driver.
11. Advance needle driver and grasp the opposite end of the suture.
12. Draw the needle back through the formed loops while placing slightly downward traction with the grasper.
13. Once both ends of the suture are free, tighten the knot by pulling the needle driver and grasper in opposite direction laterally.
14. Repeat the maneuver rotating the needle driver in the counterclockwise direction.

INSTRUMENTS FOR ENDOSCOPY

Over the last twenty years, the major advances in endoscopy have declined as a result of improved instrumentation and technically advanced equipment. Whether it was the procedures that forced equipment advancements or whether

172 GYNECOLOGIC ENDOSCOPY: Principles in Practice

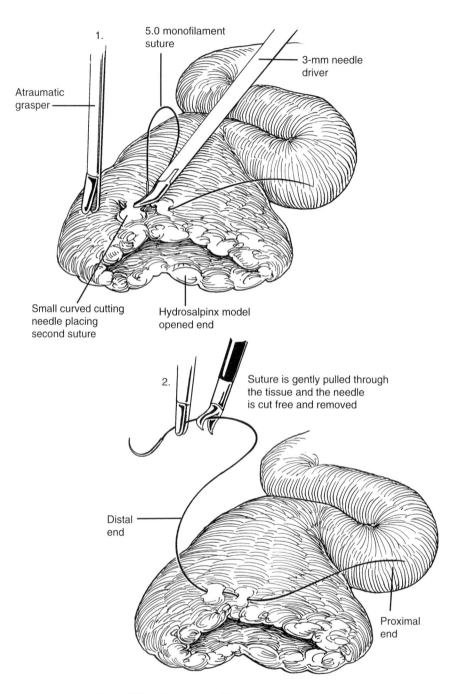

Figure 9.33. Intracorporeal knot tying—twist technique.

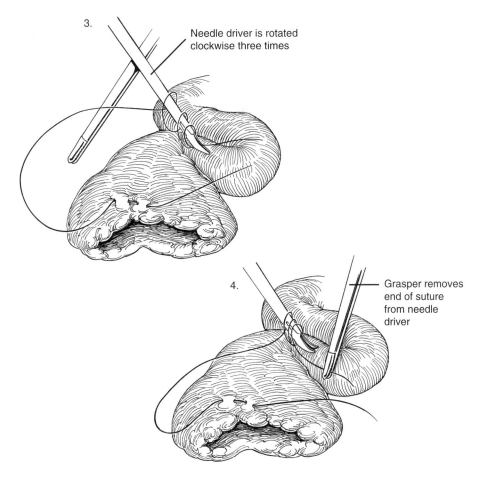

Figure 9.33. (continued)

it was the equipment availability that allowed the development of advanced procedures, is debatable. The reality is that marked changes have taken place in equipment design and availability. A selection of operating instruments should be available in the operating suite at all times during any laparoscopic procedure. Each surgeon will develop his/her preference for particular instruments. This preference will be somewhat dependent on the type and frequency of procedures preformed.

Gas and Light Source

In order to visualize the intraabdominal contents, a pneumoperitoneum must be established. Although gasless laparoscopic systems have been designed, they are not widely used and are currently expensive. Insufflation equipment should be capable of measuring intraabdominal pressure with an automatic gas cutoff at a preset value. Most surgeons prefer to use an insufflator that can deliver gas at variable rates ranging from 1 to 10 liters per minute, although insufflators are available that can deliver up to 14 liters per minute. Insufflators that

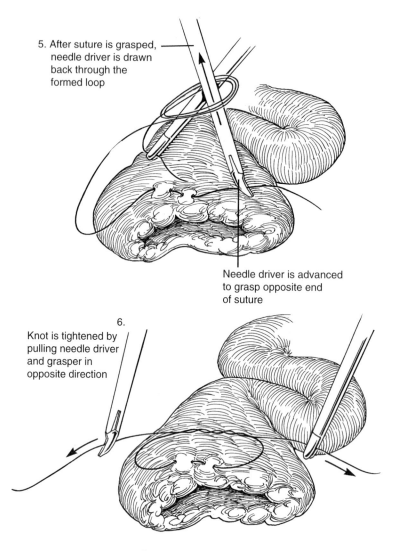

Figure 9.33. (continued)

are pressure-controlled using microprocessors are desirable for operative endoscopy. In addition, insufflation systems have been developed that will deliver gas and are also capable of smoke evacuation using a continuous recycling process. These systems are most applicable to CO_2 laser use.

Most insufflators have four gauges. The first indicates gas pressure in the major tank, the second records gas volume within the internal tank, the third indicates flow pressure (pressure within the system during insufflation), and the fourth indicates the flow rate. Insufflation tubing should have a secure attachment to the insufflator to prevent it from being dislodged during high flow rates, and should also have an inline filter. Since overinsufflation is an avoidable complication, the system's automatic shutoff mechanism should be periodically checked to ensure its accuracy. This is easily accomplished by totally occluding the insufflation tubing and examining the flow rate and the pressure gauges. The flow rate should go to zero and the intraabdominal pressure should rise markedly. Some systems are equipped with an audio alarm that sounds whenever the preset intraabdominal pressure is exceeded.

The 150-watt light sources have been replaced by xenon and halogen light sources. Xenon light sources are the most commonly used and are very reliable. The current light sources used are interfaced with the camera and allow for continuous automatic adjustment of the light intensity to reduce the amount of glare when working closely to the tissue. Light transmission has improved with the development of more efficient cables. As the number of fibers within the cable increases, so does the amount of light transmitted. Most cables can be used with several brands of light sources and laparoscopes if the necessary adapters are available. If using light sources, laparoscopes, and light cables from different manufacturers, it is best to confirm all are compatible prior to starting a case. There are also liquid light cables available. These offer the advantage of more efficient light transmission and can increase the amount of transmitted light up to 40%. Unfortunately, they have the disadvantage of an increased cost and decreased availability. They are markedly less flexible and have an increased amount of heat transmission, making them more of a potential fire hazard if the unprotected end is left unattended.

Regardless of the type of light cable used, illumination power is reduced at each junction in the system. For example, the addition of beam splitters offsets laparoscopes or angled laparoscopes; all can potentially reduce the quality of the image seen on the video monitor. Light transmission decreases as the light bundles are broken. This emphasizes the importance of careful handling of the cables, and avoiding bending and heat sterilization of the cables.

Electrosurgical Generator

The chosen electrosurgical generator should be capable of delivering both modulated and unmodulated unipolar currents, as well as bipolar applications. These waveforms have specific applications for various surgical techniques used in operative endoscopy. Of paramount importance is that the generator is compatible with the available instrumentation. The number of electrical cables needed should be kept at a minimum and readily available.

Telescopes

A variety of telescopes are available and range in size from 5 to 12 mm. The most common scope used is the 10-mm zero degree diagnostic telescope, which produces an excellent picture. Operating and laser laparoscopes have an additional port for placement of a variety of grasping and cutting instruments and are by necessity larger in caliber than those used for visualization only. Angled scopes are useful for visualizing the anterior abdominal wall during hernia repairs, but are not generally required for operative pelvic laparoscopy. Operating scopes are also available with either angled or parallel eyepieces.

Telescope warmers are available to decrease fogging of the lens. These warmers are electrical units that are controlled with a thermostat. Other solutions are available to reduce lens fogging and are generally just as useful.

Video

The single most important piece of equipment required for a successful operative laparoscopy is the camera. A high quality camera with video system is essential if one is to perform any type of operative endoscopic procedure. While some surgeons prefer using a beam splitter, the use of the beam splitter reduces light transmission and decreases the quality of the picture obtained. The use of at least two video monitors allows for a clear access for viewing for everyone during the procedure. Monitor placement is somewhat operator-dependent, but most gynecologic surgeons prefer to have these positioned caudad to maintain a similar orientation as encountered at laparotomy. Placing the video monitors on rolling stands so that they can be easily moved is also advantageous. However, wall or ceiling mounting is also available and can be just as convenient.

Uterine Cannula

A uterine cannula is used to facilitate most gynecologic laparoscopies, including all sterilization procedures. The purpose of the cannula is to manipulate the uterus and facilitate visualization of and access to the pelvic structures. Most cannulas also permit injection of a dye solution (chromopertubation), to assess tubal patency. Various types of cannulas and uterine manipulating devices are available. A cannula should not be used if the uterus is absent, anomalies exist which prevent exposure or access to the cervix, the patient is a prepubescent female, an intrauterine pregnancy is suspected, or the procedure planned includes oocyte recovery. The type of cannula chosen depends upon the type of procedure anticipated. The majority of reusable cannulas only reach into the intrauterine cavity as far as the lower uterine segment. For a normal size uterus, this is generally adequate for most procedures. If the uterus is enlarged, a cannula that reaches to the fundus is usually necessary to give the best exposure. The appropriate intrauterine cannula should carefully be chosen to meet the needs of the case. Despite the variety of devices available, all carry the risk of perforation and postoperative endometritis. Risk of a difficult insertion should always be weighed against the potential benefits.

Pneumoperitoneum Needles

Various types of pneumoperitoneum needles are available. The most frequently used is the Veress needle. Most of the pneumoperitoneum needles have an outer needle with a sharp beveled edge, combined with an inner, spring-loaded retractable blunt shaft that extends beyond the end of the needle. As the peritoneum is penetrated, the blunt shaft protrudes beyond the sharp needle. Although designed as a safety feature, the protective shaft will not prevent perforation of bowel or major vessels.

Trocars

Laparoscopic trocars are available in both reusable and disposable types, and in various diameters ranging from 3 to 12 mm to accommodate laparoscopes and instrumentation of all sizes. To date, no studies have shown that the reusable trocars with "safety shields" are safer and decrease the number of bowel or vascular injuries. Trocar tips may be either conical or pyramidal. The type chosen is generally based on the surgeon's preference, as no advantages to either type have been demonstrated. Most trocars are constructed with a hollow channel having openings at the tip as well as the top of the instrument. This permits a rush of gas to occur when the peritoneal cavity is penetrated by the trocar. When this occurs the instrument does not need to be passed farther into the abdomen. Whether to use insulated or metal sleeves is usually not an issue unless unipolar instrumentation is being used. In this case, metal sleeves offer additional safety (see Chapter 10).

Accessory Instruments

Hundreds of instruments have been developed for grasping, cutting, and placing traction on tissue and structures within the abdominal cavity. Instruments are available for biopsy and morcellation of tissue, along with atraumatic forceps, which do not crush or destroy tissue. Suction/irrigation instruments can be used for aquadissection and development of tissue planes. A new generation of instruments are available, which combine electrosurgery with cutting so that the tissue is desiccated and then cut. The design is very similar to stapling instruments that place rows of staples on either side of a structure and then ligate and divide the tissue with only one instrument placement. Other forms of stapling include individual staples, which can be used to occlude vessels or remove lymphatic tissue. The number and types of instruments that should be available depend entirely upon the anticipated procedure. A basic set of instruments that will allow the performance of most operative laparoscopic cases should always be available. Specialty instruments can be separately wrapped and available at request. In any department in which there are several endoscopic surgeons, it is best to have some uniformity in the types of basic instruments available. This will decrease confusion and subsequent frustration during cases. Equally important, the operating room personnel should be aware of what instrumentation is available and where it is located. It is often convenient to keep peel-packed individual instruments, replacement trocars, gaskets, staplers, etc. in a rolling tool cart that can be brought into the operating room. All too often, the request for additional instrumentation is answered with a flurry of instrument trays being opened in search of the requested instrumentation.

REFERENCES

1. Smith DC, Donahue LR, Waszak SJ. A hospital review of advanced gynecologic endoscopic procedures. Am J Obstet Gynecol 1994;170:1635–1642.
2. Pitkin RM. Operative laparoscopy: surgical advance or technical gimmick? Obstet Gynecol 1992:79:441–442.
3. Keye WR. Hitting a moving target: credentialing the endoscopic surgeon. Fert Steril 1994;62:1115–1117.
4. See WA, Cooper CS, Fisher RJ. Predictors of laparoscopic complications after formal training in laparoscopic surgery. JAMA 1993;270:2689–2725.
5. The American Fertility Society. Guidelines for attaining privileges in gynecologic operative endoscopy. Fert Steril 1994;62:1118–1119.

Chapter 10

Principles of Electrosurgery During Endoscopy

Richard M. Soderstrom

Despite the fact that electrophysics and its application to surgery, in particular endoscopic surgery, is a discrete science, there is little attention paid to its applied principles when surgeons receive their formal training in the technical aspects of surgery. Most training programs consider the discipline of electrosurgery as a skill that is left to the "hands on" exposure of the student, and the skills and knowledge of the average professor have been awarded through a "grandfather" process of credentials. As a result, many myths have been perpetuated over the past decades since William Bovie introduced the first electrosurgical diathermy machine using high-frequency radio waves instead of heated instruments (cautery) to destroy human tissue. Today's electrogenerators have become finely tuned instruments that offer many versatile variables for the contemporary surgeon to harness and deliver in either a discrete or broad manner to tissue to obtain a desired effect and outcome.

In the United States, gynecologic endoscopy has become one of the most common surgical procedures performed by specialists in the field. In the early 1970s, electrosurgery was the main energy source used in laparoscopy, and with great success, though at that time the majority of procedures performed were sterilizations and lysis of simple adhesions. Reports of bowel injuries, presumed to be secondary to "sparking" of monopolar energy, prompted several investigators to develop bipolar instruments, claiming these tools would reduce the bowel injuries caused by the monopolar technique. By 1980, bipolar electrosurgery had caught the fancy of the majority of endoscopic surgeons. At the same time, laser instruments designed for endoscopic procedures became available and laser endoscopy postgraduate courses were commonplace, leaving electrosurgery as a "backup" method.

Near the end of that decade, the general surgical specialty recognized the advantages of intraabdominal endoscopic surgery, especially the laparoscopic cholecystectomy, but quickly became frustrated by several limitations of contemporary lasers, returning to the electrosurgical generators for more versatility and power. The manufacturers responded quickly with solid state generators designed specifically for endoscopic use. Throughout these past two decades, the same surgical injuries attributed to monopolar energy have persisted, and no study known to this author has shown a reduction in laparoscopic injuries, especially bowel injuries, by the change to bipolar or laser technology. Each energy source capable of destroying tissue can, in specific circumstances, lead to a surgical complication which may be unique to that energy source; but one must not forget that a watt, is a watt, is a watt; when the output of energy of any source is matched for power density, power output in wattage, and the same amount of time (joules), the same tissue injury effect will occur.

I will address the issue of electrosurgery with some attention to unique characteristics and precautions when using electrosurgical techniques. A review of current literature reveals a paucity of meaningful information about electrosurgical accidents in endoscopy; most comments made are reflections of concepts addressed several decades ago. If we can assume that electrosurgical accidents are occurring, we need to address whether this is the result of the physics of electrosurgery or the method of application. To address these questions, a thorough understanding of the basic physics of electricity should be in hand. The following is meant to set such a stage.

BASIC ELECTRICITY

Electrons are particles of energy that, when pushed (or passed) through human tissue, create heat and sometimes destruction. *Voltage* is the pressure force required to push electrons. The standard unit of measure of this "electrical" pressure is 1 *volt*. Thus, if we draw the analogy of electricity to water, an electron would be analogous to a molecule of water, and voltage would be analogous to water pressure.

Whereas volume of water may be measured in cubic centimeters, the volume of electrons is measured in *coulombs*. If we push a volume of water through a conduit at a given pressure over a specific period, we create *current*. In electricity, current (measured in *amperes* or coulombs per second) means the passage of a given quantity of electrons through an area at a measured rate. With either water or electricity, as resistance increases, the flow of current decreases (given constant pressure or voltage). The difficulty of pushing the electrons through tissue or other material can be defined as *impedance* (resistance), measured in *ohms*.

As a last definition, electrical power (*watts*) is the energy produced, and energy delivered over time (quantity) is measured in *joules* (Table 10.1). The electrical power may be defined as pressure × current, or volts × current, or volts × electron flow per second.

BIOLOGICAL BEHAVIOR OF ELECTROSURGERY

At the end of an electrode, the performance depends on the shape and size of the electrode, the radio wave frequency and modulation, the peak voltage and the current coupled against an output impedance. The tissue may be cut in a smooth, deliberate fashion without arcing, or it can be burned and charred. This great variation of tissue effects is frequently ignored or misunderstood, which is

Table 10.1. Electrophysics Definitions Equated to a Hydraulic Analog

Electrical Concept	Electrical Unit	Equations	Hydraulic Analog
Energy	Joule	—	Energy
Charge	Coulomb	(6.3×10^{18} electrons)	Volume (mass)
Power	Watt	Joules/second	Power
Voltage	Volt	Joules/Coulomb	Pressure difference
Current	Ampere	Coulombs/second	Flow
Impedance	Ohm	Volts/Ampere	Resistance

why some surgeons have claimed that the laser provides better control of the energy needs and promotes better wound healing.

Electrocoagulation may be carried out in many different forms—from slow, delicate contact coagulation (*desiccation*) to the charring effects of the spray coagulation mode (*fulguration*), at times leading to carbonization. The temperature differences may vary between 100° C to over 500° C.

The essential characteristic of "CUT" waveforms is that they are continuous sine waves. That is, if the voltage output of the generator is plotted over time, a pure CUT (desiccation) waveform is a continuous sine wave alternating from positive to negative at the operating frequency of the generator, 500 to 3000 KHz (kilohertz).

The coagulation (COAG) waveform consists of short bursts of radio frequency sine waves. The important feature of the COAG waveform is the pause between each burst. If a COAG waveform had the same peak voltage as the CUT waveform, the average power delivered (energy per second) is less because the coagulation is turned off most of the time. Now suppose that the coagulation waveform had the same average voltage (RMS voltage) as the CUT waveform, and thus could deliver the same energy per second. Because the coagulation is turned off most of the time, it can only produce the same RMS voltage as the CUT by having a large peak voltage during the periods when the generator is active (Fig. 10.1).

A high voltage, coagulation waveform can spark to tissue without significant cutting effect, because the heat is widely dispersed by the long sparks (spray coag-

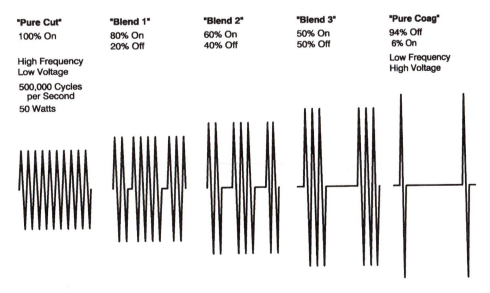

Figure 10.1. The change in voltage at a constant power output in watts when one selects a CUT, BLEND, and COAG waveform. (Courtesy of Valleylab Inc., Boulder, CO.)

ulation), and because the heating effect is intermittent. The temperature of the water in the cells does not reach the level to flash into steam. In this way the cells are dehydrated slowly but are not torn apart, which could form an incision. Because the high peak voltage is a quality of the coagulation waveform, it can drive a current through high resistances. In this way it is possible to fulgurate long after the water is driven out of the tissue and actually char it to carbon. To "coagulate" tissue is a general term that may include desiccation and/or fulguration.

Fulguration can be contrasted with desiccation in several ways. First, sparking to tissue with any practical fulguration generator always produces necrosis anywhere the sparks land. This is not surprising when you consider that each cycle of voltage produces a new spark, and each spark has an extremely high current density. For a given level of current flow, fulguration is always more efficient at producing surface necrosis, however, the depth of tissue injury is quite superficial compared to contact desiccation because, with fulguration, the sparks jump from one spot to another in a random fashion; thus the energy is "sprayed" rather than concentrated (Fig. 10.2). In desiccation, the current is no more concentrated than the area of contact between the electrode and the tissue. As a result, desiccation may or may not produce necrosis, depending on the current density delivered over time (Fig. 10.3).

For example, if an electrode is pressed against moist tissue, the electrode will begin in the desiccation mode, regardless of the waveform. The initial tissue resistance is quite low and the resulting current will be high. As the tissue dries out, its resistance rises until the electrical contact is broken. Since moist tissue is no longer touching the electrode, sparks will jump to the nearest areas of moist tissue in the fulguration mode, as long as the voltage is high enough to make a

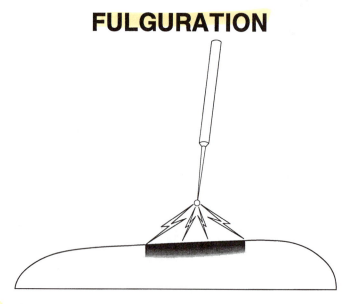

Figure 10.2. Fulguration sprays sparks to the surface of tissue, causing a surface char with only superficial heating of the deeper layers. (Courtesy of Reproductive Health Specialists, PS, Seattle, WA.)

DESICCATION

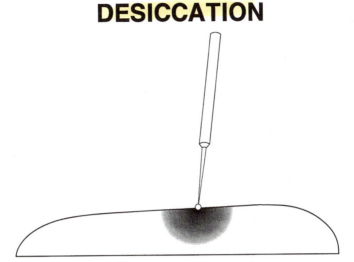

Figure 10.3. Desiccation occurs by touching the tissue before keying the generator, which creates deep penetration of heat and minimal charring of the surface tissue. (Courtesy of Reproductive Health Specialists, PS, Seattle, WA.)

spark. Eventually, the resistance of desiccated tissue will stop the flow of electrons, limiting the depth of coagulation.

CAPACITANCE IN MONOPOLAR ELECTROSURGERY

Capacitance is a physical property of monopolar energy where two conductors in close proximity, each insulated from one another, can induce an electrical current from one to the other (Fig. 10.4). The amount of this induction transfer of energy is influenced by the length of the conductors (the longer the distance the

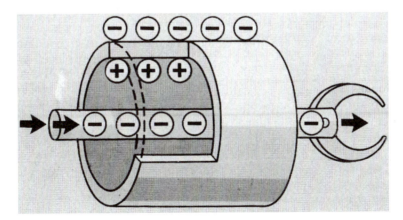

Figure 10.4. Capacitance is the induction of electrical current between two conductors separated by insulation; one conductor carries the active current and induces a separate current in the nearby conductor. (Courtesy of Reproductive Health Specialists, PS, Seattle, WA.)

more effect), the distance between the conductors (the shorter the distance the more the effect), the character of the waveform (a damped COAG waveform increases the effect) and the frequency of the waveform (the higher the frequency of the waveform the more the capacitance effect) (Table 10.2). The operating laparoscope becomes a capacitor when monopolar energy is transmitted through a long, insulated electrode with high-voltage, damped current, especially if the electrogenerator produces a frequency of three million cycles. Because the operating channel is eccentrically located in the shell of the laparoscope, the induced current can range from 50 to 80% of that current flowing through the active electrode (Fig. 10.5).

If a metal trocar sleeve is used to transport the operating laparoscope into the abdomen, the induced current is quickly transferred through the metal sleeve to the return electrode. Because the current (power) density is large (low) where the trocar sheath contacts the abdominal wall, no harm occurs. However, if the trocar sheath is nonconductive, e.g., made of fiberglass, is radiolucent, or a plastic securing collar is used (with either a metal or nonconductive trocar sleeve), the laparoscope cannot deliver the induced energy to ground. In this latter scenario, if a vital structure, e.g., bowel, touches the laparoscope, especially a small portion of its surface, the energy induced into the laparoscope may burn the organ; this may occur outside of the view of the laparoscopist. This same problem can occur when a secondary trocar sleeve is made of metal and a plastic securing collar is used, if that sleeve is used to transport a monopolar electrode.

The best way to reduce this risk is to use all metal trocar sleeves and securing collars; the next best is to use all plastic sleeves and collars. Never mix plastic with metal! Electroscope has introduced a new device that eliminates the risk of capacitance regardless of the trocar sleeve used. In addition, if there is a break in the insulation of the active electrode, this device will alert the surgeon. Electroscope has produced a device, in series with the electrical generators, to eliminate the development of capacitance (Fig. 10.6).

BIPOLAR ELECTROSURGERY

In unipolar or monopolar electrosurgery, a ground plate or return electrode carries the flowing electrons back to the generator after the electrons have passed through the patient. The electrons, which spread out after leaving a high density of energy at the point of tissue contact by the active or efferent electrode, are dispersed over the broad surface of the return electrode, which lowers the power density too low to cause tissue heating.

The bipolar system incorporates the active (efferent) electrode and the return (afferent) electrode into the forceps or two-poled instrument. This eliminates the need for a ground plate, allowing the instrument to produce a high power

Table 10.2. Physical Factors that Increase Capacitance
1. Increasing the length of the conductors
2. Decreasing the distance between the conductors
3. Using an undamped waveform (COAG)
4. Using fulguration techniques
5. Increasing the waveform frequency

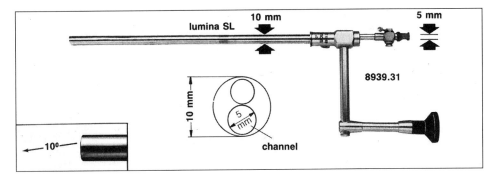

Figure 10.5. The operation laparoscope with its eccentrically placed operating channel creates a perfect model for the capacitance effect.

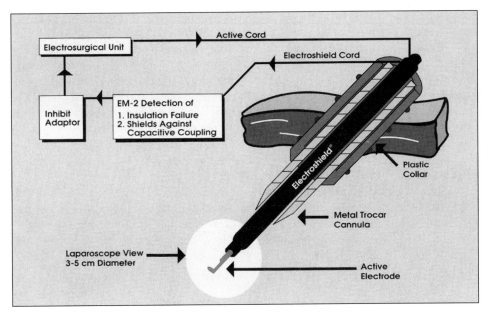

Figure 10.6. The Electroscope Device eliminates the threat of an inadvertent capacitance injury during laparoscopy. (Courtesy of Valleylab Inc., Boulder, CO.)

density at each pole of the forceps. This permits a discrete amount of desiccation confined primarily to the shape and size of the forceps in contact with the tissue, and eliminates the chance of stray or alternate pathways for current flow that might occur with monopolar activation if the ground plate was improperly applied or there was a break in the return lead.

Though these advantages over monopolar seem obvious, there are several restrictions unique to bipolar that need to be appreciated. First, the "load" of impedance that is used as a measure of power output is usually several times lower than monopolar modes in contemporary generators. If one uses a generator that has an output selection knob calibrated in numbers rather than watts, the bipolar output of energy will be many watts less than the same setting in monopolar. With those generators that read power output in watts, the impedance load is three to five times less than the load used to calibrate monopolar output such that the tissue effect may be much less than the same output reading for monopolar. Therefore, in most situations, bipolar applications are limited to a discrete area held between the forceps or scissor poles, with restricted power output but with high power density. With bipolar, only a continuous (CUT) waveform should be used. As we learn more about how to apply bipolar energy, new instruments are being developed that will broaden its applications.

EXERCISES IN ELECTROSURGICAL APPLICATIONS

Lean beef steak is an excellent model to learn certain principles of electrosurgery. If it is kept moist, its natural impedance will mimic that of the tissue that is desiccated/fulgurated in endoscopic surgery. Because of its rich color, the tissue effects are easy to see. For the "feel" of cutting through firm tissue (e.g., fibroid tumors), firm squash, turnip, or apple is preferable.

To test the cutting of tissue, choose a needle electrode and glide the electrode through the tissue using the CUT unipolar mode at a constant speed. Always "key" (activate) the generator before touching the tissue to start the microsparking, for it is the sparking that vaporizes the cells, giving the cutting effect. Next, increase the speed of the electrode's pass through tissue next to the original incision. Then, decrease the speed of the next pass through for a third incision. If the power setting and the electrode size remained constant, more desiccation of the adjacent tissue occurs where the slower electrode passed through the tissue.

Select a blade electrode and follow the same steps. Though one can still cut though the tissue, the lateral desiccation effect will be more profound. As the electrode chosen increases in size, the cutting effect will diminish and more desiccation will be seen, e.g., a large ball electrode will not cut but will deliver a uniform desiccation effect. There will be a point where the desiccation effect will be limited in depth by the impedance to flow at a fixed power setting.

Repeat the same series of events with the same electrodes using the COAG mode at the same power, but do not touch the tissue. Notice how the sparking is longer with the needle electrode, but the ball electrode "sprays" better. This fulguration technique reveals minimal depth of tissue destruction when the coagulated areas are incised open. If you touch each electrode to the tissue before you key the generator, desiccation will occur, but with more lateral charring than in the CUT mode.

To appreciate the effects of fluids on the delivery of electroenergy, irrigate the specimen with normal saline; and during the irrigation, try to desiccate and then fulgurate the surface. Next, do the same exercise using distilled water, sorbitol, or glycine. Notice how the energy was dissipated and less effective in the electrolyte solution. When one realizes that blood is saline-rich, it is easy to understand why a bloody field is hard to coagulate and stop bleeding. Irrigating with a nonelectrolyte solution or removing the blood via suction from the bleeders will improve the task.

Using a roller electrode, desiccate the surface of the specimen using a slow, rolling motion, leaving a furrow of coagulated tissue. Next to that furrow, repeat the same act of desiccation but at twice the speed. Incise through both furrows and examine the depth of desiccation. This is an exercise in the effect of time on the depth of destruction.

To test for capacitance, insert an electrode through the operating channel of an operation laparoscope or through a metal 5-mm trocar sleeve. At 100 watts, fulgurate or desiccate the tissue on the ground plate with the active electrode. Now, without touching the active electrode to the meat, touch an edge of the laparoscope or the trocar sleeve to the meat and activate the generator in each waveform at 100 watts. Run the side of its tubular shell up and down the meat gently, bouncing off and on the meat to notice the effect. Which is more profound in tissue effect, COAG or CUT?

APPLIED PHYSICS IN LAPAROSCOPY

The tissue effect of electrophysics depends on size and shape of each electrode, the chosen waveform, and power output; the challenge facing today's laparoscopists is to properly match and mix the electrodes and generators. For instance, because of the difference in the power density of the forceps as they grasp the tissue, a 5-mm grasping forceps will desiccate tissue much slower than a 3-mm forceps of similar design. A knife electrode can be used to incise tissue, yet when coagulation is needed, one can place the flat side of the electrode on the tissue, and with a cutting (undamped) waveform it will desiccate the tissue. Regardless of the waveform, a ball-shaped electrode will desiccate when pressed against tissue, but, if you hold the ball electrode away from an oozing surface, and deliver a high-voltage, coagulation waveform, you can fulgurate the bleeding area without deep tissue penetration.

As one electrode is changed to another, the surgeon should adjust the generator output to match the task at hand. This is especially important when needle electrodes are used after one has used a more blunt electrode. If not, the tissue touched by the high current density of the needle electrode may be severely damaged, and passive heat transfer may destroy the needle electrode.

When bipolar instruments are used, if a coagulation waveform is used, a sticking phenomenon is common; in general, use an undamped waveform with bipolar instruments. When performing tubal sterilization with bipolar forceps, if one uses the coagulation or damped waveform for bipolar sterilization, the center of the tube may not be destroyed because the surface of the tube is charred too quickly, rapidly increasing tissue impedance. The same problem can happen when blood vessels, surrounded by fat, i.e., mesenteric vessels, are coagulated with a bipolar instrument delivering a damped waveform; if the desiccated vessel is cut, it may bleed briskly. Using an undamped waveform, an inline current flowmeter (ammeter) is a valuable accessory to assure the surgeon that all of the tissue between the forceps has been coagulated before the tissue is transected.

As with laser surgery during operative laparoscopy, smoke accumulation can occur if fulguration techniques are used; for the most part, desiccation techniques create steam. Smoke can be reduced or eliminated by irrigating the field to be coagulated with glycine rather than saline or lactated Ringer's solution, for glycine, a nonelectrolytic solution, has a pH of 6.1, similar to lactated Ringer's solution. Several accessory instruments have been designed to allow the simultaneous delivery of glycine and electricity through an irrigation/aspiration cannula which contains an insulated, internal electrode that can protrude beyond the tip of the cannula. If one floods the field as electroenergy is being delivered, the energy is not dissipated within the solution, as it is with electrolyte-rich fluids, and in a liquid medium smoke will not develop. At the end of the procedure, any intraabdominal glycine is aspirated.

Glycine has another characteristic that is helpful. As one flushes the bleeding area, the individual bleeder will stream through the irrigating solution, giving the appearance of bleeding "snakes." The port of bleeding can be seen with ease, and quickly fulgurated. Unlike with hysteroscopy or cystoscopy, these nonelectrolytic solutions are not delivered at a pressure high enough to cause an intravascular infusion, which might lead to a water intoxication syndrome.

In the early 1980s, it was thought that the occasional bowel perforation following a laparoscopy was the result of sparking or arcing to the bowel when electrodes were used. Because the physics of fulguration will not allow an arc to be maintained in one spot, it is now understood that, at the worst, only a surface charring of the bowel could occur. To burn a hole in the bowel, the electrode must touch the bowel during the delivery of electroenergy and remain in contact with the bowel wall long enough to coagulate deep into the bowel wall. For this reason, it is best to disconnect electrodes from the generator when they are not needed for the delivery of electroenergy. To prevent one from accidentally touching the bowel with an active electrode, before keying the generator, one should withdraw the laparoscope from the operating field to create a wide, panoramic view.

At the tissue level, when the energy over time, as measured in joules, is equal between lasers and electrodes, the end result is the same. In other words, a watt, is a watt, is a watt.

APPLIED PHYSICS IN HYSTEROSCOPY

With endometrial ablation, either or both the resectoscope loop and rollerball electrode are used; a roller bar or barrel is also available. Some surgeons will shave the endometrial lining with the loop electrode; others will desiccate the endometrial lining with the roller ball or bar. A few shave first and then "paint" the shaved myometrium with a roller electrode. Unfortunately, studies on the tissue effects of different techniques, electrodes, and waveforms are few in number. Even the pressure applied to the endometrial surface will change the current (power) density; the more the pressure, the broader will be the contact surface of the electrode, creating a diminished current density. Since the speed of passage of the electrode, unique to each surgeon, is another variable, only the outcome statistics can be evaluated with any reasonable scrutiny. Some use a coagulation-only waveform at a low wattage of 30; others report success with a pure cutting waveform at 100 watts.

My personal preference is to shave the endometrium first. I use a pure, undamped waveform and drag the wire loop in a slow, deliberate motion to four millimeters deep through the tissue so there is some coagulation effect in addition to its cutting properties. By using the cutting waveform, bubble formation (hydrogen gas released from the distension fluid) on the anterior surface of the endometrial cavity is less than in the coagulation mode. I do not shave the cavity's lateral sulcus near the uterine vessels nor near the cornua of the uterine cavity.

During the "painting" phase, I continue to use an undamped waveform with a light contact of the roller electrode set at 100 watts. If the roller electrode is a bar or barrel, I will either slow up the rolling motion or increase the power output because the electrode's current density is lower than a rollerball's. At the end of the ablation procedure, I will switch to a coagulation waveform set at 75 watts. With the increased peak voltage of this waveform, skip areas will be "sought out" by the electrons pushed under higher pressure, assuring complete surface coagulation.

On seven hysterectomy specimens, histologic studies performed several months after the ablation procedure demonstrated a complete absence of the endometrial lining being replaced by cuboidal cells, and a coagulation depth into the myometrium of 3–5 mm. Still, the total amenorrhea rate using this technique in 100 cases has been only 60%. Thirty-five percent of the patients have tolerable oligomenorrhea, the failure rate being five percent. These statistics do not differ from those who use lower power settings, one electrode, and either blended or coagulation waveforms.

LITERATURE REVIEW OF ENDOSCOPIC ELECTROSURGICAL COMPLICATIONS

A search of the literature devoted to endoscopy in 1992 and much of 1993 failed to uncover studies that addressed the issues of how and why electrosurgical accidents had occurred (1–7). In some, it was clear that an electrical instrument was involved in the complication, but how and why was not mentioned. One study reviewed the histological findings of tissue heated with the Kleppinger bipolar forceps, showing that there is enough power to coagulate blood vessels up to 3 mm (8). One of the purposes of the study was to evaluate the lateral spread of energy of this instrument. Unfortunately, the alternative (monopolar) was not studied specifically, matching the power density, waveform and joules of energy.

Another clinical study evaluated the complications of laparoscopic assisted vaginal hysterectomy (LAVH) in 45 patients and states, "Equipment complications had the highest incidence; the most common type was bipolar cautery dysfunction (22 of 45)" (9). It is clear that a perceived "safety" of bipolar electrodes may lull the surgeon into a state of false security.

A review of 66 cases of bowel injuries brought to litigation have been evaluated by this author since 1985 (10). Though it was believed the cause of the injury in 58 cases was from electrical injuries, such was the case in only six (9%); the remaining were due to sharp trauma during abdominal entry with either the Veress needle, primary trocar, or the penetrating forceps or knife used in the "open" technique. Other lessons learned include:

1. All causes of injury to the bowel can present either "early" or late.
2. Blood count indices are frequently normal.
3. Emergency room personnel are poorly prepared to evaluate patients who present for care following a laparoscopy. Often, patients with increasing abdominal pain were reassured, given more pain medication, and sent home.

After laparoscopic procedures, a patient's pain pattern should improve; for it to worsen raises the question of a viscus penetration wound at the time of the procedure.
4. To resect the area of perforation is recommended; subjecting the specimen to histologic assessment with a Mallory trichrome stain, which highlights electrical injury, is good risk management when the injury is, in truth, unpreventable trauma. (This stain highlights coagulated, collagenous tissue in a distinctive blue color, confirming an injury consistent with heat damage. The absence of this finding eliminates the claim that electrical injury has occurred.)
5. Patients who have increasing pain after a laparoscopy, either early or late, have a bowel injury until proven otherwise.

SUMMARY

Electrosurgery is a method of surgery that lends itself well to endoscopic procedures. At present, the average gynecologist lacks the same basic education as devoted to lasers in the past decade. When accidents occur during laparoscopy using electrosurgical instruments, the energy source is frequently blamed. More likely than not it is due to a nonelectrical cause such as inadvertent trauma (unusually beyond the control of the surgeon), or it is an error in the direct application of the energy source to the tissue, much of which could have been prevented with in-depth education and appreciation of the nuances of electrophysics in concert with the features of the equipment used to deliver the energy. When applying the physics of good electrosurgery, the variables that affect tissue effect, such as waveform, electrode size and shape, time of application and power density, must be understood. If physicians are expected to prescribe drugs in a precise and logical manner, so should they be expected to have a similar working knowledge of the energy sources they choose to use in surgery.

REFERENCES

1. Querleu D. Complications de la chirurgie coelioscopique. J Gynecol Obstet Biol Reprod 1992;21:711.
2. Wood C, Maher P, Hill D, Selwood T. Hysterectomy: a time of change. Med J Aust 1992;157:651–653.
3. Hulka JF, Peterson HB, Phillips JM, Surrey MW. Operative laparoscopy, American Association of Gynecologic Laparoscopists 1991 membership survey. J Reprod Med 1993;38:569–571.
4. Peterson HB, Hulka JF, Phillips JM, Surrey MW. Laparoscopic sterilization, American Association of Gynecologic Laparoscopists 1991 membership survey. J Reprod Med 1993;38:574–576.
5. Capelouto CC, Kavoussi LR. Complications of laparoscopic surgery. Urology 1993;42:2–12.
6. Kavoussi LR, Sosa E, Chandhoke P, Chodak G, Clayman R, Hadley HR, Loughlin KR, Ruckle HC, Rukstalis D, Schuessler W, Segura G, Vancaillie T, Winfield HN. Complications of laparoscopic pelvic lymph node dissection. J Urol 1993;149:322–325.
7. Langebrekke A, Skar OJ, Urnes A. Laparoscopic hysterectomy, initial experience. Acta Obstet Gynecol Scand 1992;71:226–229.
8. Ryder RM, Hulka JF. Bladder and bowel injury after electrodesiccation with Kleppinger bipolar forceps, a clinicopathologic study. J Reprod Med 1993;38:595–598.
9. Schwartz RO. Complications of laparoscopic hysterectomy. Obstet Gynecol 1993;81:1022–1024.
10. Soderstrom RM. Bowel injury litigation after laparoscopy. J Am Assoc of Gynecol Laparoscopists 1993;1:74–77.

SUGGESTED READINGS

Filmar S, Jetha N, McComb P, Gomel V. A comparative histologic study on the healing process after tissue transaction I. Carbon dioxide laser and electromicrosurgery. Am J Obstet Gynecol 1989;160:1062.

Levy BS, Soderstrom RM, Dail DH. Bowel injury during laparoscopy: gross anatomy and histology. J Reprod Med 1985;30:168–172.

Luciano AA, Frishman GN, Kratka SA, Maier DB. A comparative analysis of adhesion reduction, tissue effects, and incising characteristics of electrosurgery, CO_2 laser, and Nd-Yag laser at operative laparoscopy. J Laparoendoscopy 1993;2:305–310.

Luciano AA, Whitman GF, Maier DB, Randolph JF, Maenza RM. A comparison of thermal injury, healing patterns and postoperative adhesion formation following CO_2 laser and electromicrosurgery. Fertil Steril 1987;48:1025–1029.

Odell RC. Biophysics of electrical energy. In: Soderstrom RM, ed. Operative Laparoscopy: The Master's Techniques. New York: Raven Press, 1993:35–44.

Reich H, Vancaillie TG, Soderstrom RM. Electrical techniques. In: Martin DC, ed. Manual of Endoscopy. Baltimore: Port City Press, 1990:105–111.

Voyles CR, Tucker RD. Education and engineering solutions for potential problems with monopolar electrosurgery at laparoscopy. Am J Surg 1992;164:57–61.

Chapter 11
Laparoscopic Suturing Techniques
Malcolm G. Munro

HISTORY

The history of ligatures dates to the beginning of surgery. The development of suture, surgical needles, and suturing technique was a prerequisite to the performance of both safe extirpation and effective reconstructive procedures. Furthermore, misadventures inevitably encountered in the performance of pelvic surgery, such as accidental enterotomy or cystotomy, required a suture-based method for effective repair.

With the advent of operative laparoscopy came a requisite to replicate, or substitute for, the techniques performed via open surgery. Surgical objectives include securing vascular pedicles and repairing or reconstructing damaged organs, all under endoscopic guidance. Many felt that quality laparoscopic suturing techniques were either impossible or too difficult to accomplish in a timely and cost-effective fashion. However, prescient pioneers such as Courtney Clarke of Canada and Kurt Semm of Germany demonstrated that, with creativity, practice, and patience, most, if not all, of the techniques developed for "open" surgery could be applied to endoscopically directed procedures. Clarke, in 1972, first described his set of instruments, and a technique that could be used to suture-ligate tissue and transfer standard knots, created extracorporeally, into the peritoneal cavity via endoscopic ports or cannulas (1). Semm demonstrated that pretied knots and loops could be introduced and placed around defined pedicles for secure and hemostatic ligation (2).

Unfortunately, at least in North America, these techniques and instruments were virtually ignored for almost 20 years. Instead, as operative laparoscopy became more popular, the medical device industry produced a number of stapling and clipping instruments for the acquisition or maintenance of hemostasis during the performance of extirpative procedures such as adnexectomy and hysterectomy. However, clips and staples are not effective for the closure of defects encountered if bowel or bladder are entered in the course of a laparoscopically directed procedure. Furthermore, these instruments are significantly more expensive than suture, a feature not desirable if less expensive and equally effective alternatives are available.

Consequently, in the late 1980s and early 1990s, endoscopic suturing and knot tying were rediscovered by surgeons such as Reich and Corfman (3–5). Other innovators have added to the currently available list of needle drivers, suture positioners, knot manipulators, and techniques that collectively allow for the application of suturing to virtually any procedure. While many of the techniques have been published (6–9), there are a variety of effective nonpublished variations. The recent advent of "gasless," or apneumic, laparoscopy has facilitated allowed for the use of more traditionally designed instruments to place and secure ligatures in a more conventional, but laparoscopically directed, fashion. However, at this time, the limitations of apneumic laparoscopy make its ultimate role uncertain.

TRAINING AND PRACTICE

Critical to the successful use of suturing technique at laparoscopy are appropriate training and a dedication to, as well as a facility for, practice. Many try to acquire laparoscopic suturing proficiency during the practical component of a weekend endoscopy course. Attempts to immediately apply these recently learned and poorly practiced techniques in the operating room will be inefficient at best, and inappropriate and unsafe at worst.

This should not be surprising. Most surgeons remember the hours spent learning to tie secure knots for open surgery using any of a number of surrogates including shoelaces, the drawstrings on surgical scrubs, and suture "borrowed" from an operating or delivery room. Repetition was a prerequisite for proficiency, which, in turn, had to be demonstrated before the mentor would trust the integrity of a divided vascular pedicle to the knots created by the trainee. For laparoscopic procedures it is even more important that the surgeon be facile in the placement of suture, particularly when securing vascular pedicles. The nature of minimally invasive surgery allows less opportunity for a supervisor or mentor to quickly react to, and rectify, the mistakes of the trainee or novice. Consequently, in addition to adequate instruction, the trainee requires the availability of a suitable endoscopic simulator. Even for experienced surgeons, frequent practice of techniques infrequently required at surgery will facilitate operating room efficiency and safety.

Endoscopic simulators may be complex or simple in their design. In the near future, it will be possible to simulate many endoscopic situations in computer generated environments. However, because of the complex hardware and software requirements, it is unlikely that realistic simulation of laparoscopic suturing and tying will be available soon. A useful laparoscopic simulator is depicted in Figure 11.1. For those with a home video camera, this simulator can be copied using a cardboard box and their television monitor. With the addition of suture laparoscopic cannulas and some endoscopic hand instruments, they will be able to practice at home. Wherever, the important thing is to practice.

GENERAL CONSIDERATIONS

To replicate open surgical procedures safely and effectively, laparoscopic suturing requires the same quality of technique, which is, in many ways, more difficult to achieve given the spatial limitations presented by the fixed positioning of ports, and the two-dimensional view provided by the video monitor. The latter limitation may be eliminated with the introduction of effective three-dimensional video imaging systems. In open cases the operator is presented with a variety of angles of approach to the target tissue, limited only by the degree of exposure provided by the assistants. For laparoscopically directed procedures, exposure is usually better than that obtained via open surgery. This relates to the ability of the endoscope's objective lens to be placed in close proximity to the surgical field. However the surgeon's angle of attack is determined and limited by the location and orientation of the tissue with respect to the ports through which

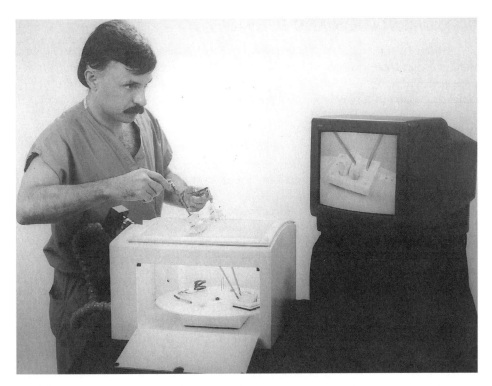

Figure 11.1. Endoscopic Simulators. Shown is a laparoscopic training simulator that has its own camera mounted on an adjustable arm, eliminating the need for an assistant, a telescope, and a medical grade endoscope camera. The box is fitted with bright neon lighting, and a removable turntable contains a number of skill stations. The simulator may be used with other inanimate tissue models.

the suturing instruments are passed. Consequently, the operator must try to anticipate the potential requirements for suturing at the beginning of the procedure, when positioning the cannulas in the abdominal wall.

The required instrumentation, needles, and suture will vary with the procedure at hand as well as the technique utilized by the surgeon. However, regardless of the technique, it is critical that the operative site be adequately exposed and centralized in the surgeon's field of view. This can require retraction, table manipulation, and/or the use of a capable assistant. The author has found that an automated laparoscope positioner is a very effective substitute for the assistant.

As noted previously, virtually any required needle may be inserted into the peritoneal cavity, provided that it is swaged onto the suture. Free ligatures may be passed *around* defined pedicles, or they may be passed *through* tissue using a ligature carrier. Suture may be secured with knots fashioned either within the peritoneal cavity (intracorporeal), or outside (extracorporeal). Extracorporeal knots must be transferred into the peritoneal cavity via a knot manipulator. Ligatures and suture may be secured by substituting clips for knots. Recently, a number of devices have been produced designed to place suture into the abdominal wall under laparoscopic guidance. Such devices may be used to secure traumatized abdominal wall vessels or prevent subsequent incisional herniation by safely closing the fascial defects produced by large caliber laparoscopic trocars.

INSTRUMENTATION AND SUPPLIES

Prior to suturing under laparoscopic guidance, the surgeon must have available, and be intimately familiar with, the necessary instrumentation and supplies. These include suture, knot manipulators, needle drivers, and other instruments used in laparoscopic suturing.

Needles and Ligatures

Types of Ligatures

The purpose of a ligature is to maintain tissue approximation until artificial support is no longer necessary for healing. While there may be no perfect ligature, the design goals include adequate strength, ease of handling, ability to hold a knot, and a lack of tissue reactivity. Tissue reactivity creates inflammation in the suture track and can affect the strength of the ligature and the ultimate strength of the healed incision. Because there is no ideal ligature, there are a wide variety of options that may excel in one or more of the desired features. Ligatures vary in their composition, construction, caliber, and length. Proper selection depends upon the tissue and the procedure to be performed.

Caliber. Ligatures are sized by a convention described in Figure 11.2. At laparoscopy, it is difficult to work with suture that is finer in caliber than 6-0. Newer, finer instruments will soon be available that will allow effective manipulation of needles attached to 8-0 suture. In general, for a given composition and

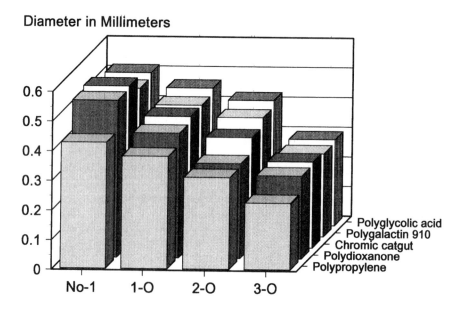

Figure 11.2. Ligature Size. Ligatures vary in caliber from 10-0 (fine) to No. 2 (thick). Demonstrated are the actual diameters of 3-0 to 1-0 suture made of five commonly used materials. (Adapted from von Fraunhofer JA, Storey RS, Stone IK, Masterson BJ. Tensile strength of suture materials. J Biomed Mater Res 1985;19:596.)

construction, smaller caliber ligatures are associated with weaker suture lines, but less tissue reaction. Conversely, large caliber ligatures will generally cause more tissue reaction but will be more secure. However, this may be a specious concept as larger caliber ligatures may cause more tissue reaction, both because they may be tied tighter, causing more necrosis, and because their larger caliber incites more local inflammatory response. The increased inflammatory response may, in turn, decrease the life of the suture itself.

Composition. Ligatures may be composed of nonabsorbable materials, staying permanently in the body unless removed, or they may be fashioned from biodegradable materials that allow their eventual resorption. In general, biodegradable suture is associated with more tissue reaction than are permanent ligatures.

The first biodegradable ligatures were spun from animal gut, and, not surprisingly, and probably because of their antigenicity, they were associated with a significant degree of tissue reaction. More recently, synthetic biodegradable ligatures have been introduced. These have been found to contribute less tissue reaction than a similar caliber gut suture. Furthermore, because these ligatures are stronger, the surgeon may use smaller caliber suture, which, in turn, results in even less tissue reaction. Braided synthetic sutures of polyglycolic acid (Dexon, Polysorb) or polyglactin 910 (Vicryl) will maintain strength for about one month. Monofilament synthetics like polydioxanone (PDS) and polyglyconate (Maxon) will provide approximately three months of significant strength until they break down.

The original permanent sutures were made from cotton and silk. While still used by many, they have been largely replaced with synthetics such as nylon and polypropylene. While the latter may be useful for skin closure, their value in laparoscopic procedures is limited.

Construction. The third variable that contributes to the feel and function of a ligature is its construction. There are basically two types of construction, monofilament and polyfilament, where a number of fine monofilaments are braided to form the ligature. In general, the smooth surface of monofilament suture is less traumatic as it is pulled through the tissue. However, these ligatures generally do not hold knots as well as do braided varieties, making it necessary to fashion more throws. On the other hand, polyfilamentous suture is easier to tie, with fewer knots, but somewhat more traumatic as it is passed through tissue. Such trauma can lead to the suture "sawing" through the tissue being sewn. Manufacturers continue to try to develop ligature that balances the atraumatic nature of monofilamentous designs with the feel and knot holding ability of the braided sutures.

Suture Absorption. Not surprisingly, all three of the above variables contribute to the rate of absorption of a biodegradable suture. Of interest to the surgeon are two endpoints—the time when strength is lost and the time until complete absorption. The accompanying graph helps to reveal the characteristics of specific materials and construction (Fig. 11.3).

The composition of the ligature is perhaps the most relevant variable. The

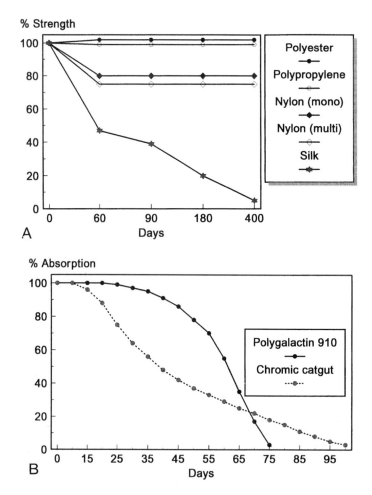

Figure 11.3. Suture Absorption and Strength. Loss of suture strength varies with composition and caliber. **A.** Nonabsorbable sutures such as polyester (Ethibond and Mersilene), and Polypropylene (Prolene) retain 100% of their strength at 400 days. Monofilament nylon (Ethilon) loses about 20% in the same time, while multifilament nylon loses slightly more of its strength. Silk loses 50% by two months and has virtually no strength at 400 days. **B.** Absorbable sutures ideally maintain optimal strength until healing occurs, then dissolve. In this typical instance 4-0 synthetic absorbable (polyglactin 910; Vicryl) maintains strength longer, and then dissolves faster than 4-0 chromic catgut. The fact that synthetic absorbable suture is considerably stronger than gut, and associated with less tissue reaction, is a significant advantage in the majority of instances. (Adapted from Salthouse TN. Biologic response to sutures. Otolaryngol Head Neck Surg 1980;88:658–664.)

most rapidly absorbed material is plain gut, which loses most of its strength in a matter of a few days, and is completely absorbed soon thereafter. Such material is inappropriate for use in fascial closure. On the other end of the spectrum are the synthetic absorbables that maintain strength for weeks, and can often be found in the body months later.

Construction also affects absorption. For a given caliber of suture, constructed from the same material, monofilamentous varieties will lose maximal strength earlier, and will stay in the body longer than their braided counterparts.

This is likely because only the surface of the monofilament is available for biodegradation—it has less total surface area than do the multiple strands of the polyfilamentous ligature.

The final variable is the caliber of the suture. It is self-evident that, for sutures of equal composition and construction, larger caliber varieties will, in most instances, remain stronger longer and will take longer to be absorbed.

Ligature and Needle Selection

The surgeon can select ligatures from one of two sources: (*a*) the wide variety of suture ligatures readily available and originally designed for use at "open" surgery, and (*b*) those sutures that have been designed specifically for laparoscopic surgery. Suture ligatures created for laparoscopic surgery may possess a number of conveniences for the surgeon; the appropriate ligature length, needle designs that facilitate entry and removal, and, in some instances, pretied knots and/or integrated knot manipulators. While these packages may represent conveniences for some surgeons in some situations, total reliance on "laparoscopic sutures" greatly limits the ability of the surgeon to perform a wide variety of tasks. Consequently, it behooves the trainee to become familiar with both and to become confident with introduction, manipulation, and extraction of virtually any suture thought appropriate for a given situation.

Selection of needles and suture depends upon the task at hand and the preferences of the surgeon. For *extracorporeal ties* the suture must be long enough to pass into the peritoneal cavity, around the target tissue, and back out again, with enough additional length to allow the surgeon comfort in fashioning the knot. Consequently, ligature should be at least 30 inches (75 cm) long. In general, suture caliber should be 2-0 or larger, for finer suture is more likely either to break or to shear tissue. Braided absorbable suture is generally preferable to monofilament ligatures, but either may be used.

When a ligature carrier is used, or when a pedicle is already isolated, a swaged-on needle is unnecessary. However, in other circumstances, as when suture ligating the uterine vessels, a needle is mandatory. There are three basic needle configurations: straight, curved, and the so-called "ski-tip," designed to offer the advantage of a curved needle while still capable of introduction into the peritoneal cavity through 5-mm laparoscopic ports (Fig. 11.4). Curved needles are still far more versatile and there exist a number of methods by which even relatively large diameter versions may be efficiently passed into and out of the peritoneal cavity. In general, undesirable twisting of needles in the needle holder is reduced with the selection of versions that possess a flat edge on the internal curve of their circumference (Fig. 11.5). Prepackaged suture ligatures are available with attached straight, ski-tipped, or curved needles and integrated Type IV knot manipulators. The end of the suture is already loaded into the central channel of the knot manipulator and fixed to its scored proximal end, which may be easily snap-separated, freeing the ligature, allowing transfer of the knot into the peritoneal cavity. Specific suggestions regarding suture selection will be provided in the subsequent discussion on technique.

When fashioning intracorporeal knots, shorter sutures are used. For running closures, such as those used for the repair of a defect in the uterus or an

200 GYNECOLOGIC ENDOSCOPY: Principles in Practice

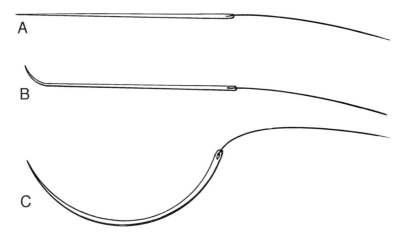

Figure 11.4. Surgical Needles. **A.** Straight. **B.** Ski-tipped. **C.** Curved.

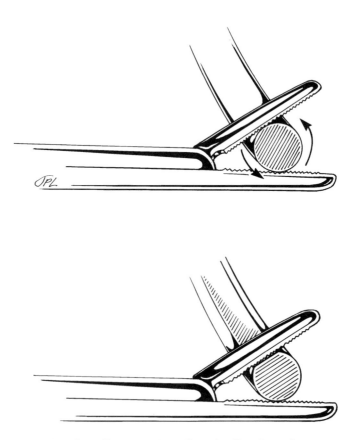

Figure 11.5. Prevention of Needle Torque. A needle with a flat edge will resist torque, particularly when grasped by an alligator-jawed needle driver.

ovary, a noose positioned at the end of the suture may function as an anchor knot (6). Such knots may be created with standard suture ligatures or they may be purchased pretied. Straight, ski-tipped, or curved needles may be selected at the discretion of the surgeon and depending on the task at hand.

Knot Manipulators

The incisions created at laparoscopic surgery are too small to allow for the transfer of extracorporeally tied knots into the peritoneal cavity using the surgeon's hands. The purpose of a knot manipulator is to act as a surrogate for the human finger in both the transfer of such knots into the peritoneal cavity and for securing them in place. There are essentially four basic types of knot manipulators, although there are a number of varieties of each. *Type I* manipulators are open ended or forked, *Type II* possess a closed loop, *Type III* have a side notch, and *Type IV* have a channel running their entire length.

Type I—Open Ended

In the opinion of the author, the most practical and useful devices are those patterned after the instrument originally designed and reported by H. Courtney Clarke in 1972 (1). These devices, just under 4 mm in diameter, are designed to transfer standard half hitch knots through cannulas with inside diameters no less than 5 mm. The additional space is required to allow the suture to pass through the cannula, beside the knot manipulator, and into the peritoneal cavity. The open end of the device allows easy loading of the ligature and even permits the tightening of several knots in sequence (Fig. 11.6). A number of similar devices have been designed and marketed, both disposable and nondisposable in nature (Fig. 11.7). A variation of this knot manipulator was recently described by Clarke (10). While possessing the same open end, the distal tip of the device may be opened, forming two arms, making it easier to apply the lateral force necessary to secure knots on smooth surfaces. In addition, the device possesses an integrated cutting tool.

Type II—Loop End

Open ended designs allow the suture to slip out of the device, a circumstance that may be problematic when it occurs in the cannula, for, in such instances, it is difficult to retrieve the knot. For this reason some prefer the device to be modified into a closed loop, a feature that obviates some of the advantages of the open instrument, but one that ensures that the suture stays connected to the end of the device (Fig. 11.8). In addition, with such an instrument, it may be easier to transfer a surgeon's knot into the peritoneal cavity.

Type III—Notched

The third type of knot manipulator is one designed for slip knots, such as the Roeder or the Weston. These are essentially notched probes that catch the relatively large mass of the knot and the short end of the suture, so that together they can be transferred into the peritoneal cavity and secured in place (Fig. 11.9).

202 GYNECOLOGIC ENDOSCOPY: Principles in Practice

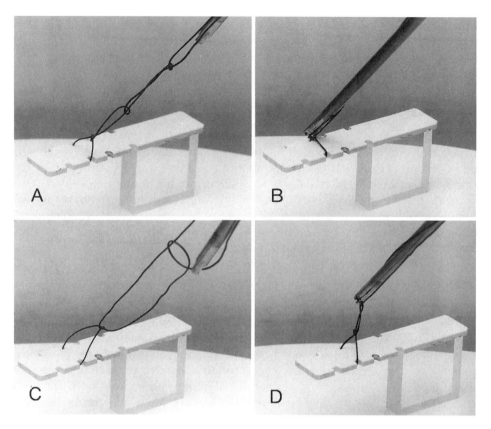

Figure 11.6. Sequential Knots. Type I knot manipulators may be used to tighten a series of knots. **A.** A series of three knots is placed into the peritoneal cavity with at least 2 cm between each. **B–D.** The knots are sequentially caught in the manipulator and tightened.

Type IV—Channeled

Another device, designed for either standard half hitches or slip knots, is a simple probe that contains a channel bored for its entire length. To use the device, a narrow caliber wire with a loop on one end is fed into the channel. Then the suture is loaded by passing one end through the loop and, with traction placed on the wire, it is drawn into and through the channel. The knot may be formed either before or after passing the suture through the channel. The other end of the suture remains outside of the knot manipulator. While this device is available in nondisposable forms (Fig. 11.10), the most widely used varieties are single use units that are packaged with pretied fisherman's or Weston slip knots (Fig. 11.11).

Needle Drivers

For tissue apposition using swaged needles, it is necessary to grasp and manipulate the needle with an instrument. For laparoscopy performed within an insufflated peritoneal cavity, the needle driver must conform to the dimensions of the laparoscopic cannulas. Consequently, it is more difficult to design instruments that effectively hold the needle. In addition, function is compromised by the fact

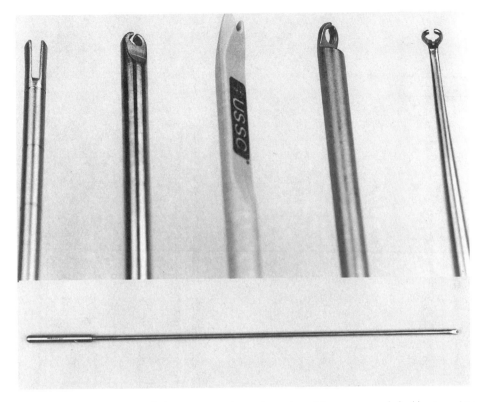

Figure 11.7. Type I (Open Ended) Knot Manipulators. A number of 4-mm open or forked knot manipulators are available. From the *left*, Reznick Inc.; Clarke-Reich (Marlow Surgical Inc.); Disposable (United States Surgical Corp.); Clarke (Marlow Surgical Inc.); Right angled (Karl Storz Inc.).

that the ports are fixed with respect to their orientation to the target tissue. With gasless, or apneumic, laparoscopy, the instruments designed for open surgery may be inserted directly into the peritoneal cavity via the small abdominal incisions.

There exists a variety of laparoscopic needle driver designs, each of which may provide some advantage for certain surgeons or in specific situations. Variation occurs in the design of the user interface, or handles, as well as the *end effector*, or the mechanism employed in grasping the needle itself. Most of these instruments are designed to be passed through 5-mm cannulas, although some are available in 3-mm designs. More recently, a number of instruments have been introduced that automate at least some aspect of the sewing process, features that for some may further facilitate the process of suturing and/or tying.

Handles

The handles of a needle driver are important because they are the interface with the surgeon. Because surgeons vary in their hand size, their dexterity, and the procedures they perform, there exist a variety of handle designs. The most obvious variable is the orientation of the handle to the shaft. There are two basic configurations, one an offset grip, the other aligned in the same axis as the shaft, or "inline" (Fig. 11.12). While inline instruments are generally better designed to

204 GYNECOLOGIC ENDOSCOPY: Principles in Practice

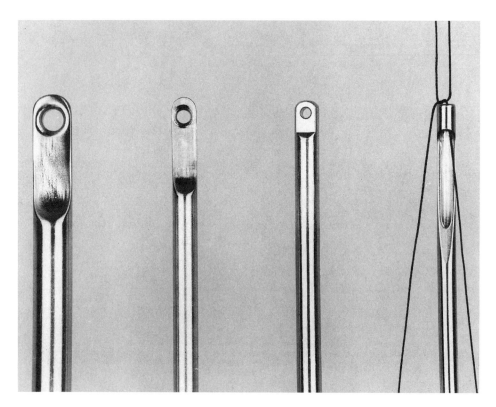

Figure 11.8.   Type II (Loop End) Knot Manipulators. From *left* to *right*: Jarit Inc; Marlow Surgical Inc; 5 mm and 10 mm, Sharpe Endosurgical Inc.

translate wrist rotation to the needle, they may be awkward in situations where the surgeon must operate with the hand and arm extended (Fig. 11.13). In such instances the offset handle designs may be preferable. There are available a number of variations in both inline and offset handle design, each of which may provide a degree of comfort or ease of use in different situations (Figs. 11.14, 11.15).

An important aspect of handles is the way in which they are manipulated to place pressure on the needle at the other end of the device. This may be accomplished directly, or the mechanism may be spring loaded to exert pressure passively, when the hand is relaxed. Most needle drivers possess some sort of locking mechanism that fixes the needle in position in the end effector. Needle drivers designed for open surgery, and familiar to most surgeons, allow direct translation of hand pressure, and lock with a ratcheted mechanism when this pressure is maximized. Similar devices designed for laparoscopic surgery, available with all of the described mechanisms, translate pressure to the needle directly, passively, and while configured in a locked mode.

End Effector

At the opposite end of the device is the end effector, the component of the instrument that is in direct contact with the needle. In open surgery the only widely used end effectors are those that are based upon an "alligator jaw" design.

Chapter 11: Laparoscopic Suturing Techniques   205

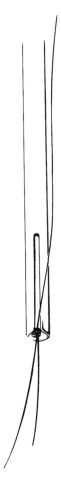

Figure 11.9. Type III (Notched) Knot Manipulator. These devices are used for the transfer of slip knots into the peritoneal cavity. The notch is used to catch the bulk of the knot, sliding it until it tightens.

The jaws may be aligned with the shaft of the instrument or they may be angled to allow easier manipulation in narrow recesses (e.g., Heaney design). Such instruments are also available for use at laparoscopy and represent the most commonly used format (Fig. 11.16). Included are needle drivers designed for the manipulation of the fine needles and suture necessary for the performance of laparoscopic microsurgery (Fig. 11.17). Most trainees will be initially attracted to such needle drivers, and, indeed, this basic design is preferable for the complex manipulation of suture and needles within the peritoneal cavity.

There are a number of end effector design characteristics that may affect the performance of an alligator-jawed needle driver. Instruments that possess mechanical components that project beyond the diameter of the shaft may interfere with the performance of intracorporeal knot tying. Suture looped around the shaft, above the projecting components, may be caught when the knot is completed (Fig. 11.18).

Design constraints result in alligator-jawed instruments that exert a limited

206   GYNECOLOGIC ENDOSCOPY: Principles in Practice

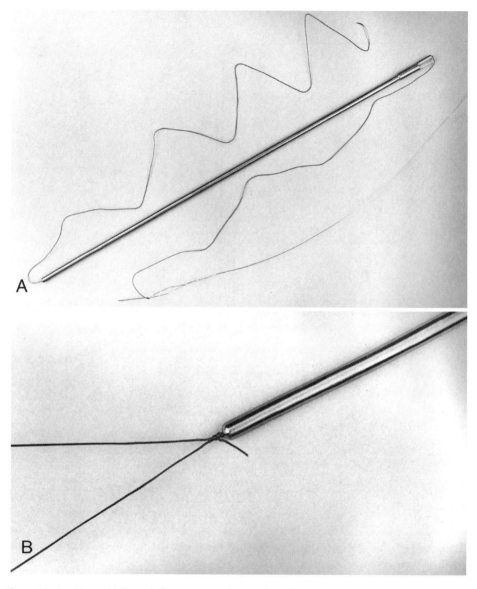

Figure 11.10. Type IV (Channeled) Knot Manipulators. These devices are available in both disposable and nondisposable forms (pictured). **A, B.** The device may be loaded either before or after the ligature or suture has been positioned. **C, D.** Withdrawal of the wire loads the ligature through the channel.

amount of pressure upon the needle, allowing it to twist with a relatively mild degree of torque. Such an undesirable result may be minimized with the selection of needles with a flat edge, reducing the tendency to rotate while gripped. The jaw's surface characteristics may affect function. Those needle drivers with grooved jaws may be less able to hold a needle securely when it is positioned anywhere but aligned with the grooves.

The limitations of alligator jaw designs have spawned the development of a variety of means by which the needle may be affixed to the end of the driver.

Chapter 11: Laparoscopic Suturing Techniques 207

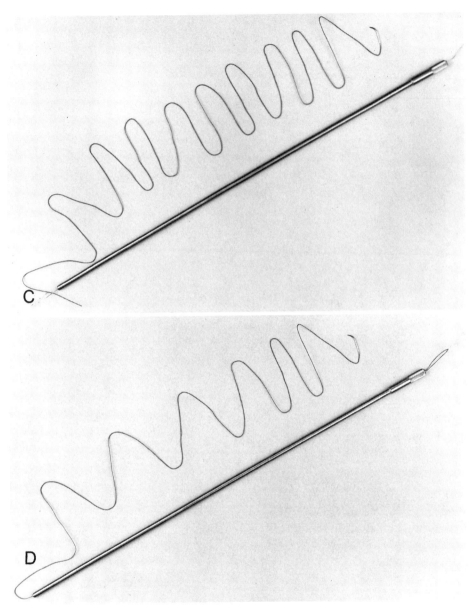

Figure 11.10. (continued)

Most of the newer designs are based upon a side loading mechanism. Such an end effector may effectively fix the needle in a way that is more resistant to torsion because it exploits the curve of the needle to create a stable mount. Consequently, such drivers may be preferable when passing needles at difficult angles, or through tough tissue such as the ileopectinate (Cooper's) ligament. However, these needle drivers have some limitations. The needle can be loaded at only one angle to the shaft and the spring is very stiff, a feature that most can

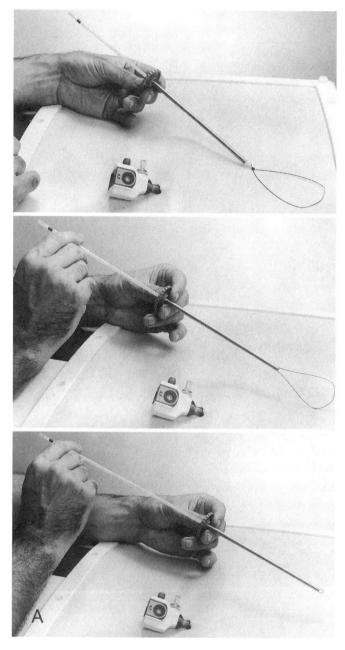

Figure 11.11. Pretied Loop Ligatures. **A.** The device is backloaded into an introducer sleeve. **B.** Then the assembly is inserted into the peritoneal cavity via a laparoscopic cannula. **C** and **D.** A suitable grasping forceps is passed through the loop to grasp the pedicle. The loop is slipped over the pedicle and the knot positioned by the manipulator in the desired location. **E.** The end of the manipulator is snapped, freeing the main body to be advanced, thereby closing the loop. **F.** Moderate traction is applied for about 8 seconds, and excess ligature is cut with laparoscopic scissors.

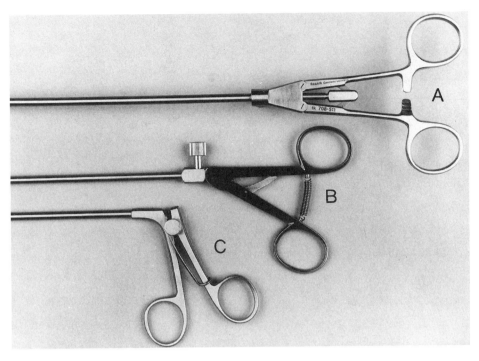

Figure 11.12. Needle Driver Handle Alignment. **A.** Inline. **B.** Partial offset. **C.** Offset.

adapt to, but which may present difficulties to those with small hands. However, the devices are available in left- and right-handed designs as well as two angles, 90° and about 45° (Fig. 11.19). As a result, if, when using a side loading driver, it becomes necessary to position the needle at an angle, a separate needle driver is required. In addition, care must be exercised when manipulating sutures, as they may be cut by the Cook driver's end effector.

Shaft

The shaft of a laparoscopic needle driver joins the handle to the end effector and contains the mechanism for transmitting the movement of the handle to the end effector. Most needle drivers contain an irrigation port near to or in the handle to facilitate cleaning of this mechanism. Laparoscopic needle driver shafts vary in their length and diameter. Most have a length that ranges between 31 and 34 cm. In some situations needle drivers with shafts less than 30 cm may be too short. Although there are a number of 10-mm shafts available, there are few applications where such a design is of additional value. An exception may be the Laurus needle driver (described later). While 5-mm diameter shafts are, in general, more sturdy than the 3-mm variety, the latter may, by virtue of the smaller end effector, be more useful for smaller needles and finer ligatures. Another advantage of 3-mm designs is the ability to directly transfer suture with ski-tipped or small curved needles into the peritoneal cavity through a 5-mm diameter cannula. There is not enough room between the shaft of a 5-mm driver and a 5- to 5.5-mm cannula to allow such a maneuver.

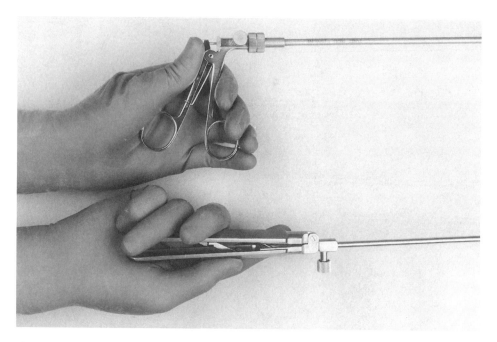

Figure 11.13. Needle Driver Handle Alignment. The more commonly used offset alignment (*top*) offers a mechanical advantage when the surgeon's arm must be extended. The inline variety (*bottom*) is better designed to transfer wrist rotation to the end effector and may be especially helpful when sewing near the anterior abdominal wall.

Needle Driver Alternatives

Ligature Carriers

An alternative method for passing suture through tissue is the laparoscopic ligature carrier first described by Clarke (1). Such an instrument is displayed in Figure 11.20. A free ligature is passed through an "eye" or opening in the sharpened tip and then transferred into the peritoneal cavity via the laparoscopic cannula. Then the tip is driven through the target tissue, carrying the suture with it. After both ends of the suture have been externalized, a knot is fashioned extracorporeally. Other ligature carriers have been designed or modified for use in repair of lacerated abdominal wall vessels such as the deep inferior epigastrics, or for the reapposition of fascial defects created by large laparoscopic cannulas (Fig. 11.21). Some are simple ligature carriers requiring more complicated maneuvers on the part of the surgeon, while others are more complex devices designed to simplify the suturing process.

Mechanical Suturing Devices

These devices have only recently been introduced and have not yet experienced widespread use. Nevertheless, by automating some or several aspects of the suturing process they may provide particular advantages in at least some instances.

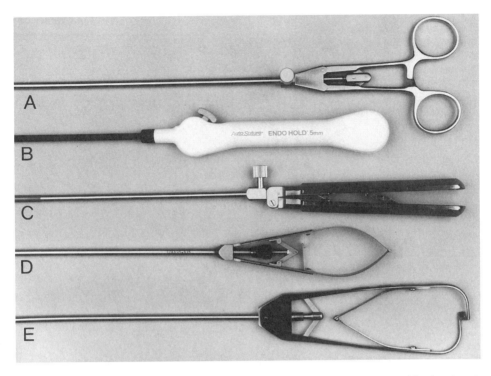

Figure 11.14. Inline Handles. **A.** Classical ratcheted design (Reznik Inc.). **B.** Disposable, thumb activated (United States Surgical Corp.). **C.** Locking handle (Karl Storz Inc.). **D.** Modified ratcheted spring handle (Cabot Inc.). **E.** Castro-Vieho design, ratcheted (Jarit Inc.).

A device with a mechanized end effector design has recently been released by Laurus Medical Corporation and Ethicon Endosurgery. This device, when loaded, will transfer a standard curved needle (Davis & Geck T-19, Ethicon CT-2, United States Surgical Corp. GS-22), into the peritoneal cavity, which, in turn, is driven into tissue by squeezing the plunger in the inline handle. Such a device may be particularly advantageous in instances where a curved needle driver would be used in open surgery or for specific situations, such as the placement of suture in Cooper's ligament (Fig. 11.22*A*).

Borrowing from the technology of the sewing machine, the United States Surgical Corp. "Endo-Stitch" device uses special sutures, but facilitates the performance of running suture, and even may be used to tie intracorporeal knots. The device is pictured in Figure 11.22*B*.

Introducer Sleeves

When transferring needles, suture, or extracorporeal knots into the peritoneal cavity, valved laparoscopic ports may interfere with effective performance of the technique. The needles and instruments can become caught in the valves and the suture may dislodge from the knot manipulator. One solution is to use cannulas without internal valves. However, another option is the use of an introducer sleeve, a hollow cannula that fits inside the laparoscopic port, holding the valve open, but designed wide enough to allow the easy passage of the needle

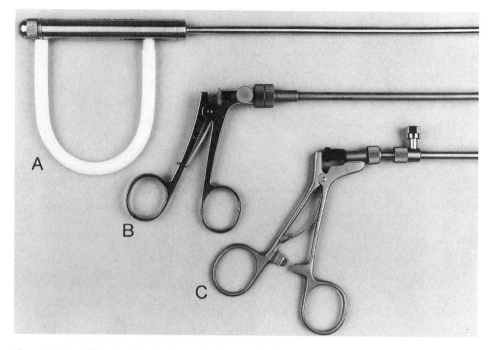

Figure 11.15. Offset Handles. **A.** Spring handle (side loading) from Cook Surgical Inc. **B.** Nonratcheted (Marlow Surgical, Inc.). **C.** Ratcheted (Ethicon).

driver or knot manipulator and accompanying needles or ligatures (Fig. 11.23). Many prepackaged suturing kits containing preformed loops or designed for extracorporeal knotting, include an introducer sleeve.

Clips and Clip Applicators

Clips are an alternative to knots for anchoring or finishing continuous suture. A specific, disposable clip, called *Lapraty*, has been developed by Ethicon-Endosurgery Inc. of Cincinnati, OH. Application of the clips is performed with a nondisposable clip applicator that must be inserted through a cannula 10 mm in diameter or larger (Fig. 11.24). The clips, made of absorbable polyglactin, are designed to secure suture that ranges from 2-0 to 4-0 in caliber.

KNOTS

This section will deal with the basics of knots as they are utilized in laparoscopic surgery. There are basically two types—overhand knots and slip knots. Overhand knots are conceptually simple to understand, can be formed both outside of and within the peritoneal cavity (extracorporeal; intracorporeal), but can sometimes be more difficult to tighten securely. On the other hand, slip knots are more complex than overhand knots, and, practically, can only be fashioned extracorporeally. However, a single slip knot, properly fashioned and tightened, can securely hold a pedicle. The knots also differ in their applicability to delicate tis-

Chapter 11: Laparoscopic Suturing Techniques 213

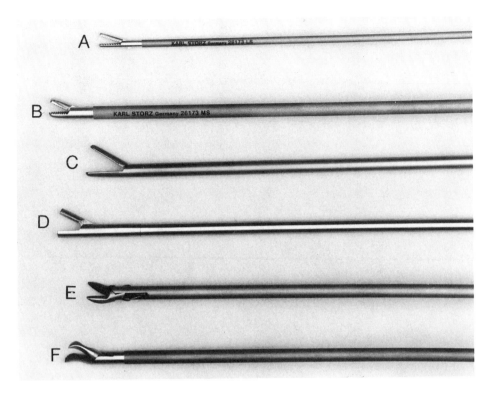

Figure 11.16. Alligator Jaw End Effectors. **A.** 3-mm straight (Karl Storz Inc.). **B.** 5-mm straight (Karl Storz Inc.). **C.** 5-mm straight (Cabot Inc.). **D.** 5-mm straight convex/concave (Resnick). **E.** 5-mm angled Reddick-Saye (Marlow Inc.). **F.** 5-mm angled (Karl Storz).

sue or fine suture, as well as the types of knot manipulators required for their extracorporeal-to-intracorporeal transfer.

Overhand Knots

Even novices are familiar with at least some versions of overhand knots, for they are widely used in sewing and for fastening clothing and shoes. To create a secure fastening, overhand knots are repeated a number of times, depending upon the knot, the tension on the tissue, and the nature of the suture used. Overhand knots may be tied either within the peritoneal cavity (intracorporeal) or outside (extracorporeal) from where they must be transferred to the operative field with a Type I, II, or IV knot manipulator.

Half Hitch

The *half hitch* knot is probably the first knot that anyone learns, and its mechanics form the basis for many other knots used at surgery. In essence, once the tie is secured around the desired object, one end is passed over (or under) the other forming a loop (Fig. 11.25A). When sewing skin, or in most nonsurgical situations, lateral tension on the two ends will result in the loop sliding to, and tightening around, the objective. In most surgery there is an additional need to direct the knot

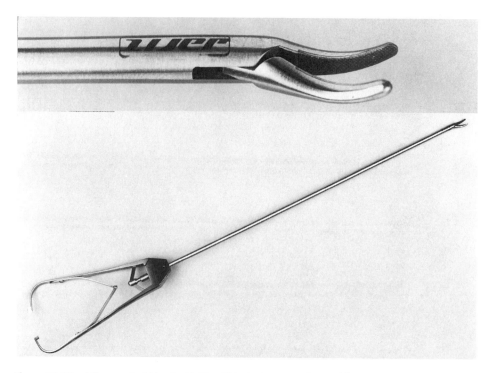

Figure 11.17. Microsurgical Needle Holder. This device, manufactured by Jarit Inc., is capable of securely holding needles swaged onto 5-0 and 6-0 suture for microsurgical work.

to the objective, minimizing the upward tension that could avulse the ligature or shear the tissue. For open surgery this is accomplished by using the index finger on one strand to "push" the knot down, while applying opposing upward traction with the other hand on the other strand. The index finger is actually positioned to facilitate application of force in two opposing vectors, resulting in direction of the knot to the desired site (Fig. 11.26). When a knot manipulator is applied laparoscopically, it is positioned in a fashion that results in the same vectors of force.

Square Knot

A single half hitch is inadequate in itself to secure, for example, a vascular pedicle. Consequently, additional throws are required. The square knot is a series of two half hitches, where the second is formed in the opposite direction to the first (Fig. 11.25B). For example, if the first half hitch is formed "left over right," a square knot is created by fashioning the second hitch "right over left." The square knot is characterized by the fact that both ends come out of the loops on the same side as they "enter" the knot. Gut and silk sutures will generally be made secure with three throws, each of the latter two fashioning square knots.

Granny Knot

A *granny knot* is created if two consecutive half hitches are made in the same direction (Fig. 11.25C). Such knots are more secure than a half hitch alone, but far

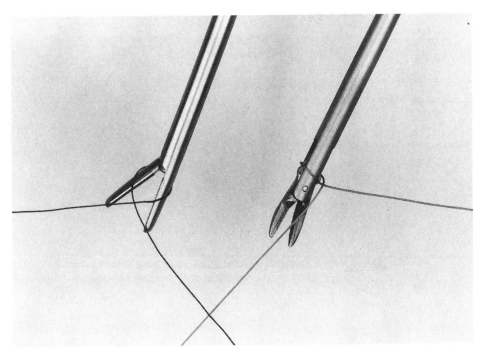

Figure 11.18. Mechanical Impediments to Intracorporeal Knot Tying. Mechanical projections may catch suture, interfering with the mechanics of knot tying. The driver on the *left*, while restricted to one articulating jaw, does not have such a mechanism and therefore may be better designed for intracorporeal tying.

less reliable than a square knot. However, they do not "lock" as a square knot does, a feature that, if premature, compromises the ability of the knot to securely occlude a blood vessel or appose tissue. The advantage of the granny lies in the fact that it can be tightened after it is formed. Consequently, granny knots have a place, but their use should be restricted to the temporary fixation of a ligature, prior to being secured by overlying square knots. This is especially applicable to braided synthetic sutures such as Vicryl (Ethicon Inc.), Dexon (Davis & Geck), and Polysorb (United States Surgical Corp.). This type of ligature can be tied with an initial granny knot, followed by two square knots, making a total of four overhand throws necessary for knot security.

Surgeon's Knot

A *surgeon's knot* is formed by creating a half hitch, then repeating the maneuver one more time in the same direction—a double throw (Fig. 11.25D). The surgeon's knot is more secure than the half hitch, and, like the granny knot, is generally adequate for temporary fixation of the ligature while additional square knots are fashioned to secure it in place.

Slip Knots

Most individuals have had limited experience with the formation of slip knots. Consequently, this unfamiliarity, together with the complexity of the knots,

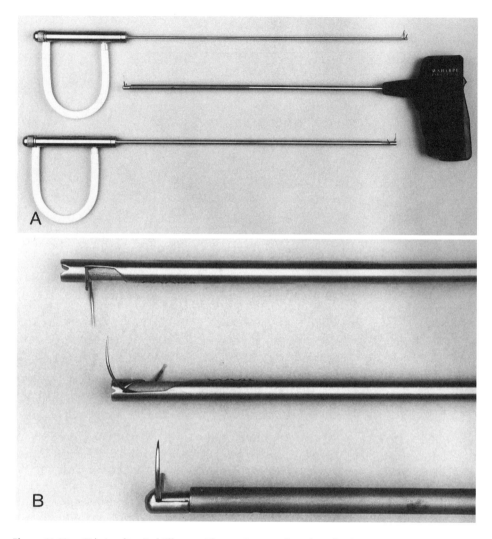

Figure 11.19. Side Loading End Effectors. There exist a number of needle drivers with side loading end effectors. **A.** *Top*, 3-mm Cook Surgical Inc; *middle*, 5-mm Sharpe; *bottom*, Cook Surgical 5-mm. **B.** End Effectors: *Top*, Cook 90°; Cook 45°, Sharpe 90°.

often act as sources of frustration for the novice. Because of their complexity, slip knots are not commonly fashioned within the peritoneal cavity. Instead, they are usually tied extracorporeally and then, using either a Type III or Type IV knot manipulator, transferred into the peritoneal cavity and secured in place. While there exist a number of slip knots that have value in specific surgical situations, each can be slid into place yet remain securely in position.

Roeder Loop

The first slip knot demonstrated safe for laparoscopic surgery was the *Roeder loop*, designed for tonsillectomy, but applied by Semm to vascular pedicles (2). The knot is described in Figure 11.27A and is transferred to the desired loca-

Chapter 11: Laparoscopic Suturing Techniques 217

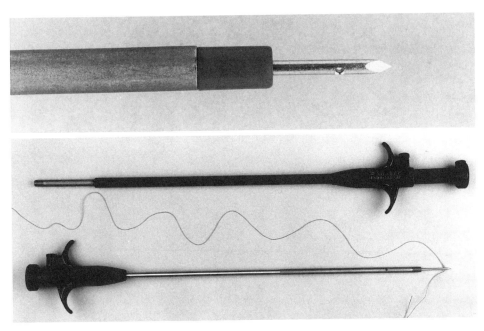

Figure 11.20. Ligature Carriers. Sharpe Endosurgical retractable ligature carrier in 10-mm (*top*) and 5-mm (*middle*) formats. The fenestration on a deployed 5-mm device is shown (*bottom inset*). These devices may be used to fix ligatures in tissue without swaged-on needles. Some of the advantage of this approach is lost by the reduction in manipulation flexibility created by the straight end effector.

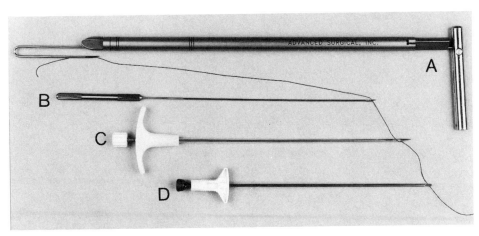

Figure 11.21. Abdominal Wall Suturing Devices. These instruments are ligature carriers that have been designed or modified to close the laparoscopic incisions or ligate bleeding deep inferior epigastric vessels. In all instances the suturing should be directed by a small caliber laparoscope (8 mm or less) in a small diameter port. **A.** Advanced Surgical's device that requires no intracorporeal manipulation of suture. **B.** Nondisposable ligature carrier and snare (Reznik Inc.). The closed eye of the device may be used to pass the ligature into the peritoneal cavity while the open eye snares the end intracorporeally so that it completes the loop. **C.** Medical Concepts; these devices possess side notches that are used to fix the ligature for insertion. Then they are reloaded inside the peritoneal cavity after positioning the other side of the closure. **D.** Endoknot, patterned after the Veress needle (United States Surgical Corp.).

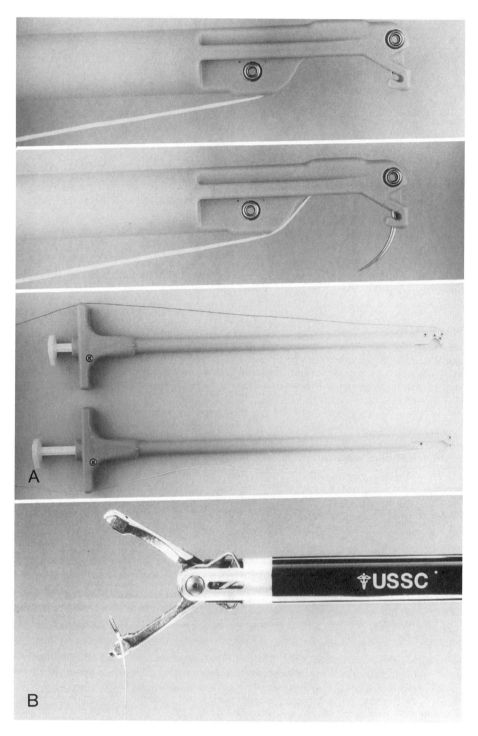

Figure 11.22. Mechanized Suturing Devices. **A.** Laurus medical device designed to place curved needles of a predetermined configuration (e.g., Ethicon Inc. CT-2). Designed for Cooper's ligament, the device can simulate the action of a Heaney needle driver. **B.** United States Surgical's Endo-Stitch can form running closures with specially designed needles. The instrument can be used to tie as well.

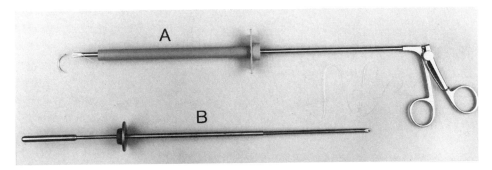

Figure 11.23. Introducer Sleeves. The introducer sleeve bypasses any valves that could catch instruments, needles, or suture. **A.** The device can also be used to backload a needle and needle driver (prior to inserting the whole assembly into the cannula); or (**B**) allow easier transfer of an extracorporeal knot into the peritoneal cavity with a knot manipulator.

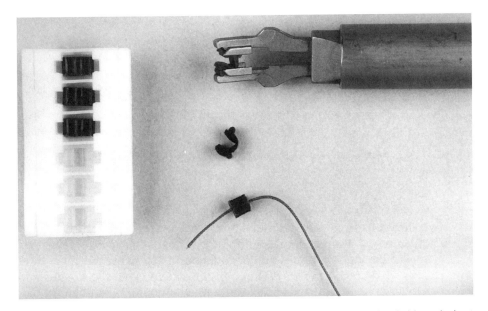

Figure 11.24. The Ethicon Lapraty System. Cartridges containing synthetic, absorbable, polyglactin clips are loaded singly into the specially designed 10-mm diameter reusable, hand activated applicator. The clips may be applied securely to suture ranging from 2-0 to 4-0 in caliber.

tion with a Type III (notched) or Type IV (channeled) knot manipulator. The amount of tension applied is important, as too little will result in inadequate compression on the pedicle, while too much can cause breakdown of the knot, or breakage of the suture. Moderate pressure for about 6 to 8 seconds is ideal; more may actually decrease knot security (11). This knot should be relied upon only if fashioned out of gut. When used for braided or monofilament suture, the knot is not as secure (4, 12). The slippage may be reduced by adding a half hitch after the Roeder knot is positioned satisfactorily.

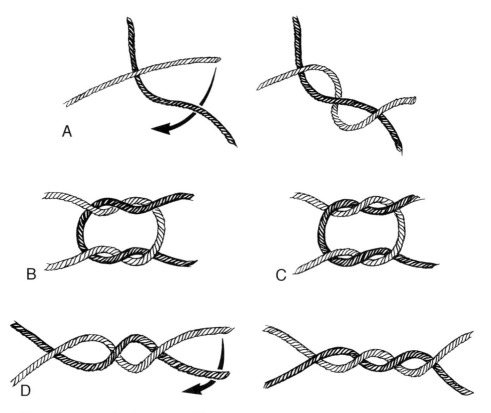

Figure 11.25. Overhead Knots. **A.** Half hitch. **B.** Square knot. **C.** Granny knot. **D.** Surgeon's knot.

Other

Two slip knots have been described that may be superior to the Roeder loop for monofilament or braided suture (Fig. 11.27A). The *Weston knot* (9) starts in a fashion identical to the Roeder but differs dramatically following the initial throw (Fig. 11.27B). This knot is transferred in a fashion identical to the Roeder knot. The *Duncan loop* is also reported secure for braided ligature. With either of these knots, an additional half hitch may provide an added degree of security (Fig. 11.27C). Hasson has described the use of a noose knot useful for anchoring running sutures or to replace the first throw of an interrupted knot (6).

LAPAROSCOPIC SUTURING TECHNIQUE

Suturing techniques may be used to ligate blood vessels for the purpose of hemostasis, for reconstructive surgery, or to repair intentional or accidental incisions. The competent laparoscopic surgeon should have the skills to pass needles and ligatures into the peritoneal cavity, position them in or around the target tissue, and then to fasten them securely.

The selection of instruments, needles, and suture depends upon the task to be performed and the individual preferences of the surgeon. In addition, there are generally a number of methods by which a given task can be successfully and

Chapter 11: Laparoscopic Suturing Techniques   221

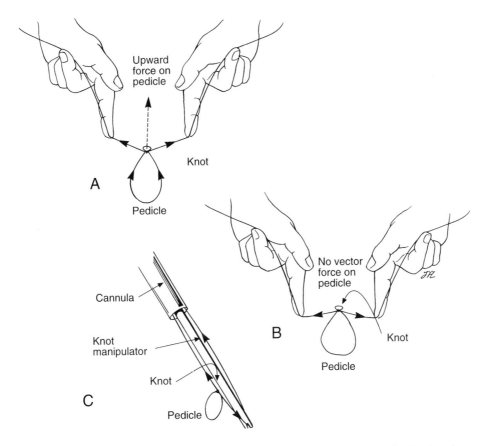

Figure 11.26. Direction of Traction When Securing an Overhead Knot. Closure and tightening of overhand knots requires opposing force applied to each end of the ligature. If the target is not aligned with the vectors of force (**A**) the ligature may avulse or shear the tissue. Instead, both vectors of force and the target are best maintained in the same plane, using fingers (**B**) or using a knot manipulator (**C**).

effectively completed. Because there are so many alternatives, the novice is often bewildered, drifting among a number of techniques and mastering none. Consequently, it is generally preferable to become facile at the performance of a single technique, and then experiment with other methods that may seem to have merit. In this section, the reader will be presented with a limited number of options, that, in the opinion of the author, will allow the surgeon the ability to meet any task likely to require the use of suture. In order to establish convention, the descriptions of technique will assume that the surgeon is right handed and is standing on the patient's left side, viewing a television monitor located at the foot of the operating table.

Preparation and Tissue Orientation

When beginning a laparoscopic procedure where suturing is to be contemplated, it is important to select appropriate ancillary cannulas and to position them in an optimal location. If relatively large needles are to be used, large diam-

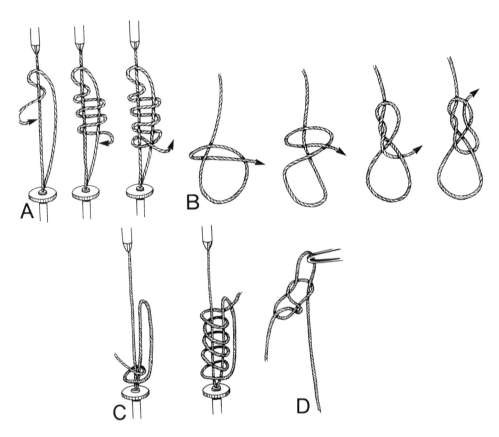

Figure 11.27. Slip Knots. **A.** The *Roeder loop* is started with a half hitch, then the short end of the ligature is wrapped around both itself and the long end three times, the last in the form of a second half hitch, around the long end. **B.** The *Weston clinch knot* starts with a half hitch around the long end of the suture, forming a loop. Then the short end is thrown in the opposite direction around the other side of the loop in a half hitch. Subsequently, it is passed over and around the long end and the short end and then back through the loop, so that both short and long ends "enter" the loop on the same side. **C.** The *Duncan knot* is fashioned by wrapping the short or free end of the suture around both ends, from bottom to top four times. **D.** The *Noose knot* is formed by creating a half hitch near the end of the suture with an important variation—instead of drawing the whole long end through, a portion is doubled up to form a loop which is passed through the loop of the half hitch, forming a noose.

eter ports will be required. Alternatively, if, for cosmetic reasons, small caliber cannulas are utilized instead, care should be taken to position them lateral to the rectus muscles in areas where subcutaneous tissue is minimal. Prior to suturing, it is necessary to orient the tissue to the visual field of the surgeon. The laparoscope should be stabilized by an assistant or a suitable positioning device. Adequate exposure of the tissue must be obtained, either by manipulation of the patient's position by adjusting the table, or by the use of an assistant providing intraperitoneal retraction. The needle drivers should be inserted through ports that are as close as possible to being equidistant from the target tissue that, in turn, should be centralized in the surgeon's field of view (Fig. 11.28).

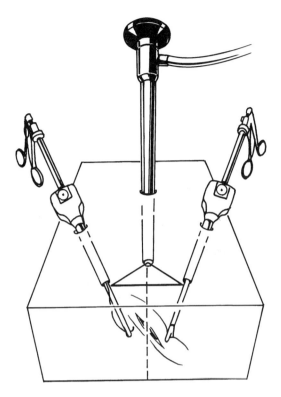

Figure 11.28. Triangulation of Instruments. The two needle manipulators and the laparoscope should ideally form an isosceles triangle, with the target tissue distal to, but equidistant from, the two hand instruments.

Insertion of Needles into the Peritoneal Cavity

Needles with swaged-on suture must be passed into the peritoneal cavity prior to use. *Straight needles* are the easiest to insert. They may be introduced directly into the peritoneal cavity via the laparoscopic port after grasping the suture near the attachment point with the needle. Then, the needle driver is passed through the cannula and into the abdomen, dragging the needle with it (Fig. 11.29). For this technique, the diameter of the needle driver must be comfortably less than that of the cannula to allow the free passage of the needle into the peritoneal cavity. Catching of the needle on the valves of the cannula may be eliminated with the use of valveless cannulas or an introducer sleeve (Fig. 11.23). Some surgeons prefer to backload the needle into the introducer sleeve prior to inserting the assembly into the peritoneal cavity via the laparoscopic cannula. *Ski-tipped* designs may be inserted by an identical technique but, to allow passage of the bent portion of the needle, require slightly more room between the needle driver and the cannula sleeve.

Curved needles are, in general, more difficult to pass into and out of the peritoneal cavity. Relatively small needles may be directly inserted in a fashion identical to that described above for the straight and ski-tipped varieties. Slightly larger diameter curved needles may be directly inserted via larger laparoscopic

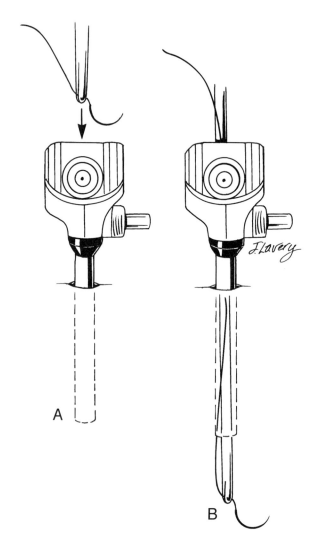

Figure 11.29. Direct Intraperitoneal Insertion of Straight or Curved Needles. **A.** The suture is grasped near its attachment to the needle before the needle driver is inserted into the cannula. **B.** Then the needle driver is passed into the peritoneal cavity, drawing the needle with it. The process is facilitated with the use of an introducer sleeve or a valveless cannula.

ports, preferably using those without valves or, alternatively, via a suitable introducer sleeve. The insertion may be facilitated by carefully bending the needle to a diameter that allows its insertion via the cannula.

Virtually any large curved needles may be passed into, and removed from, the peritoneal cavity through a 5-mm incision, provided they are swaged onto the suture. For this method to be effective, the cannula locations should be in the thinner aspect of the abdomen lateral to the rectus muscles, as the skin track is more likely to stay open, allowing easier reinsertion of the needle driver (Fig. 11.30).

Chapter 11: Laparoscopic Suturing Techniques 225

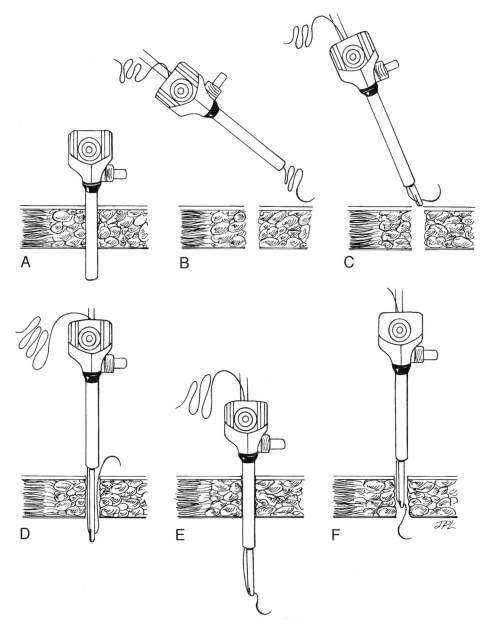

Figure 11.30. Intraperitoneal Insertion and Removal of Curved Needles Through Small Caliber Ports. **A.** Cannulas should be placed lateral to the rectus abdominus muscle. The cannula is removed from the abdominal wall. **B.** Then the needle driver is passed back into and through the cannula to grasp the long end, which is pulled through the cannula. **C.** Now, the end of the ligature is released and the driver is passed back into and through the cannula, where it is used to regrasp the suture at a point proximal to the needle. This should be approximately 2 cm more than the thickness of the abdominal wall. **D.** Then the needle driver, grasping the suture, with the laparoscopic cannula hanging like a collar, is inserted through the now empty incision into the peritoneal cavity, dragging the needle with it. **E.** The cannula may now be slid into place over the driver, using it as a guide. **F, G.** After positioning the suture, the needle is removed by grasping the suture with the needle driver at the same location. Then the cannula is removed so that the suture and attached needle are removed by the needle driver.

Suture, Needle, and Needle Driver Selection

To preserve flexibility in the intracorporeal manipulation of needles, two identical needle drivers are preferred, suitable in design for the task at hand, bearing in mind the tissue, the needle, and the suture. In some instances, such as when side-loading drivers are used, it will be necessary to use instruments that differ from each other in their design. However, use of dissimilar devices adds an unnecessary degree of potential confusion and technical complexity, as each hand must behave differently to achieve the same mechanical result. If intracorporeal tying is to be performed, alligator-jawed needle drivers are preferred. Not infrequently, manipulation of the tissue with a needle driver is unsatisfactory. In such instances, a toothed grasping forceps may be used, with a handle design similar to the needle driver. Care should be exercised when using such a device to manipulate needles, as it is less effective and more prone to damage.

If fine suture (5-0 or 6-0 caliber) is used, a needle driver specifically designed for small caliber needles is preferred (Fig. 11.17). Larger caliber suture and needles will require the use of more sturdy needle drivers. However, in most instances, it is preferred that larger caliber sutures, such as the 0 or 2-0 varieties, be used to ligate vascular pedicles using an extracorporeal technique. Other advantages and disadvantages of the various types of needle drivers were described previously.

The type and caliber of suture selected will depend upon a number of factors, including the tissue being opposed and the preferences of the surgeon. For intracorporeal overhead knots, braided suture is generally preferred over the monofilament variety because it is easier to tie securely. However, monofilament ligature can be secured satisfactorily using extracorporeal techniques to fashion either overhand or slip knots. At the present time, it is difficult to work with suture finer in caliber than 6-0, given the available instruments and considering the resolution of current television monitors. New microsurgical instruments are forthcoming, capable of securely holding 8-0 needles.

The length of the suture should be the minimal amount necessary to accomplish the task. While this minimizes the chance for entanglement of the suture, too little suture will prevent the surgeon from accomplishing an intracorporeal tie. For a single intracorporeal stitch, about five inches (13 cm) is usually appropriate; for running stitches, the allowance should be about ½ to 1 inch (1–2 cm) per pass depending upon the distance from the tissue edge and between bites. An additional length of suture should be accounted for (2–5 inches; 5–13 cm) depending upon the selected method for finishing the stitch. Ligatures for extracorporeal knotting must be at least 75 cm in length for overhand ties, and 100 cm or more for slip knots, accounting for the distance between the ligature site and the surgeon's hands, and allowing adequate length to form the knot.

Needle Manipulation

These maneuvers are described pictorially in Figure 11.31. The surgeon should strive for an economy of movement, anticipating moves several steps in advance of actually performing them. Orientation of the needle in the driver is

Chapter 11: Laparoscopic Suturing Techniques 227

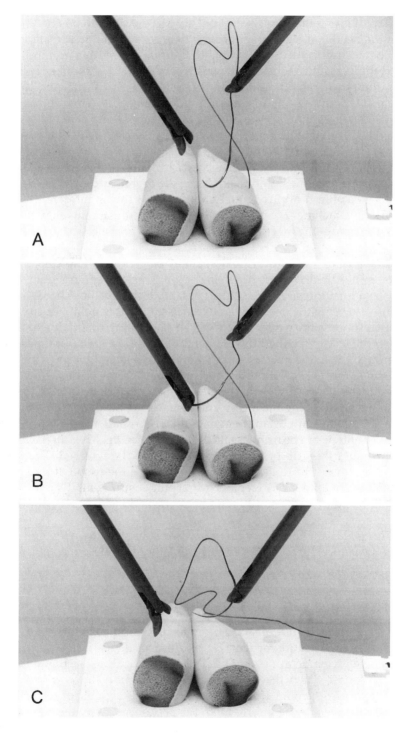

Figure 11.31. Intracorporeal Needle Manipulation. *Right-Left-Right.* **A.** The *right* needle driver grasps the suture near the swaged-on point. **B.** Is transferred to the *left* needle driver, grasping the needle near its tip. **C.** The needle is transferred back to the *right* side where it is grasped in an appropriate location by the right driver.

the first step. It is generally easier, but not always possible, to position the plane or axis of the needle at right angles to the long axis of the driver, allowing the needle to be positioned at a right angle to the shaft. With this in mind, the following "right-left-right" series of steps is recommended. First, the *right* needle driver continues to grasp the suture in the fashion used to enter the peritoneal cavity near the point where it is swaged onto the needle. Then the *left* needle driver is used to grasp the needle near its distal end, taking care not to damage the pointed tip. The right driver is now used, if necessary, to orient the needle for its eventual transfer, either by nudging the needle itself, or by altering its position by tugging on the suture. When a satisfactory position is achieved, the needle is transferred from the left to the *right* needle driver, and fixed in the desired position by grasping it approximately one-third of the circumference as measured from the attachment to the suture. Any final adjustments may be accomplished by tapping the needle with the left driver before the handles are squeezed or locked.

Prior to placing the suture, the tissue may be grasped, if necessary, with either the other needle driver or a toothed grasping instrument, orienting and stabilizing it in a position suitable for the passage of the needle. The right needle driver is used to bring the needle close to the tissue. At this point, for curved needles, in open surgery, the driver is "cocked" by pronating (palm down) the right wrist. Then the wrist is rotated toward a supine position (palm up), passing the needle through the tissue in a fashion that minimizes lateral torque. However, in laparoscopic surgery, such motions may not only be impossible, they can be counterproductive. In many instances, it is more appropriate to push the needle through tissue, minimizing the arc by grasping the needle closer to the midpoint of the arc. It is always important to maintain a grip on the needle with the right needle driver until it can be firmly secured with the needle driver in the left hand. Only then should the grip of the right needle driver be released. Then the left driver may be employed to draw the needle through the tissue. If the device in the left hand is not a needle driver, but a grasping instrument, it should be used only to stabilize the needle until it can be regrasped by the driver in the right hand.

Knotting and anchoring will be described subsequently. However, if after anchoring the suture, further bites are required, the steps described above are repeated as necessary.

Ligature Carriers

An alternate to the use of swaged-on needles and needle drivers is the use of free ligatures and ligature carriers (Fig. 11.20). This device is best suited for use in association with extracorporeal tying. The desired ligature is fed into the eye of the ligature carrier. Then the instrument is passed into the peritoneal cavity through a laparoscopic port. If the tip of the carrier is capable of retraction into the shaft, the device may be inserted into the peritoneal cavity through any type of cannula. However, ideally, the device is passed into the peritoneal cavity via an introducer sleeve or a valveless cannula. Then as the target is oriented, preferably with a pointed and/or toothed grasping forceps, the tip of the ligature carrier is passed through the tissue. The process is depicted in Figure 11.32.

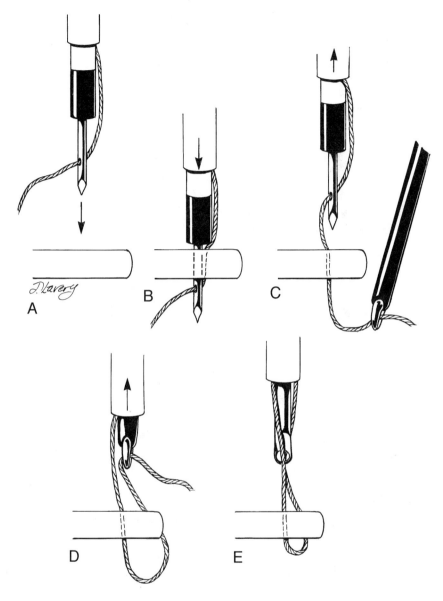

Figure 11.32. Use of a Ligature Carrier. **A** and **B.** The loaded ligature carrier is passed through the target tissue. **C.** A grasping forceps is used to hold and stabilize the ligature while the ligature carrier is removed. **D.** A second grasper retrieves the intracorporeal end and externalizes it while the first grasper feeds ligature into the peritoneal cavity to prevent shearing of the pedicle. **E.** Then the pedicle is secured with a knot tied extracorporeally and secured with a suitable knot manipulator.

Laparoscopic Knotting

Intracorporeal Ties

These ties may be used to anchor a running stitch or may be applied in interrupted fashion. The concept is identical to the technique learned and used by many for suturing skin lacerations or wounds (Fig. 11.33).

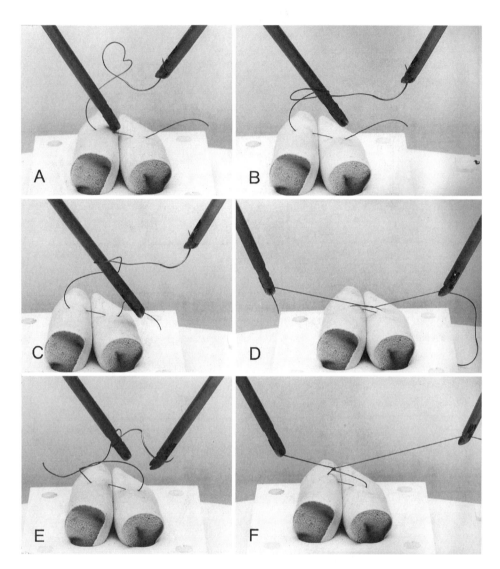

Figure 11.33. Intracorporeal Overhand Tie. First the suture is positioned, as desired, in tissue. **A.** The needle is held in the right with the concave surface up and the heel of the needle to the left. **B.** The heel of the needle is used to wrap the suture over and under the left needle driver once, forming a half hitch. **C.** The left driver picks up the short end of the suture, which is pulled through the loop. **D.** The knot is tightened. **E** and **F.** To form a square knot the procedure is repeated in the opposite direction under and over.

Half Hitches and Variations

Required Materials:

- Short suture ligature, about 12 cm long.
- Two laparoscopic ports, at least 5 mm diameter.
- Introducer sleeve (or valveless cannula).
- Laparoscopic scissors.
- Laparoscopic needle drivers × 2.

Transfer into the peritoneal cavity and positioning of the suture has been described above. It is assumed that the needle has been passed from right to left. A short end, or tail, about one inch long (2–3 cm) is left so that it can be easily seen in the surgeon's field of view. One driver is held in each hand with the end effectors near the site where the ligature is to be secured. The first tie is started by holding the needle with the right driver, near its tip, so that the concavity (if curved or ski-tipped) is directed upward. Then, with the right hand, the suture is loosely wrapped around the distal end of the left driver. If additional knot security is desired, a double wrap is fashioned around the needle driver, a maneuver that will result in the formation of a surgeon's knot. Following this, the left driver is directed toward the short end of the suture, while the right side maintains its grasp on the needle. The short end is grasped by the right needle driver and is drawn through the loop forming the half hitch or surgeon's knot. With the two needle drivers applying traction in opposite directions, the knot is secured. If a long suture is used, as for a running closure, the above steps remain the same. However, it will be necessary to tie the knot by holding suture in the right, without the benefit of the mechanical advantage provided by the needle. For this reason, the author usually anchors running closures with the noose knot described below.

If a half hitch is used, the second throw should be a half hitch formed in the same direction, forming a "granny" knot. The advantage of this is that any slippage of the first knot can be corrected with traction. Two subsequent throws should be fashioned in opposite directions, forming a secure square knot. If a surgeon's knot is the first hitch thrown, the subsequent throws are thrown in opposite directions.

Noose Knots. Noose knots can be fashioned in the field (Fig. 11.34), or purchased pretied. They may be used effectively and efficiently to anchor a running suture or to function as the first knot in an interrupted stitch. The principal value of these sutures is the ability to cinch a knot with a limited number of movements.

Required Materials:

- Short suture ligature, about 15–20 cm.
- Two laparoscopic ports, at least 5-mm diameter.
- Introducer sleeve or valveless cannula.
- Laparoscopic scissors.
- Laparoscopic needle drivers × 2.

A suture of appropriate composition, caliber, and length is prepared with a noose knot at the end and is inserted into the peritoneal cavity via one of the ports. The needle is used to position the suture in tissue and then is passed through the open loop, pulling the suture with it, and applying traction until the loop closes. If the suture is to be of the running variety, the surgeon may proceed directly to complete the closure. If an interrupted stitch is to be performed, additional throws are fashioned, ends are cut with scissors, and the needle removed.

Finishing Knots. Running sutures can be finished with intracorporeal knotting techniques, as well as the clips described below. The most simple ap-

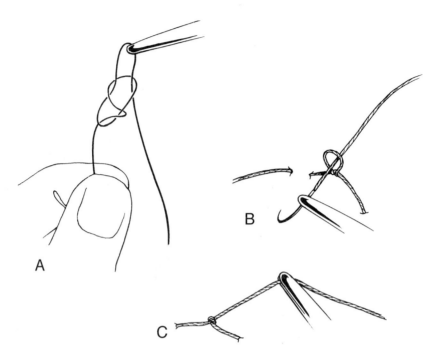

Figure 11.34. Pretied Noose Knots. **A.** The noose knot is fashioned at the end of the suture. **B** and **C.** Once the stitch is placed, the needle is drawn through the loop, tightening it until secure.

proach is to double back to the original anchoring knot, finishing with overhand square knots. Alternatively, the second to last stitch may be doubled with a loop and tied in an overhand fashion to the single end, an approach often taken in open surgery. A novel technique is a form of slip knot call the *Aberdeen knot* or crochet knot, a secure double-looped version of a slip knot (Fig. 11.35).

Clip Ties. The securing of a ligature with a clip is a method that may save time, particularly for the novice. It is important to understand that only specially designed clips should be used for this purpose, for the closure may not be as secure with other clips (Fig. 11.24). In addition, the available clips are designed to secure only those ligatures that range from 4-0 to 2-0 in caliber. The method may be used at either end of a running closure or to secure interrupted stitches.

Required Materials:

- Adequate length of 2-0 to 4-0 caliber suture ligature.
- Two ancillary laparoscopic ports, one 5 mm in diameter, the other at least 10 mm in diameter.
- Absorbable clips designed to secure suture (Lapraty, Ethicon, Inc.).
- Dedicated clip applicator (10-mm diameter).
- Two laparoscopic needle drivers or one driver and one grasping forceps.
- 10-mm introducer sleeve.
- Laparoscopic scissors.

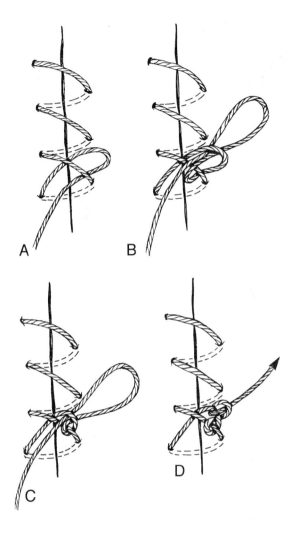

Figure 11.35. *Aberdeen* Finishing Knot. **A.** The end of the suture is looped through the loop formed by the last stitch. **B.** A second loop is passed through the first. **C.** The first loop is tightened before the free end of the suture is passed through the second loop **D**, which is tightened with traction, finishing the knot.

The suture is prepared by attaching a clip to its free end with the clip applicator (Fig. 11.36). Then the needle driver is passed through the introducer sleeve, grasping the suture near the attachment with the needle. After withdrawing the needle driver and the ligature into the sleeve (backloading), the assembly is inserted into the large cannula. The driver is advanced, placing the suture with attached needle in the peritoneal cavity, where it is positioned in the tissue as described previously. If a running suture is to be created, the suture is drawn through the tissue to the location of the clip, which now serves as an anchor. At the end of the running closure, the applicator is used intraperitoneally to affix the second anchoring clip. If, instead, an interrupted stitch is to be fashioned, the suture is pulled tightly as the clip applicator is used to apply a second clip, thus securing the stitch in place.

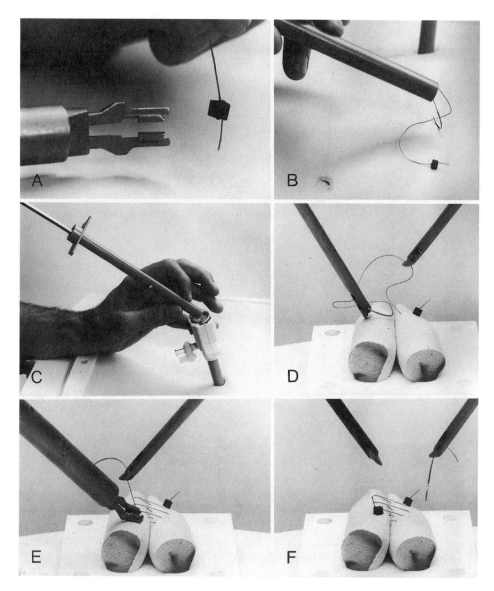

Figure 11.36. Clip Ligatures and Stitches. **A–C.** The first clip is attached extracorporeally to the end of the suture and then inserted into the peritoneal cavity, using a needle driver and an introducer sleeve. **D.** A running stitch is created, using the clip as an anchor. **E** and **F.** A second clip is added to secure the closure.

Extracorporeal Ties

Extracorporeal ties are used when the required amount of knot tension cannot be applied predictably via intracorporeal techniques. Examples include securing vascular pedicles like the uterine vessels or when tying sutures used for retropubic suspension of the bladder. Generally, large caliber suture is used and the surgeon must take care not to shear the target tissue during the ligature manipulation.

Half Hitches and Surgeons Knots

Required Materials:

- Long ligature, at least 75 cm.
- Two ancillary laparoscopic ports, at least 5 mm in diameter.
- Type I (open ended) or Type II (closed) knot manipulator.
- Introducer sleeve or valveless cannula.
- Laparoscopic scissors.
- Two laparoscopic needle drivers or grasping forceps.

Preparation:

The cannulas are preferably positioned to form an isosceles triangle, the apex of which is defined by the site of entrance of the laparoscope into the peritoneal cavity (Fig. 11.28). If curved needles are to be passed into the peritoneal cavity (described previously), care should be taken to locate the cannulas lateral to the lateral edge of the rectus muscles. Suture manipulation is facilitated if the target tissue is located caudal to the base of the triangle and near the line that bisects the angle at the apex—therefore equidistant from the two ancillary ports. Prior to passing a free ligature, the target pedicle is identified, isolated, and stabilized.

Passing the Ligature Around the Pedicle:

The steps employed in passing the ligature are depicted in Figure 11.37. First, the introducer sleeve is passed through the laparoscopic cannula. This step is not absolutely necessary, particularly if a cannula without internal valves is used. Then one end of the ligature is grasped with a laparoscopic needle driver or suitable grasping forceps and passed through the port into the peritoneal cavity. The ligature is fed around the pedicle, with the aid of a second grasper or needle driver passed through the other ancillary cannula. The suture is then brought back out through the first cannula while, simultaneously, the second forceps is used to feed the rest of its length into the peritoneal cavity. This prevents traction on, or shearing of, the pedicle by the braided suture. Both ends of the ligature are now externalized through the same port. When an adequate length has been exteriorized, the knot can be hand tied.

Tying, Transferring, and Securing the Knot:

The knot-tying steps are shown in Figure 11.38. Either a half hitch or a surgeon's knot may be used, although with the Type I manipulator the former version is more easily transferred. The knot manipulator is held in one hand, while, with the other hand, a mild degree of traction is exerted on both ends of the suture. One end is hooked over the index and one over the little finger. The knot is advanced toward the pedicle, still holding the ends of the suture in one hand, and simultaneously using the other hand to apply the necessary traction with the manipulator. Tightening is achieved by applying traction on the two strands, varying the tension on the two by rocking the hand at the wrist, simultaneously using the manipulator as a pulley, located distal to the pedicle, thereby creating the opposing vectors of force necessary for securing the knot. Once the knot is tightened sufficiently, the manipulator is removed. Additional hitches can be added as re-

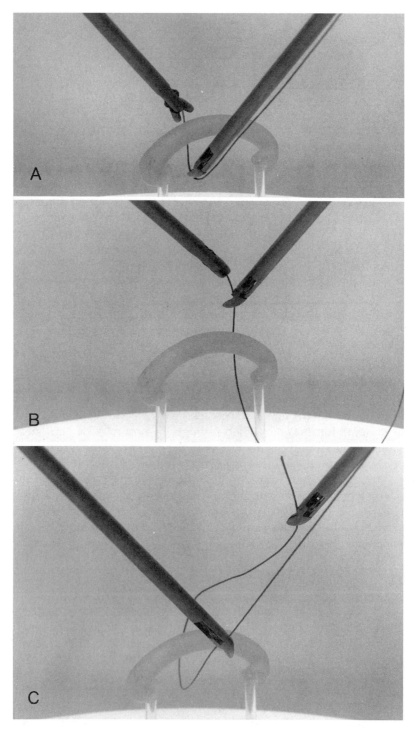

Figure 11.37. Passing a Ligature Around a Pedicle. **A–C.** Feeding the ligature around the pedicle. One end of the suture is fed into the peritoneal cavity as the other is withdrawn to reduce shearing and trauma on the pedicle.

Chapter 11: Laparoscopic Suturing Techniques 237

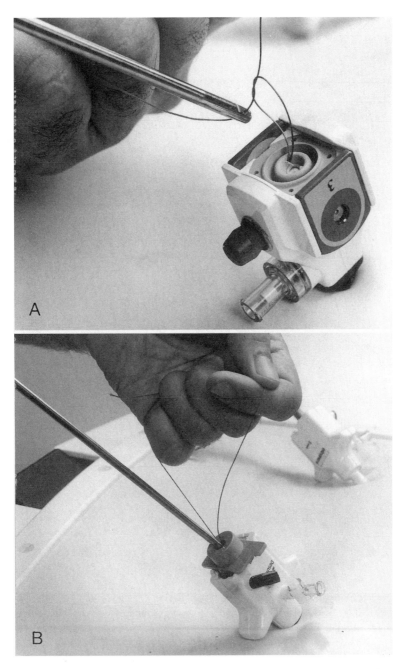

Figure 11.38. Extracorporeal Tie with Type I Knot Manipulator. The ligature is already positioned around the target tissue with both ends externalized. **A.** A half hitch knot is created and the knot manipulator is positioned to the side and above the knot. **B.** The knot is transferred into the cannula or introducer sheath, keeping a slight degree of tension on the ligature ends, and advanced into the peritoneal cavity.

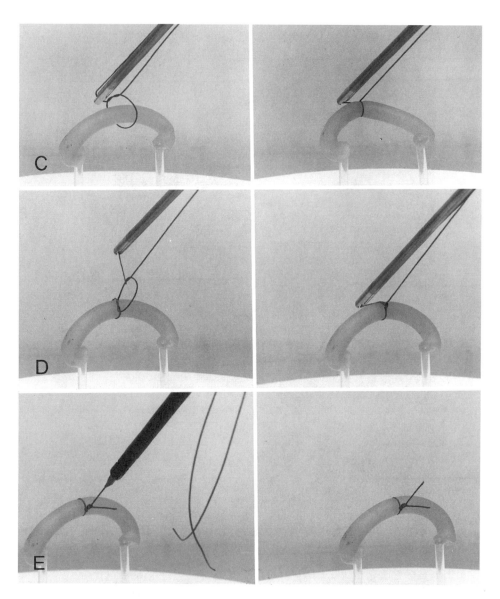

Figure 11.38. **C.** Tension is applied equally to both ends—this can be accomplished by holding them on opposite sides of the same hand. **D.** Additional throws are added as necessary—it is recommended that the first be a granny knot. **E.** The excess ligature is cut with scissors.

quired—four for braided polygalactide sutures, three for silk or gut, and five or more for monofilament absorbable or nonabsorbable ligatures. The ends of the suture are then cut with scissors, which can be passed into the peritoneal cavity through either cannula.

Sequential Knots:

A series of knots may be created and left extracorporeally or transferred loosely into the peritoneal cavity. Then, using a Type I manipulator (open ended), the knots can be tightened in sequence (Fig. 11.6). Such a maneuver may reduce the chance of slippage between throws caused by extracorporeal manipulation.

Slip Knots. Slip knots have been described previously (Fig. 11.27). The short end is cut short and an appropriate manipulator (Type III or IV) must be used for the purposes of transferring and tightening the knot. In practiced hands they may be used effectively, particularly the loops that may be used for open pedicles like an appendix.

Required Materials:

- Pretied loop ligatures or long suture, about 120 cm long.
- Two ancillary laparoscopic ports, at least 5-mm diameter.
- Type III (notched) or Type IV (channeled) knot manipulator (unless prepackaged loop ligatures used).
- Introducer sleeve (5-mm diameter variety included with many pretied kits).
- Laparoscopic scissors.
- Suitable grasping forceps.

Preparation:

The cannulas, including that used for the laparoscope, are preferably positioned to form an isosceles triangle as for the hitches described above. If a loop ligature is to be fashioned and/or used, the narrowest plane of the structure to be removed must fit through the loop and the pedicle must be narrow enough to allow transfer of knot pressure adequate to occlude the underlying vessel(s). Gut sutures are secured with the Roeder knot while the Weston or Duncan modification is considered preferable for monofilament or braided polyglactin ligatures. There exist a number of prepackaged products that include the suture, the knot pusher, and the introducer sleeve.

Technique:

Description of the creations of various types of extracorporeal slip knots are provided in Figure 11.27. It is critical that the surgeon practice these knots extensively prior to utilizing them for laparoscopic procedures. Loop ligatures may be created prior to entry into the peritoneal cavity, but for closed pedicles such as the infundibulopelvic ligament, the knot can only be created after positioning the ligature around a pedicle.

The necessary steps for positioning the knot are described in Figure 11.11. After backloading the loop into the introducer sleeve, the assembly is inserted into the laparoscopic port and advanced, passing the loop into the peritoneal cavity under direct vision. A suitable laparoscopic forceps is used to grasp the pedicle *through* the preformed loop. Care must be taken to ensure that too much tissue is not included in the ligated pedicle, as an artery or vein may be inadequately compressed and subsequently bleed. For disposable units, the perforated end of the Type IV manipulator is snapped, allowing the suture to be pulled through the central channel. Prior to tightening the loop, the knot is held at the desired spot on the pedicle with the manipulator. Then, the loop is tightened by pulling on the externalized end of the suture. Traction should be placed on the knot for about 6 to 8 seconds. The suture is severed with laparoscopic scissors that may be passed through the same cannula.

To secure closed pedicles the ligature is passed around the pedicle and externalized through the same port as described in Figure 11.38. Then a slip knot is fashioned and transferred into the peritoneal cavity with a Type III or Type IV knot manipulator (Figs. 11.9, 11.10).

ABDOMINAL WALL SUTURING

It is apparent that laparoscopic surgeons must be competent with positioning suture in the abdominal wall under laparoscopic guidance. Injury to the deep inferior epigastric vessels may cause significant bleeding. The increased frequency of incisional dehiscence or hernia, particularly in association with the use of large diameter cannulas, has led to a requirement to repair these defects (see Chapter 12). There exist a number of methods by which hemostasis can be achieved and incisional repairs made.

One approach is to pass large needles through the abdomen to ligate the vessels or reapproximate fascia. Long, straight, "Keith" needles can be inserted into the peritoneal cavity under laparoscopic guidance and then, after turning them around intracorporeally, they can be passed back out, completing the stitch. Such an approach is generally effective in patients with thin abdominal walls, but for even the mildly obese, it is often difficult to transfer the needle out of the abdomen with precision and without injuring the finger of the surgeon. For inferior epigastric artery bleeding, some surgeons use large curved needles to pass suture through all abdominal layers, tying the suture externally. However, the suture must be removed in a delayed fashion and its presence is uncomfortable and inconvenient for the patient. If such an approach is performed for fascial closure of the last incision, bowel could become incorporated in the closure.

Most incisions can be repaired using a standard needle driver to drive a small circumference, but sturdy urological needle such as the UR-6 (Ethicon, Inc.), the TT-20 (Davis & Geck), or the GU-46 (United States Surgical Corp.). A narrow caliber laparoscope is used through a port that does not require closure (less than 10 mm) to ensure that bowel is not caught in the wound. The suture is tied extracorporeally. If there is difficulty inserting the finger in the wound to securely tighten the knot, a Type I or II knot manipulator may be used. The fascia can also be reapproximated using any of the instruments and techniques described for ligation of the inferior epigastric vessels.

The inferior epigastric vessels can be occluded temporarily with a Foley balloon or, occasionally, with unipolar or bipolar desiccation. However, in most instances, suture ligation is preferred. Ligature carriers such as the Peyerra device can be utilized to aid in securing lacerated blood vessels. First the ligature is passed into the peritoneal cavity, through the original incision, directed to one side and inferior to the vessel, then it is externalized after inserting the empty ligature carrier on the other side of the vessel and loading it intracorporeally with a grasping instrument. Following externalization of the suture it can be tied, if necessary with the aid of a knot manipulator.

Unfortunately, threading the closed eye of the Peyerra ligature carrier is somewhat difficult under laparoscopic guidance. As a result, a number of devices

Chapter 11: Laparoscopic Suturing Techniques 241

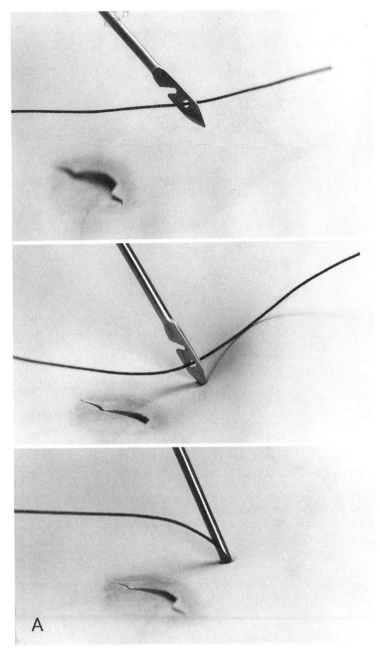

Figure 11.39. Simple Ligature Carrier for Abdominal Wall. This ligature carrier is depicted occluding a blood vessel. **A.** The ligature is passed into the peritoneal cavity on one side of the vessel.

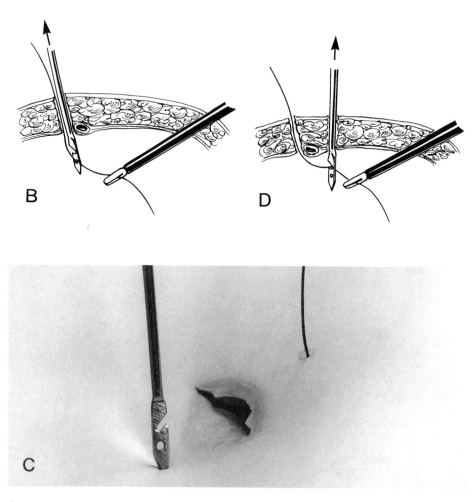

Figure 11.39. **B.** A grasping instrument is used to secure the ligature while the carrier is removed. **C.** The empty carrier is reinserted in the desired spot on the other side of the vessel. **D.** It is loaded usually with the assistance of a grasping forceps. **E** and **F.** The ligature is externalized and tied.

have been developed for use in these circumstances (Fig. 11.21). The simplest devices are ligature carriers that are used to pass the suture into the peritoneal cavity, like the Peyerra device. However, loading these devices for ligature removal is easier as the fixed "eye" has been replaced by a notch designed to catch the suture, preferably with the aid of a grasping device (Fig. 11.39). Other devices have been designed, obviating the need for manipulation with the needle driver (Fig. 11.21*A*).

Chapter 11: Laparoscopic Suturing Techniques

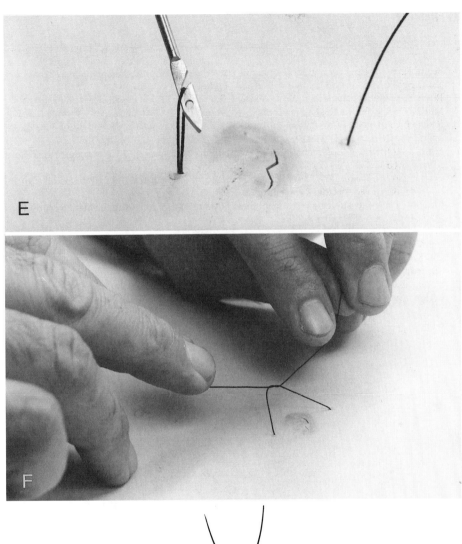

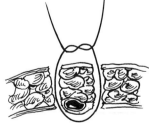

Figure 11.39. (continued)

REFERENCES

1. Clarke HC. Laparoscopy—new instruments for suturing and ligation. Fertil Steril 1972;23: 274–277.
2. Semm K. Tissue puncher and loop-ligation—new ideas for surgical therapeutic pelviscopy (laparoscopy) endoscopic intraabdominal surgery. Endoscopy 1978;10:119–124.
3. Reich H, McGlynn F. Laparoscopic repair of bladder injury. Obstet Gynecol 1990;76:909–910.
4. Marrero MA, Corfman RS. Laparoscopic use of sutures. Clin Obstet Gynecol 1991;34:387–394.
5. Reich H, Clarke HC, Sekel L. A simple method for ligating with straight and curved needles in operative laparoscopy. Obstet Gynecol 1992;79:143–147.
6. Hasson HM. Suture loop techniques to facilitate microsurgical and laparoscopic procedures. J Repro Med 1987;32:765–767.
7. Nathanson LK, Easter DW, Cuschieri A. Ligation of the structures of the cystic pedicle during laparoscopic cholecystectomy. Am J Surg 1991;161:350–354.
8. McComb PF. A new suturing instrument that allows the use of microsuture at laparoscopy. Fertil Steril 1992;57:936–938.
9. Weston PV. A new clinch knot. Obstet Gynecol 1991;78:144–147.
10. Clarke HC. An improved ligator in operative laparoscopy. Obstet Gynecol 1994;83:299–300.
11. Hay DL, Levine RL, von Fraunhofer JA, Masterson BJ. Chromic gut pelviscopic loop ligature. Effect of the number of pulls on the tensile strength. J Repro Med 1990;35:260–262.
12. Nathanson LK, Nathanson PDK, Cuschieri A. Safety of vessel ligation in laparoscopic surgery. Endoscopy 1991;23:206–209.

Chapter 12

Complications of Laparoscopy
Malcolm G. Munro

Laparoscopic procedures do not always turn out as anticipated. As is the case with any intervention, and despite all efforts to the contrary, adverse clinical outcomes may occur. Some complications are minor, and have little effect on the patient's short- or long-term surgical result. However, others may be of greater consequence and undermine the expectations of the patient and the health care provider. Given the current and likely future state of surgical art, such shortcomings are likely to continue, to a degree, at least for some time to come.

When a procedure results in morbidity, be it hemorrhagic, traumatic, or infectious, there occur both measurable and insidious manifestations that have an impact upon quality of life, and the individual and systemic costs of providing health care. Most patients, as well as their employers, their relatives, and their physicians, find such an outcome difficult to tolerate. Consequently, prevention, or at least early detection and appropriate management, are the hallmarks of ideal surgical care. In this chapter we will deal with the issue of complications and their prevention. For, while the innate imperfections in the human condition make total prevention impossible, failure to try must be considered indefensible.

Many of the complications associated with diagnostic and operative laparoscopy are known but, as yet, few have been widely reported. Consequently, in most instances, their incidence can only be estimated. Such estimations are difficult given the rapid increase in the number of procedures, types of equipment, and the plethora of new technicians. This review will address the known complications with respect to prevention, detection, and appropriate management.

As with any surgical intervention, laparoscopic procedures can be complicated by infectious, traumatic, or hemorrhagic morbidity. Because of the closed nature of the cases, the incidence of infection seems to be drastically reduced compared to procedures performed via laparotomy. On the other hand, problems associated with visualization of the operative field, together with the change in anatomical perspective, individually or collectively may increase the likelihood of damage to blood vessels or vital structures such as the bowel, the ureter, or the bladder. As laparoscopically directed dissections extend farther outside of the peritoneal cavity, the incidence of neurologic trauma will no doubt increase.

There are other complications that may be more unique to laparoscopy than with procedures performed via laparotomy or via the vaginal route. The instillation of large amounts of fluid into the peritoneal cavity may contribute to electrolyte disturbances or volume overload. The prolonged use of intraperitoneal gas under pressure may have significant metabolic effects or may adversely affect cardiorespiratory function. The intraperitoneal use of electrical or laser energy creates the potential for a variety of complications that can be minimized with a combination of sound knowledge of the energy source and meticulous care and maintenance of the instrumentation.

Gynecologists have been performing laparoscopic procedures longer and in greater volume than any other group of physicians. As a result there is a relatively large body of literature reflecting this experience, which is principally comprised of diagnostic and minor operative procedures, most notably female sterilization. The reported incidence of minor and major complications ranges from 1 to 4% and 0.3 to 2.8%, respectively (1–5). However, many of these reports are voluntary surveys of a given population of surgeons, a feature that potentially biases the data. In addition, the fact that most of these studies focus on diagnostic and minor operative procedures could underestimate the complication risk for the more advanced and complicated operative procedures introduced to North America in the 1980s. This concern seems to be validated by a recently published evaluation of the experience with operative endoscopy at a community hospital in a major metropolitan center in the United States. In this report, the incidence of complications associated with operative procedures like removal of ectopic gestation, adhesiolysis and laparoscopic hysterectomy were 13%, 55% and 60%, respectively; far greater that what would be expected from the literature (6). One possible explanation lies in the fact that many of these complications were experienced by patients of surgeons with little experience with the procedures performed.

The German literature may provide a glimpse into the future as, in that country, operative laparoscopy has enjoyed a longer history of use. From 1949 to 1988 the death rate has steadily declined from 0.09% (1949–1977) to 0.008% (1986–1988). The serious complication risk started at 3.56% between the years 1949–1977 but now ranges from 1.93 to 2.36%. However, again, these data are collected by self-reporting techniques that may not accurately reflect risk (7).

For the patient contemplating a laparoscopic procedure, such data are not very helpful. They are not procedure specific, nor do they reflect the experience of the specific surgeon or institution. Where possible in this section, the reader will be provided available case-specific complication information. However, the validity of such information is clouded by the shortcomings described above.

ANESTHETIC AND MEDICAL COMPLICATIONS

Anesthetic complications include those that are more common in association with laparoscopic surgery as well as those that can occur in any procedure requiring general anesthetics. One-third of the deaths associated with minor laparoscopic procedures such as sterilization are secondary to complications of anesthesia (8).

Among the potential complications of all general anesthetics are hypoventilation, esophageal intubation, gastroesophageal reflux, bronchospasm, hypotension, narcotic overdose, cardiac arrhythmias, and cardiac arrest. Gynecologic laparoscopy poses a number of inherent features that can enhance some of these risks. For example, the head down (Trendelenburg) position, in combination with the increased intraperitoneal pressure provided by pneumoperitoneum, places greater pressure on the diaphragm, potentiating hypoventilation, resulting hypercarbia, and metabolic acidosis. This position, combined with anesthetic agents that relax the esophageal sphincter, facilitates regurgitation of gastric content, which, in turn, often leads to aspiration and its attendant complications of bronchospasm, pneumonitis, and pneumonia.

Parameters of cardiopulmonary function associated with both CO_2 and N_2O insufflation include reduced pO_2, O_2 saturation, tidal volume and minute ventilation, as well as an increased respiratory rate. The use of intraperitoneal CO_2 as a distension medium is associated with an increase in pCO_2 and a decrease in pH. Elevation of the diaphragm may be associated with basilar atelectasis, a resulting right-to-left shunt and a ventilation perfusion mismatch (9, 10).

Despite the fact that during laparoscopy the patient's anesthetic care is in the hands of the anesthesiologist, it is important for the surgeon to understand the prevention and management of anesthetic complications. Such insight fosters an attitude of cooperation between the members of the operating room team, a circumstance that is essential to consistently achieving optimal patient outcome.

Carbon Dioxide Embolus

Carbon dioxide is the most widely used peritoneal distension medium. Part of the reason for this selection is the ready absorption of CO_2 in blood. Consequently, the vast majority of frequent microemboli that do occur are absorbed, usually by the splanchnic vascular system, quickly and without incident. However, if large amounts of CO_2 gain access to the central venous circulation, if there is peripheral vasoconstriction, or if the splanchnic blood flow is decreased by excessively high intraperitoneal pressure, severe cardiorespiratory compromise may result.

Diagnosis

Among the presenting signs of CO_2 embolus are sudden, otherwise unexplained hypotension, cardiac arrhythmia, cyanosis and the development of the classical "mill-wheel" heart murmur. The end tidal CO_2 may increase and findings consistent with pulmonary edema may manifest. Accelerating pulmonary hypertension may also occur, resulting in right-sided heart failure.

Risk Reduction

Because gas embolism may occur as a result of direct intravascular injection via an insufflation needle, the surgeon should ensure that blood is not emanating from the needle prior to the initiation of insufflation. Gynecologic surgeons can uniformly reduce the risk of CO_2 embolus by operating in an environment where the intraperitoneal pressure is maintained at less than 20 mm Hg. In most instances, excepting the initial placement of trocars in an insufflated peritoneum, the surgeon should be able to function comfortably with the intraperitoneal pressure between 8 and 12 mm Hg. Such pressures may also provide protection from many of the other adverse cardiopulmonary events described below. The risk of CO_2 embolus is also reduced by the meticulous maintenance of hemostasis, for open venous channels are the portal of entry for gas into the systemic circulation. Another option is the use of "gasless" or "apneumic" laparoscopy, where extra or intraperitoneal lifting mechanisms are used to create a working space for the surgeon. However, limitations of these devices have, to date, precluded their wide acceptance by surgeons.

The anesthesiologist should continuously monitor the patient's color, blood pressure, heart sounds, electrocardiogram, and end-tidal CO_2 so that the signs of CO_2 embolus are recognized early.

Management

If CO_2 embolus is suspected or diagnosed, the operating room team must act quickly. The surgeon must evacuate CO_2 from the peritoneal cavity and should place the patient in the Durant, or left lateral decubitus position, with the head below the level of the right atrium. A large bore central venous line should be immediately established to allow aspiration of gas from the heart. Because the findings are nonspecific, other causes of cardiovascular collapse should be considered.

Cardiovascular Complications

Cardiac arrhythmias occur relatively frequently during the performance of laparoscopic surgery and are related to a number of factors, the most significant of which is hypercarbia and the resulting acidemia. Early reports of laparoscopy-associated arrhythmia were in association with spontaneous respiration. Consequently, most anesthesiologists have adopted the universal practice of mechanical ventilation during laparoscopic surgery. There are also a number of pharmacological considerations that lead the anesthesiologist to select agents that limit the risk of cardiac arrhythmia. The surgeon may aid in reducing the incidence of hypercarbia by operating with intraperitoneal pressures that are less than 12 mm Hg (11).

The use of an alternate intraperitoneal gas is another method by which the risk of cardiac arrhythmia may be reduced. However, while nitrous oxide is associated with a decreased incidence of arrhythmia, it increases the severity of shoulder tip pain, and, more importantly, is insoluble in blood. External lifting systems (apneumic laparoscopy) are another option that can provide protection against cardiac arrhythmia.

Hypotension can also occur secondary to excessively increased intraperitoneal pressure resulting in decreased venous return, and resulting decreased cardiac output. This undesirable result may be potentiated if the patient is volume depleted. Hypotension secondary to cardiac arrhythmias may also be a consequence of vagal discharge in response to increased intraperitoneal pressure (12). All of these side effects will be more dangerous for the patient with preexisting cardiovascular compromise.

Gastric Reflux

Gastric regurgitation and aspiration are complications potentiated by laparoscopic surgery. Some patients are at increased risk, including those with obesity, gastroparesis, hiatal hernia or any type of gastric outlet obstruction. In such patients it is important to quickly secure the airway with a cuffed endotracheal tube and to routinely decompress the stomach with a nasogastric or orogastric tube. The surgeon can contribute to aspiration prophylaxis by operating at the lowest necessary intraperitoneal pressure. Patients should be taken out of the Trendelenburg position prior to being extubated. The adverse effects of aspiration may be minimized with the routine preoperative administration of metoclopramide, H2 blockers, and nonparticulate antacids.

EXTRAPERITONEAL GAS

A number of the complications associated with pneumoperitoneum or its achievement are described in the vascular, gastroenterologic, urologic, and anesthetic sections. However, the problem of extraperitoneal placement or extravasation of gas has not been considered. In some instances, this complication occurs as a result of deficient technique (incorrect placement of insufflation needles; excessive intraperitoneal pressure), while in others the extravasation is related to gas tracking around the ports or along the dissection planes themselves.

Subcutaneous emphysema most commonly results from preperitoneal placement of an insufflation needle or leakage of CO_2 around the cannula sites, the latter frequently because of excessive intraperitoneal pressure. The condition is usually mild and limited to the abdominal wall. However, subcutaneous emphysema can become extensive, involving the extremities, the neck, and the mediastinum. Another relatively common location for emphysema is the omentum or mesentery, a circumstance that the surgeon may mistake for preperitoneal insufflation.

Diagnosis

Usually the diagnosis will not be a surprise, for the surgeon will have had difficulty in positioning the primary cannula within the peritoneal cavity. Subcutaneous emphysema may be readily identified by the palpation of crepitus, usually in the abdominal wall. In some instances, it can extend along contiguous fascial planes to the neck, where it can be visualized directly. Such a finding may reflect the development of mediastinal emphysema. If mediastinal emphysema is severe, or if pneumothorax is developing, the anesthesiologist may report difficulty in maintaining a normal pCO_2, a feature that may indicate impending cardiovascular collapse.

Risk Reduction

The risk of subcutaneous emphysema is reduced by proper positioning of an insufflation needle, if it is used. Such positioning has been described elsewhere (Chapter 9). To summarize, prior to insertion, it is important to check the insufflation needle for proper function and patency and to establish the baseline flow pressure by attaching it to the insufflation apparatus. The best position for insertion is at the base of the umbilicus, where the abdominal wall is the thinnest. The angle of insertion varies from 45° to near 90°, depending upon the patient's weight, as described in the section on prevention of vascular injuries. The insertion action should be smooth and firm until the surgeon, observing and listening to the device passing through the layers—two (fascia and peritoneum) in the umbilicus and three (two layers of fascia; one peritoneum) in the left upper quadrant—feels that placement is intraperitoneal.

No one test is absolutely reliable at predicting intraperitoneal placement—instead, a number of tests should be used. Of course, aspiration of the insufflation needle should precede all other evaluations. Two tests depend upon the preinflation intraperitoneal pressure. If a drop of water is placed on the open end of the insufflation needle, it should be drawn into the low-pressure intraperitoneal environment of the peritoneal cavity. Although some disagree, the author feels that elevation of the anterior abdominal wall is a reasonable way of creating a negative intraperitoneal pressure. Perhaps a more quantitative way of demonstrating the same principle is to attach the tubing to the needle after insertion but prior to initiating the flow of gas. Elevation of the abdominal wall should result in the creation of a low or negative intraperitoneal pressure (-1 to -4 mm Hg). Insufflation should be initiated at a low flow rate of about 1 liter per minute until the surgeon has confidence that proper placement has been achieved. Loss of liver dullness should occur when about 500 mL of gas has entered the peritoneal cavity. The measured intraperitoneal pressure should be below 10 mm Hg—but up to 14 mm Hg if the patient is obese. Abdominal distension should be symmetrical. If, at any time, the surgeon feels that the needle is not located intraperitoneally, it should be withdrawn and reinserted. Once the peritoneal cavity has been insufflated with an adequate volume of gas, the primary trocar is introduced. The laparoscope is introduced, and, if the cannula is satisfactorily located, the tubing is attached to the appropriate port.

The risk of subcutaneous emphysema may be reduced by maintaining a low intraperitoneal pressure following the placement of the desired cannulas. The author always operates below 15 mm Hg and usually works at about 10 mm Hg. Other approaches that reduce the chance of subcutaneous emphysema include open laparoscopy and the abdominal wall lifting systems that render gas unnecessary. Although primary blind insertion of sharp trocars has been demonstrated to be as safe as secondary insertion following pneumoinsufflation, the relative incidence of subcutaneous emphysema is unknown (13–15).

Management

If the surgeon finds that the insufflation has occurred extraperitoneally, there exist a number of management options. While removing the laparoscope and repeating the insufflation is possible, it may be made more difficult because of the new configuration of the anterior peritoneum. Open laparoscopy or the use of an alternate site such as the left upper quadrant should be considered options. One attractive approach is to leave the laparoscope in the expanded preperitoneal space while the insufflation needle is reinserted through the peritoneal membrane, caudad to the tip of the laparoscope under direct vision (16).

For mild cases of subcutaneous emphysema, no specific intra or postoperative therapy is required, as the findings, in at least mild cases, quickly resolve following evacuation of the pneumoperitoneum. When the extravasation extends to involve the neck, it is usually preferable to terminate the procedure, as pneumomediastinum, pneumothorax, hypercarbia and cardiovascular collapse may result (17–20). Following the end of the procedure it is prudent to obtain a chest x-ray. The patient should be managed expectantly unless a tension pneumothorax results, when immediate evacuation must be performed, using a chest tube or a wide bore needle (14–16 gauge) inserted in the second intercostal space in the midclavicular line.

COMPLICATIONS ASSOCIATED WITH THE USE OF ELECTRICITY

Complications of electrosurgery occur secondary to thermal injury from one of three basic causes. The first is thermal trauma from unintended or inappropriate use of the active electrode(s). The second results from current diverting to another, undesirable path, causing injury remote from the immediate operative field. Third is injury at the site of the "return" or dispersive electrode. Active electrode injury can occur with either unipolar or bipolar instruments, while trauma secondary to current diversion or dispersive electrode accidents only occurs with the unipolar technique. Complications of electrosurgery are reduced with strict adherence to safety protocols coupled with a sound understanding of the circumstances that can lead to undesirable effects on tissue.

Active Electrode Trauma

Unintended activation is one of the more common mechanisms by which the active electrode causes complications. Such a complication frequently occurs when an electrode, left untended within the peritoneal cavity, is inadvertently activated by compression of the hand switch or depression of the foot pedal (21). Control of the electrosurgical unit or generator (ESU) by someone other than the operating surgeon is also a source of accidental activation of the electrode.

Direct extension is another mechanism by which the active electrode(s) cause complications. The zone of vaporization or coagulation may extend to involve large blood vessels or vital structures such as the bladder, ureter, or bowel. Bipolar current reduces, but does not eliminate, the risk of thermal injury to adjacent tissue (22). Consequently, care must be taken to isolate blood vessels prior to desiccation, especially when near vital structures, and to apply appropriate amounts of energy in a fashion that allows an adequate margin of noninjured tissue.

Diagnosis

The diagnosis of direct thermal visceral injury may be suspected or confirmed intraoperatively. Careful evaluation of nearby intraperitoneal structures should be made if unintended activation of the electrode occurs. The visual appearance will depend upon a number of factors including the type of the electrode, its proximity to tissue, the output of the generator, and the duration of its activation. High power density activations will often result in vaporization injury, and will be more easily recognized than lower power density lesions that result in desiccation and coagulation.

The diagnosis of visceral thermal injury is often delayed until the signs and symptoms of fistula or peritonitis present. This will be particularly true with desiccation injury. Because these complications may not present until two to at least ten days following surgery, long after discharge, both the patient and the physician must be made aware of the possible consequences. Consequently, patients should be advised to report any fever or increasing abdominal pain experienced postoperatively.

Risk Reduction

These kinds of injury are largely prevented if (a) the surgeon is always in direct control of electrode activation, and (b) all electrosurgical hand instruments are removed from the peritoneal cavity when not in use. When removed from the peritoneal cavity, the instruments should be detached from the electrosurgical generator or they should be stored in an insulated pouch near to the operative field. These measures prevent damage to the patient's skin if the foot pedal is accidentally depressed.

Management

Thermal injury to bowel, bladder, or ureter, recognized at the time of laparoscopy, should immediately be managed appropriately, considering the potential extent of the zone of coagulative necrosis. The extent of thermal trauma will depend upon the characteristics of the energy transferred to tissue. An electrosurgical incision made with the focused energy from a pointed electrode will be associated with a minimal amount of surrounding thermal injury, and may be repaired in a fashion identical to one created mechanically. However, with desiccation injury created as a result of prolonged contact with a relatively large caliber electrode, the thermal necrosis may extend centimeters from the point of contact. In such instances, wide excision or resection will be necessary.

Current Diversion

Current diversion can occur when an electrical current finds a direct path out of the patient's body via grounded sites other than the dispersive electrode. Alternatively, the current can be diverted directly to other tissue before it reaches the tip of the active electrode. In either instance, if the power density becomes high enough, unintended and severe thermal injury can result.

Alternate Ground Site Burns

These injuries can only occur with ground-referenced ESUs because they lack an isolated circuit (see Chapter 10). In such generators, when the dispersive electrode becomes detached, unplugged, or otherwise ineffective, the current will seek any grounded conductor. If the conductor has a small surface area, the current or power density may become high enough to cause thermal injury (Fig. 12.1). Examples include electrocardiograph patch electrodes or the conductive metal components of the operating table.

Modern ESUs are designed and built with isolated circuits and impedance monitoring systems. Consequently, if any part of the circuit is broken, an alarm sounds, and/or the machine "shuts down," thereby preventing electrode activation. Since the widespread introduction of such generators, the incidence of burns to alternate sites has become largely confined to cases involving the few remaining ground-referenced machines. Nevertheless, many such machines are still in existence. As a result, it is important for the surgeon to establish the type of machine(s) available in their operating rooms before surgery.

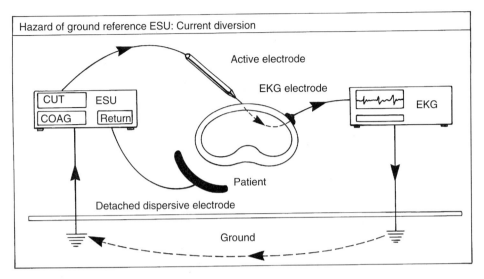

Figure 12.1. Current Diversion: Detached Dispersive Electrode. Ground-referenced electrosurgical generators will not detect breaks in the circuit such as a detached dispersive electrode. In this example, the circuit is completed through the EKG electrode, which, because of its relatively small surface area, concentrates the current to a degree adequate to result in thermal injury to skin.

Insulation Defects

Defects in the insulation coating the shaft of a laparoscopic electrosurgical electrode can allow current diversion to adjacent tissue. The high power density resulting from such small points of contact fosters the creation of a significant injury (Fig. 12.2). During laparoscopic procedures, bowel is frequently the tissue near to, or in contact with, the shaft of the electrode, making it the organ most susceptible to this type of electrosurgical injury. The fact that the whole shaft of the electrode is frequently not encompassed by the surgeon's visual field at laparoscopy makes it possible that such an injury can occur unbeknown to the operator.

Prevention of these complications starts with the selection and care of electrosurgical hand instruments. Loose instrument bins should be replaced with containers designed to keep the instruments from damaging each other. The instruments should be examined prior to each case, searching for worn or obviously defective insulation. When found, the damaged instrument should be removed and repaired or replaced. Despite all efforts, unobserved breaks in insulation may rarely occur. While the use of disposable instruments is often claimed as a way of reducing the incidence of insulation failure, there is no guarantee that this is the case, as invisible defects may occur in the manufacturing process. Furthermore, the insulation on disposable electrodes is thinner and more susceptible to trauma. Consequently, when applying unipolar electrical energy, the shaft of the instrument should be kept free of vital structures and, if possible, totally visible in the operative field.

Direct Coupling

Direct coupling occurs when an activated electrode touches and energizes another metal conductor such as a laparoscope, cannula, or other instrument. If

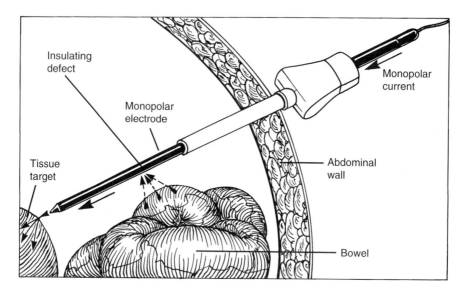

Figure 12.2. Current Diversion: Insulation Defect. Defects in the insulation of monopolar electrodes may result in thermal injury to nearby tissue. Because these defects are difficult to detect, care should be taken to avoid contact of the shaft of the electrode with tissue, and to keep the entire shaft in view when activating the electrode.

the conductor is near to, or in contact with, other tissue, a thermal injury can result (Fig. 12.3). Such accidents often happen following unintentional activation of an electrode. Prevention of direct coupling is facilitated by removal of the electrodes when not in use, and visually confirming that the electrode is not in inappropriate contact with other conductive instruments prior to activation.

Capacitive Coupling

Capacitance reflects the ability of a conductor to establish an electrical current in an unconnected but nearby circuit. An electrical field is established around the shaft of any activated laparoscopic unipolar electrode, a circumstance that makes the electrode a capacitor. This field is harmless if the circuit is completed via a dispersive, low power density pathway (Fig. 12.4A). For example, if capacitive coupling occurs between the laparoscopic electrode and a metal cannula positioned in the abdominal wall, the current harmlessly "returns" to the abdominal wall where it traverses to the dispersive electrode (Fig. 12.4B). However, if the metal cannula is anchored to the skin by a nonconductive plastic retaining sleeve, or anchor (a hybrid system), the current will not return to the abdominal wall because the sleeve acts as an insulator. Instead, the capacitor will have to "look" elsewhere to complete the circuit. Consequently, bowel, or any other nearby conductor, can become the target of a relatively high power density discharge (Fig. 12.4C). The risk is greater with high voltage currents, such as the coagulation output on an electrosurgical generator. This mechanism is also more likely to occur when a unipolar electrode is inserted through an operating laparoscope that, in turn, is passed through a plastic laparoscopic port. In this configuration, the plastic port acts as the insulator. If the electrode capacitively couples

Chapter 12: Complications of Laparoscopy 255

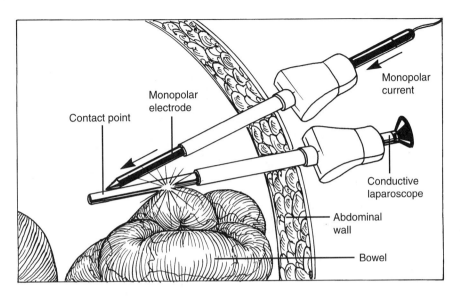

Figure 12.3. Current Diversion: Direct Coupling. When an activated electrode comes in contact with a conductor, such as an uninsulated grasping instrument, or, in this case an uninsulated endoscope, the current can be diverted to tissue touching the conductor. If the current is concentrated the direct coupling can result in thermal injury.

with the metal laparoscope, nearby bowel will be at risk for significant thermal injury (23, 24).

Prevention of capacitive coupling can largely be accomplished by avoiding the use of hybrid laparoscope cannula systems that contain a mixture of conductive and nonconductive elements. Instead, it is preferred that all-plastic or all-metal cannula systems be used. When and if operating laparoscopes are employed, all-metal cannula systems should be the rule unless there is no intent to perform unipolar electrosurgical procedures through the operating channel. Furthermore, the risk is minimized if low voltage radiofrequency current (cutting) is used, and when the high voltage outputs are avoided.

Dispersive Electrode Burns

As noted previously, the use of isolated circuit generators with return electrode monitors has all but eliminated dispersive electrode related thermal injury. Return electrode monitoring (REM) is actually accomplished by measuring the impedance (sometimes called resistance) in the dispersive electrode, which should always be low because of the large surface area. To accomplish this, most return electrode monitors actually are divided into two electrodes, allowing the generator to compare the impedance from the two sides of the pad. If the overall impedance is high, or if there is a significant difference between the two sides, as is the case with partial detachment, the active electrode cannot be activated. Without such devices, partial detachment of the patient pad could result in a thermal injury because reducing the surface area of the electrode raises the current density (Fig. 12.5).

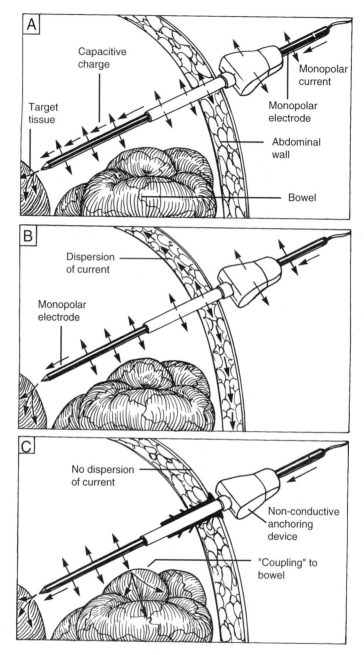

Figure 12.4. Current Diversion: Capacitive Coupling. **A.** Every conductor, including this activated unipolar laparoscopic electrode, develops a surrounding electromagnetic charge, capable of completing the circuit in a nearby conductor. **B.** If the nearby conductor disperses the current, in this case to the dispersive electrode via the conductive metal cannula and the abdominal wall, no concentration of current will occur and no thermal injury will result. **C.** On the other hand, if conduction to the abdominal wall is impeded by a nonconductive plastic anchoring sleeve, the charge builds on the metal cannula and will "seek" ground elsewhere, in this case by arcing to the nearby bowel. A similar circumstance occurs when a unipolar electrode is activated in a conductive operating laparoscope, which, in turn, is within a nonconductive laparoscope cannula.

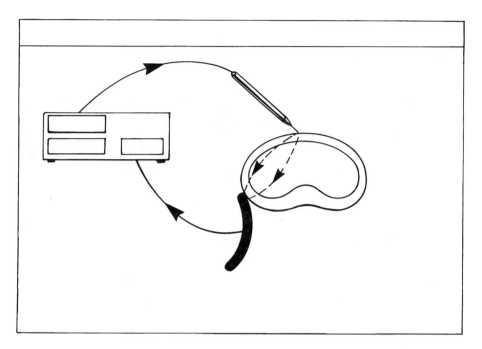

Figure 12.5. Dispersive Electrode Burns. If the dispersive electrode becomes partially detached from the skin, the current or power density may be adequate to cause thermal injury, given adequate activation time. Impedance monitoring systems will prevent such injuries by shutting off the power from the generator.

It is important for the surgeon to establish what type of ESU is being used in each case. Absence of a REM system is a reason for increased scrutiny of the positioning of the dispersive electrode, both before the surgery begins, and as the operation progresses.

Electrode Shields and Monitors

A United States-based company, (Electroscope Inc., Boulder, CO) markets a system that helps to reduce further the chance of direct or capacitive coupling (Fig. 12.6). A reusable shield is passed over the shaft of the laparoscopic electrode prior to its insertion into the peritoneal cavity. This shield protects against insulation failure and detects the presence of significant capacitance. Should an insulation break occur, or when capacitance becomes threatening, the integrated monitoring system automatically shuts down the generator. The shield enlarges the effective diameter of the electrode by about 2 mm, making it necessary to use larger caliber laparoscopic ports.

Summary

Despite perceptions to the contrary, electrosurgery has been rendered a safe modality for use in surgical procedures. However, safe and effective application of electrical energy requires an adequate understanding and implementation of basic principles (Chapter 10) as well as the availability of modern electrosurgical

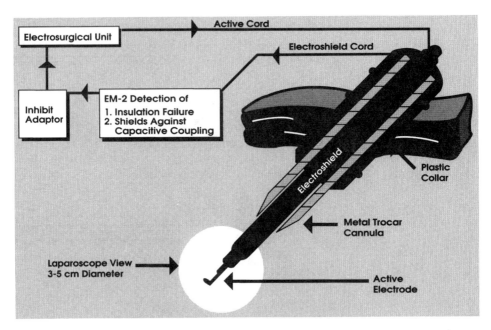

Figure 12.6. Capacitance Monitoring. The Electroshield monitor system detects capacitance, shutting off the generator if the risk of capacitive coupling becomes great. In addition, the sheath for the electrode protects against injury from direct coupling and insulation defects. (Courtesy of Valleylab Inc., Boulder, CO.)

generators and appropriate education of medical and support staff. To optimize safety, there are a number of principles that must be observed.

The equipment must meet acceptable standards. Electrosurgical generators ideally are designed with isolated circuits and return electrode monitors. While digital displays allow for more precise calculation of power output, they are not essential for safety. The operating instruments should be in good working condition with intact insulation. The risk of capacitive coupling may be reduced by minimizing the use of high voltage "coagulation" current and by eliminating the use of unipolar electrosurgical instruments through an operating laparoscope. For bipolar instruments, the use of a serial ammeter better identifies the endpoint of desiccation and may reduce problems associated with excessive (e.g., visceral) injury or inadequate desiccation of the fallopian tube or of severed blood vessels.

Proper application of the dispersive electrode to an appropriate site is important. When attached to large body scars even transmission of electrical current is impaired and thermal injury can result. Instead, the electrode should be applied over normal skin, away from joints, but near to the operative site, without intervening potential sources of grounding such as EKG electrodes. For gynecological laparoscopy, an ideal site is the medial aspect of the thigh. To avoid accidental injury to both intra and extraperitoneal structures by inadvertent activation of the active electrode, instruments not in use should be carefully placed in plastic holsters or detached from the electrosurgical generator, which, in turn, should be always in the control of the operating surgeon—not an assistant.

Care and prudence must be exercised when utilizing electricity within the peritoneal cavity. The zone of significant thermal injury usually extends beyond that of the visible injury, a feature that must be borne in mind when operating in close proximity to vital structures such as bowel, bladder, ureter, and large and important blood vessels. It is equally important to impart the minimal amount of thermal injury (if any) necessary to accomplish the task at hand, even around nonvital structures, by using the ideal power output and the appropriate active electrodes.

HEMORRHAGIC COMPLICATIONS

Hemorrhagic complications may occur as a consequence of entry into the peritoneal cavity, or as a result of trauma incurred to blood vessels encountered during the course of the procedure.

Hemorrhage Associated with Peritoneal Entry

Great Vessel Injury

The most dangerous hemorrhagic complications of entry are to the great vessels, including the aorta and vena cava as well as the common iliac vessels and their branches, the internal and external iliac arteries and veins. The incidence of major vascular injury is probably underreported, but has been estimated to range widely from 0.93 to 9 per 10,000 cases (7, 25–27). The trauma most often occurs secondary to insertion of an insufflation needle, but may be created by the tip of the trocar (25, 28). However, not uncommonly, the injury is associated with the insertion of ancillary laparoscopic ports into the lower quadrants. The vessels most frequently damaged are the aorta and the right common iliac artery, which branches from the aorta in the midline. The anatomically more posterior location of the vena cava and the iliac veins provides relative protection, but not immunity, from injury (28). While most of these injuries are small, amenable to repair with suture, some have been larger, requiring ligation with or without the insertion of a vascular graft. Not surprisingly, death has been reported in a number of instances.

Recognition. Most often the problem presents as profound hypotension with or without the appearance of a significant volume of blood within the peritoneal cavity. In some instances, the surgeon aspirates blood via the insufflation needle, prior to introduction of distension gas. Frequently, the bleeding may be contained in the retroperitoneal space, a feature that usually delays the diagnosis. Consequently, the development of hypovolemic shock in the recovery room may well be secondary to otherwise unrecognized laceration to a great vessel. To avoid the specter of late recognition, it is important to evaluate the course of each great vessel prior to completing the procedure.

Risk Reduction. There are a number of ways by which the incidence of large vessel trauma can be minimized. Certainly it is essential that the positioning of ancillary, or secondary, trocars in the lower quadrants be performed under direct vision. This is more difficult for the primary cannula. It has been suggested that the use of "open laparoscopy" for the initial port entirely avoids the issue of great vessel injury secondary to insufflation needles and trocars (29). However, open laparoscopy has its own potential drawbacks such as increased operating time, the need for larger incisions, and a greater chance of wound infection, all without eliminating the incidence of bowel injury at entry.

The risk of large vessel injury should be reduced if careful attention is paid to equipment and technique. If used, both insufflation needles and the trocar should be kept sharp or should be disposable. The safety sheath of the insufflation needle should be checked to ensure that both the spring and the sliding mechanism are functioning normally. Many disposable trocar-cannula systems are constructed with a safety mechanism that covers or retracts the trocar following passage through the fascia and peritoneum. However, there are currently no available data that demonstrate a reduction in the incidence of major vessel injury with the use of these devices.

The application of appropriate technique is based upon a sound understanding of the normal anatomic relationships between the commonly used entry points and the great vessels. A "safety zone" exists inferior to the sacral promontory in the area bounded superiorly by the bifurcation of the aorta, posteriorly by the sacral curve, and laterally by the iliac vessels (Fig. 12.7). Safe insertion of the insufflation needle mandates that the instrument be maintained in a midline, sagittal plane while the operator directs the tip between the iliac vessels, anterior to the sacrum but inferior to the bifurcation of the aorta and the proximal aspect of the vena cava. Such positioning requires elevation of the abdominal wall while angling the insufflation needle about 45° to horizontal. The tactile and visual feedback created when the needle passes through the fascial and peritoneal layers of the abdominal wall, if recognized and heeded, may prevent overaggressive insertion attempts. Such proprioceptive feedback is diminished with disposable needles as compared to the classic Veress model. Instead, the surgeon must listen to the "clicks" as the needle obturator retracts when it passes through the rectus fascia and the peritoneum. The needle should never be forced.

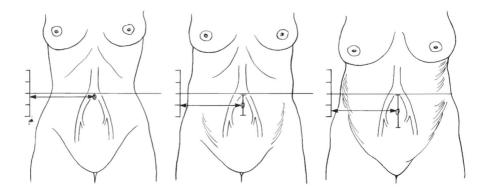

Figure 12.7. Relationship of Aortic Bifurcation to Umbilicus. In women of normal weight for height the bifurcation is, on average, 0.4 cm cephalad to and 6 cm (±3) beneath the umbilicus. For overweight women, the distances are 2.4 and 10 cm (±2), respectively. In obese women, the umbilicus is 2.9 cm inferior to the bifurcation and 13 cm (±4) anterior to the level of the aorta.

It is critical to note that these anatomic relationships may vary with body type and with the orientation of the patient to the horizontal position. In women of normal weight and body habitus, in the horizontal recumbent position, the bifurcation of the aorta is located immediately beneath the umbilicus. However, in obese individuals the umbilicus may be positioned up to 2 or more cm below the bifurcation (Fig. 12.7). Fortunately, this circumstance allows the insufflation needle to be directed in a more vertical position—those between 160 to 200 pounds between 45° and 90°, while those women over 200 pounds at nearly 90°. Women placed in a "head-down" position (Trendelenburg's position) will shift their great vessels more superiorly and anteriorly in a fashion that may make them more vulnerable to an entry injury. Consequently, positioning of the insufflation needle, and at least the initial trocar and cannula, should be accomplished with the patient in a horizontal position. This approach additionally facilitates the evaluation of the upper abdomen, an exercise that is limited if the intraperitoneal content is shifted cephalad by the patient's head-down position.

The risk of great vessel injury is likely reduced by insufflating the peritoneal cavity to adequate pressure. An intraperitoneal pressure of 20 mm Hg, while not desirable for prolonged periods of time, can aid in separating the abdominal wall from the great vessels during the process of insertion of a sharp trocar.

Management. If blood is withdrawn from the insufflation needle, it should be left in place while immediate preparations are made to obtain blood products and perform laparotomy. If the diagnosis of hemoperitoneum is made upon initial visualization of the peritoneal cavity, a grasping instrument may be used, if possible, to temporarily occlude the vessel. While it is unlikely that significant injury can predictably be repaired by laparoscopically directed technique, if temporary hemostasis can be obtained, and the laceration visualized, selected, localized lesions can be repaired, with suture, under laparoscopic guidance. Such an attempt should not be made by any other than experienced and technically adept surgeons. Even if such an instance exists, fine judgment should be used so as not to delay the institution of life-saving, open surgical repair.

Most surgeons should gain immediate entry into the peritoneal cavity, and immediately compress the aorta and vena cava just below the level of the renal vessels, gaining at least temporary control of blood loss. At that juncture, the most appropriate course of action, including the need for vascular surgical consultation, will become more apparent.

Abdominal Wall Vessels

By far the most commonly injured abdominal wall vessels are the superficial inferior epigastrics as they branch from the femoral artery and course cephalad in each lower quadrant. They are invariably damaged by the initial passage of an ancillary trocar, or when a wider device is introduced later in the procedure. The problem may be recognized immediately by the observation of blood dripping along the cannula or out through the incision. However, it is not uncommon for the cannula itself to obstruct the bleeding until withdrawal at the end of the case.

More sinister are injuries to the deep inferior epigastric vessels, branches of the external iliac artery and vein that also course cephalad but are deep to the rectus fascia and often deep to the muscles themselves. More laterally located are the deep circumflex iliac vessels that are uncommonly encountered in laparoscopic surgery. Laceration of these vessels may cause profound blood loss, particularly when the trauma is unrecognized and causes extraperitoneal bleeding.

Recognition. Recognition is by visualization of the blood dripping down the cannula, or by the postoperative appearance of shock, abdominal wall discoloration, and/or a hematoma located near to the incision. In some instances the blood may track to a more distant site, presenting as a pararectal or vulvar mass. Delayed diagnosis may be prevented at the end of the procedure by laparoscopically evaluating each peritoneal incision following removal of the cannula.

Risk Reduction. Transillumination of the abdominal wall from within will, at least in most thin women, allow for identification of the superficial inferior epigastric vessels. However, the deep inferior epigastric vessels cannot be identified by this mechanism because of their location deep to the rectus sheath. Consequently, prevention of deep inferior epigastric vessel injury requires that the surgeon understand the anatomic course of these vessels (Fig. 12.8).

The most consistent landmarks are the median umbilical ligaments (obliterated umbilical arteries) and the entry point of the round ligament into the inguinal canal. At the pubic crest, the deep inferior epigastric vessels begin their course cephalad between the medially located medial umbilical ligament and the laterally positioned exit point of the round ligament. The trocar should be inserted medial or lateral to the vessels, if they are visualized. If the vessels cannot be seen, and it is necessary to position the trocar laterally, it should be positioned 3–4 cm lateral to the median umbilical ligament, or lateral to the lateral margin of the rectus abdominis muscle. Too lateral an insertion will endanger the deep circumflex epigastric artery. The operator may further limit risk of injury by placing a No. 22 spinal needle though the skin at the desired location, directly observing the entry via the laparoscope. This not only provides more reassurance that a safe location has been identified, but the easily visualized peritoneal needle hole gives the surgeon a target for inserting the trocar with greater precision.

A common mistake is to fashion the incision appropriately, only to direct the trocar medially in its course through the abdominal wall, thereby injuring the vessels. Another factor that may contribute to the risk of injury is the use of large diameter trocars. Consequently, for this and other reasons, it behooves the surgeon to use the smallest trocars necessary for performance of the procedure.

Management. Superficial inferior epigastric artery lacerations usually respond to expectant management. Rotation of the cannula to a position where compression is possible is also helpful. Rarely is a suture necessary.

We have found that the use of a straight ligature carrier, like the Peyerra device, is most useful for the ligation of lacerated deep inferior epigastric vessels. A number of other devices and techniques have been introduced that facilitate the accomplishment of this task, and have been described elsewhere in this text (see Fig. 11.21). To summarize, the trocar and cannula are removed. Then, under laparoscopic visualization, and using a ligature carrier, a ligature is placed through

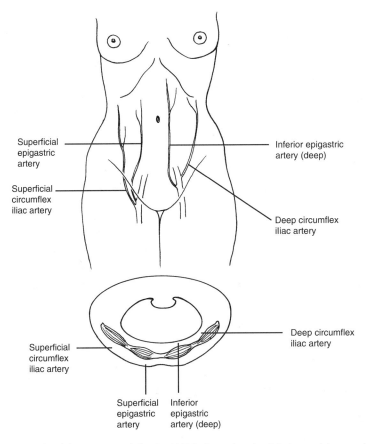

Figure 12.8. Vessels of the Anterior Abdominal Wall. Frontal and axial views of the usual location of the superficial and deep vessels of the anterior abdominal wall. The deep inferior epigastric vessels run cephalad, within 3 cm lateral to the obliterated umbilical vessels (median umbilical ligaments).

the incision and directed laterally and inferiorly, where it is held by a grasping forceps. The ligature carrier is removed and subsequently passed through the incision again, without a suture, but this time medial and inferior to the lacerated vessels. The suture is threaded into the carrier from within the peritoneal cavity, and is then externalized and tied. For small incisions, narrower than the diameter of the surgeon's finger, the knot may be tightened with a knot manipulator.

There are other, less uniformly successful methods for attaining hemostasis from a lacerated deep inferior epigastric vessel. The most obvious is the placement of large, through-and-through mattress sutures. These are usually removed about 48 hours later. Electrodesiccation may be successful. Either a unipolar or bipolar grasping forceps is passed through another ancillary cannula taking care to identify, grasp, and adequately desiccate the vessel. Either continuous or "blended" current is used at appropriate power outputs for the machine and the electrode. Another method that has enjoyed some success is temporary compression with the balloon of a Foley catheter, passed through the incision into the peritoneal cavity, then secured and tightened externally with a clamp. While some suggest that the balloon should be left in place for 24 hours, the delicate channel may be damaged by the clamp, making it impossible to deflate the balloon. For this reason, the author does not recommend this option.

If the lacerated vessel presents postoperatively as a hematoma, the initial efforts should be with local compression. The temptation to open or aspirate the hematoma should be resisted, as such a maneuver may inhibit the tamponade effect and could increase the risk of abscess formation (30). However, if the mass continues to enlarge, or if the patient demonstrates signs of hypovolemia, wound exploration is indicated.

Intraperitoneal Vessel Injury

As with any intraperitoneal surgical procedure, hemorrhage may occur from vessels encountered in the course of the surgical dissection. The bleeding may result from inadvertent entry into a vessel, failure of a specific occlusive technique, or human error in the application of the selected technique. Furthermore, in addition to the problem of delayed hemorrhage inherent in transection of arteries, there may be further delay in diagnosis at laparoscopy because of the restricted visual field and the temporary occlusive pressure exerted by the CO_2 within the peritoneal cavity.

Recognition

Inadvertent division of an artery or vein will usually become immediately self-evident. However, in some instances, transected arteries will go into spasm only to begin bleeding minutes to hours later, an event that may temporarily go unnoticed due to the limited field of view presented by the laparoscope. Consequently, at the end of the procedure, all areas of dissection should be carefully examined. In addition, the CO_2 should be vented, decreasing the intraperitoneal pressure to about 5 mm Hg, allowing recognition of vessels occluded by the higher pressure.

Risk Reduction

Attention to meticulous technique is at least as important in laparoscopically directed surgery as it is for open or vaginal cases. During dissection, vessels should be identified and occluded prior to division, a task made more simple by the magnification afforded by the laparoscope. If suture is used to occlude a vessel, it must be of the appropriate caliber, positioned with an adequate pedicle, and tied snugly with a secure knot. Electrosurgery, if used, should be applied in the appropriate waveform and power density (see Chapter 10), and for a time adequate to allow for sufficient tissue desiccation. Clips should be of a size appropriate for the vessel, and they must be applied in a secure fashion, also with an adequate pedicle of tissue. Care should be exercised to avoid manipulation of pedicles secured with clips or suture, as such trauma could adversely affect the security of the closure. When linear stapling devices are employed, the appropriate staple size should be selected and the tissue encompassed in the staple line should be of uniform thickness. Failure to maintain relatively uniform tissue thickness may result in inadequate compression of blood vessels that course through the thinner areas of the pedicle.

Management

Transected vessels should be secured immediately. If electrosurgical desiccation is used to maintain or achieve hemostasis, the use of a serial ammeter is useful to demonstrate the endpoint of energy application. There is evidence that arteries larger in diameter than 3 mm are less reliably occluded with desiccation than are those 3 mm or less (31). Care must be exerted to avoid blind clamping and electrosurgical desiccation, even with bipolar instruments, especially when less than 1 cm from ureter or bowel (31). When a vessel is in such a location, it is usually preferable to secure it with a clip.

Identification of small vessel bleeding and ooze is often facilitated by the use of copious irrigation and even underwater examination. Capillary ooze may be managed with higher voltage fulguration currents using electrodes with a bulbous tip. When using electrosurgery for this purpose, the use of electrolyte-containing solutions should be avoided, as they disperse current, rendering the technique ineffective. Instead the low viscosity fluids like glycine are recommended as, in addition to being nonconductive, they may facilitate localization of the vessels.

GASTROINTESTINAL COMPLICATIONS

Following laparoscopy, it is not uncommon for the patient to experience nausea. However, in some instances the problem becomes severe. Gastrointestinal viscera potentially injured during the performance of gynecologic laparoscopy include the stomach, the small bowel, and the colon. The incidence of gastrointestinal injury has been reported to range from 1.0 to 2.7 per 1000 procedures (32, 33). Again, most of these data include a large number of diagnostic and simple operative procedures, although the American Association of Gynecologic Laparoscopists (AAGL) does publish the results of its operative laparoscopy survey separately (5). However, a survey of the general surgical experience with laparoscopic cholecystectomy (4292 hospitals; 77,604 cases) suggests that the incidence of penetrating bowel injury is 1.4 per 1000 cases, similar to that reported for gynecology (34).

Insufflation Needle Injuries

Needle entry into the stomach almost invariably happens in the presence of gastric distension. While this may occur secondary to aerophagia, the complication is frequently related to difficult or improper intubation or to the use of mask induction with an inhalation anesthetic. Mechanical entry into large or small bowel may occur in any instance, but is up to 10 times more common when laparoscopy is performed on patients with previous intraperitoneal inflammation or abdominal surgery (35–37). In such instances, loops of intestine can adhere to the abdominal wall under the insertion site. Perforation may also occur following an overly aggressive attempt to insert the insufflation needle.

Recognition

Recognition of gastric entry by the insufflation needle may follow identification of any or all of the signs of extraperitoneal entry, including increased filling pressure, asymmetric distension of the peritoneal cavity, or the aspiration of gastric particulate matter through the lumen of the needle. However, the hollow, capacious nature of the stomach may allow the initial insufflation pressure to remain normal. Unfortunately, in some instances, the problem is not identified until the trocar is inserted and the gastric mucosa identified by direct vision. Recognition of bowel entry usually follows observation of the signs described above for gastric injury, with the addition of feculent odor to the list of findings.

Risk Reduction

Prevention of insufflation needle injury to the gastrointestinal tract is important because such measures largely eliminate the risk of more sinister trocar trauma. Gastric perforation can largely be eliminated with the selective use of preoperative oral or nasogastric suction. The surgeon should request that this be performed if there has been difficulty with intubation or when the needle is intentionally inserted near to the stomach in the left upper quadrant.

Many have suggested that "open laparoscopy" is the most appropriate and effective way to reduce the incidence of intestinal injury in a patient at risk because of previous lower abdominal surgery. However, there are no studies that prove this to be the case. Indeed, there exists evidence that open laparoscopy is itself associated with intestinal injury (29). Consequently, many surgeons have suggested the use of left upper quadrant insertion with a properly decompressed stomach (38, 39).

Although not strictly a prophylactic measure, the routine use of preoperative mechanical bowel preparation, at least in selected, high-risk cases, will diminish the need for laparotomy and/or colostomy if large bowel entry occurs.

Management

The management of any trauma to the gastrointestinal tract depends in part upon the nature of the injury and in part upon the organ(s) involved. In general, insufflation needle punctures that have not resulted in a defect significantly larger than their diameter may be handled expectantly. Larger defects should be repaired or resected, by laparoscopic or laparotomy-based technique, depending upon the skill of the operator and the extent of the lesion.

If, following insertion of an insufflation needle, particulate debris are identified, the needle should be left in place and an alternate insertion site identified, such as the left upper quadrant. If the insufflation needle possesses a removable obturator, a narrow caliber optical fiber or laparoscope may be passed to evaluate the location of the tip and to aid in later identification of the puncture site. Immediately following successful entry into the peritoneal cavity, the site of injury is identified. Unless significant injury or bleeding is identified, the situation may be handled expectantly. If there is unexpected extension of the laceration, it should be managed similarly to a trocar injury.

Trocar Injuries

Damage caused by sharp trocar penetration is usually more serious than when needle injury occurs. Most often, the injury is created by the primary trocar, because of its blind insertion. However, inadequate attention paid to the insertion of ancillary cannulas may also result in visceral injury.

Recognition

If a primary trocar penetrates bowel, the diagnosis is usually made when the surgeon visualizes the mucosal lining of the gastrointestinal structure following insertion of the laparoscope. If large bowel is entered, feculent odor may be noted. However, in some instances, the injury may not immediately be recognized as the cannula may not stay within, or it may pass through, the lumen and out the other side of the viscus. Such injuries usually occur when a single loop of bowel is adhered to the anterior abdominal wall near to the entry point. Consequently, it is important at the end of the procedure to directly view the removal of the primary cannula, either through the cannula itself or via an ancillary port. Routine direct visualization of primary port incisional closure will facilitate the accomplishment of this task.

Unfortunately, the injury may go unrecognized until it presents postoperatively as peritonitis, abscess, enterocutaneous fistula, or death (34, 40).

Risk Reduction

Despite the widespread use of retractable trocars or safety sheaths, injury to bowel or other structures may occur. As stated above, many employ, routinely or selectively, the concept of "open" laparoscopy, where the peritoneal cavity is entered directly via an intra or infraumbilical incision. Despite the apparent virtues of this approach, bowel entry may still occur (29). An alternative approach, especially when entering an abdomen with previous laparotomy scars, is the insertion of a narrow caliber cannula in the left upper quadrant following decompression of the stomach. It is unusual for a patient to have had previous surgery in this location. Following placement of the cannula, usually just below the costal margin in the midclavicular line, a narrow diameter laparoscope may be passed, allowing a direct view of the abdominal wall under the umbilicus or other planned site of insertion. If necessary, the small laparoscope may be used to direct the dissection of intestine from under the insertion site. This approach gains additional value with the introduction of a fiber laparoscope small enough to fit through the lumen of an insufflation needle.

Stomach injuries, as described above, most frequently occur when there has been difficulty in intubation, and may be more common following left upper quadrant insertion if the stomach has not previously been decompressed. Consequently, liberal use of oral or nasogastric decompression will likely reduce the incidence of trocar injury to the stomach.

Bowel injuries usually occur when the intestine is adherent to the abdominal wall under the site of trocar insertion. Adherence is usually secondary to previous surgery. Consequently, in such patients open laparoscopy or left upper quadrant entry may be used. Preoperative mechanical bowel preparation should be employed in high-risk patients to facilitate repair of colonic defects without the need to perform a laparotomy.

Management

Trocar injuries to bowel require repair. If it can be ascertained that the injury is isolated, and if the operator is capable, the lesion may be sutured under laparoscopic guidance with a double layer of running 2-0 or 3-0 synthetic absorbable suture. Extensive lesions may require resection and reanastomosis. In well trained and experienced hands this may be performed under laparoscopic direction. However, in most instances, laparotomy will be required. Regardless of the method of repair, copious irrigation should be employed and the patient admitted for postoperative observation. The patient is kept without oral intake and nasogastric decompression should be liberally used at the discretion of the surgeon. If the injury is to the sigmoid colon, primary repair may be attempted if the bowel has been mechanically prepared preoperatively. Otherwise, colostomy should be considered, with the possible exception of ascending colon lesions. If uncertainty exists regarding the extent of injury, laparotomy is always indicated.

Dissection and Thermal Injury

Recognition

Recognition of injury to the bowel incurred during the course of dissection may be more straightforward. Any length of dissected bowel should be carefully examined prior to proceeding further with the procedure. This is, if anything, more important during laparoscopic operations in comparison to those performed via laparotomy, for comprehensive "running" of the bowel near the end of the case is far more difficult under endoscopic guidance.

There has been confusion in the past regarding the frequency of thermal injury to bowel following the use of electrical energy. Formerly, many injuries actually caused by mechanical trauma were erroneously attributed to electrosurgical accidents, a feature that, in 1981, led the AAGL to erroneously recommend the cessation of monopolar laparoscopic electrosurgical technique (41, 42). Fortunately, Levy and Soderstrom demonstrated that it is generally easy to distinguish between electrosurgical and mechanical trauma, and that the incidence of electrical bowel injury at laparoscopy had been vastly overestimated (43). This revelation caused the AAGL to rescind its previous position in 1985 (44).

Thermal injury to bowel may be more difficult to diagnose intraoperatively, particularly if created with electrical or laser energy, a feature that makes careful adherence to safety protocols a surgeon's imperative. Even if thermal injury is recognized, it is difficult to estimate the extent of the damage by visual inspection, as the zone of desiccation may exceed the area of visual damage. An understanding of the differing impacts of the various types of electrical current is essential for estimation of the extent of injury. In some instances, diagnosis is delayed until the development of peritonitis and fever, usually a few days later, but occasionally not for several weeks.

Risk Reduction

Total prevention of dissection or thermal injury is impossible, but the incidence of penetrating or energy-based enteric complications may be reduced with patience, prudence, and meticulous technique. A sound understanding of the principles of electrosurgery is critical to reducing the incidence of electrical trauma.

When dissecting, exposure of the operative field must be accomplished with a combination of good visualization and adequate traction and, if necessary, countertraction applied by forceps. In many instances it will be necessary to enlist the aid of a competent assistant. Dissection close to bowel should be performed mechanically, using sharp scissors, not with electrical or laser energy sources. Occlusion of blood vessels near to bowel is preferably accomplished with clips, but may be performed with *bipolar* current, provided that there is an adequate margin of tissue, a circumstance that usually requires skeletonization of the vessel. There is no certainty about the proper distance to maintain between the electrode and the bowel serosa. Animal histological studies, using the rather large caliber Kleppinger forceps, have demonstrated that desiccation injury begins to affect bowel serosa and muscularis between 5 and 10 mm away (31). It is likely that the zone of safety is less for instruments that compress tissue well or that use electrodes with a smaller surface area. Regardless, if the difficulty of the dissection makes the surgeon uncomfortable, alternative methods for hemostasis should be used. If this is not feasible, the aid of more experienced colleagues should be sought, the procedure abandoned, or converted into an open case.

Management

The treatment of mechanical bowel trauma recognized during the dissection follows the principles described above for trocar injury. If the diagnosis is delayed until the postoperative recognition of peritonitis, surgical consultation should be obtained and laparotomy arranged.

Thermal injury may be handled expectantly, if, in the estimation of the surgeon, the lesion is superficial and confined. Wheeless reported a series of 33 individuals with such injuries who were followed expectantly in the hospital. Only two required laparotomy for perforation (45). It is possible to estimate the degree of tissue injury if the nature of the current and other parameters are known, such as the wattage, current density, and duration of contact with tissue. For example, fulguration current, arcing to bowel, is unlikely to cause thermal injury more than 1 mm deep, even with rather prolonged exposure. On the other hand, the high power density provided by a sharp electrode will quickly cause penetrating injury of the bowel. Such lesions will have relatively little collateral thermal injury and may be repaired as if they were created by mechanical means. This is a circumstance vastly different from that occurring when there is direct, and even relatively short, duration of contact (seconds) with a low power density electrode. The significant thermal injury that results will often mandate wide excision of the lesion or local resection of the injured segment of bowel.

UROLOGIC INJURY

Laparoscopy associated damage to the bladder or ureter may occur secondary to mechanical or thermal trauma. The AAGL estimates that the incidence of unintended laparotomy to repair urinary tract injury at 1.6 per 1000 procedures (5). Vesical injury is often secondary to a trocar entering the undrained bladder, but may also occur during dissection of the bladder, either from other adhered structures or from the anterior aspect of the uterus (46, 47). The proliferation of laparoscopically directed retropubic suspension for urinary incontinence will likely be associated with bladder injury. Ureteric injury is more commonly encountered secondary to thermal damage (21, 22, 48). However, more recently, there have been descriptions of ureteric trauma secondary to other causes, such as mechanical dissection or the use of linear stapling devices (49, 50). The author is aware of many other unreported cases of ureteric trauma.

Recognition

Intraoperative identification of the injury is the most important aspect of management. The surgeon may be cognizant of entering a hollow viscus or may note the presence of urine in the operative field. If an indwelling catheter is in place, hematuria or pneumaturia (CO_2 in the indwelling drainage system) may be noted. Existence of a bladder laceration may be confirmed with the injection of sterile milk or a dilute methylene blue solution via a catheter. Thermal injury to the bladder may not be initially apparent, presenting later in the patient's postoperative course.

Unfortunately, although intraoperative recognition of ureteric injury has been described (21, 51), diagnosis is usually delayed until some time following the procedure. Ureteric lacerations may be proven intraoperatively with the injection of indigo carmine. Thermal injury will present 24 hours to 14 days following surgery with one or a combination of fever, abdominal or flank pain, and the clinical findings of peritonitis. A leukocytosis may be present and an intravenous pyelogram (IVP) will demonstrate extravasation of urine or a urinoma. Intraoperative recognition of mechanical obstruction, with staples or a suture, will be made only by direct visualization. Not surprisingly, cases of laparoscopy associated ureteric obstruction seem to present at a time similar to those that follow laparotomy-based procedures a few days to a week following the operation (50). These patients present with flank pain and may have fever. The diagnosis may be suggested by abdominal ultrasound, but an IVP can be more precise at identifying the site and completeness of the obstruction.

Uretero or vesicovaginal fistula will present in a delayed fashion with incontinence or discharge. Confirmation of bladder fistula will be by direct visualization and/or the leakage of instilled methylene blue onto a tampon. Ureterovaginal fistula will not pass the methylene blue from the bladder, but will be demonstrated with the intravenous injection of indigo carmine.

Risk Reduction

Trocar-related cystotomies are generally preventable with routine preoperative bladder drainage. Additional caution must be exercised in the patient previously exposed to abdominal or pelvic surgery, where there is a tendency for the bladder to be pulled above the level of the symphysis pubis. The urachus, although rarely patent, should be avoided if possible. It is likely that the placement of an indwelling catheter, at least for prolonged or difficult cases, will reduce the incidence of injury resulting from dissection. Surgical separation of the bladder from the uterus or other adherent structures requires good visualization, appropriate retraction, and excellent surgical technique. Sharp mechanical dissection is preferred, particularly when relatively dense adhesions are present.

Knowledge of the anatomy of the ureter as it courses through the pelvis is a prerequisite to reducing the risk of injury. It is essential to understand the proximity of the ureter to the uterine artery, the cervix, and the uterosacral ligaments, and that any of these relationships may be distorted by previous surgical dissection or by disease such as endometriosis or leiomyomas.

If the surgeon cannot, with assurance, steer a wide path from its course, the ureter must be directly visualized. This is especially true when laser, electrosurgical, or stapling techniques are employed. Frequently, the ureter can be seen through the peritoneum of the pelvic sidewall between the pelvic brim and the attachment of the broad ligament. However, because of patient variation, or the presence of pathology, the location of the ureter can become obscured. In such instances, the ureter can usually be visualized through the peritoneum at the pelvic brim, although the maneuver is slightly more difficult on the left because of the location of the sigmoid mesentery. If CO_2 laser energy is to be employed, fluid injected at an appropriate location between the peritoneal surface and the ureter can provide a degree of protection from thermal injury (52).

If entry into the retroperitoneal space is required for exposure, there should be no hesitation to undertake such dissection. The surface of the peritoneum should be breached with scissors at the closest level proximal, and anterior, to the most distal site of planned dissection where the location of the ureter is known or anticipated. If the ureter is seen through the peritoneum, it may be grasped with a Babcock forceps to minimize trauma while the peritoneum is incised. Careful sharp and blunt dissection then may be applied to provide adequate exposure in the operative field. If the ureter cannot be seen through the peritoneal surface, a fine, toothed forceps should be employed to grasp and elevate the peritoneum allowing careful entry into the retroperitoneal space.

The techniques used for retroperitoneal dissection are also important in reducing the risk of ureteric injury. A number of authors have suggested that blunt dissection can be facilitated with the instillation of fluid into the retroperitoneal space under pressure (52). Others have advocated the selective preoperative placement of ureteric stents, including those that are illuminated, to provide additional safety. The author prefers instead the use of mechanical (sharp or blunt) dissection with sharp-curved scissors and a narrow, pointed grasping forceps attached to an electrosurgical generator. The assistant is provided with a narrow, pointed, and toothed grasping forceps as well as a suction irrigation system to use, as requested, through an ancillary cannula. Dissection proceeds, respecting the blood supply of the ureter by minimizing direct manipulation and by preserving the integrity of its sheath. If electrical energy is used, it must be applied judiciously, at safe distances from the ureter and its blood supply. The narrow, pointed grasping forceps facilitates precise and safe desiccation of small caliber blood vessels.

Treatment

Very small caliber injuries to the bladder (1–2 mm) may be treated expectantly, with prolonged catheterization for 7 to 14 days. However, in such cases the duration of catheterization can be reduced or eliminated if repair is undertaken intraoperatively. When a more significant injury to the bladder is identified, it may often be repaired under laparoscopic direction, provided the presence of adequate surgical skill and a location that is amenable to laparoscopic technique (46,

47). Further evaluation of the location and extent of the laceration may be provided by direct laparoscopic examination of the mucosal surface of the bladder. Should the laceration be near to or involve the trigone, open repair may be preferable. In making this evaluation the mechanism of injury should be considered, as desiccation resulting from electrical energy may extend beyond the visible limits of the lesion.

For relatively small lesions, a purse-string closure may be fashioned using any of a number of synthetic absorbable sutures of 2-0 to 3-0 caliber, tying the knot either intra or extracorporeally (see Chapter 11). For linear lacerations, the defect is preferably closed in two layers. If there is significant thermal injury, it may be valuable to excise the coagulated segment. Postoperative catheterization with either a large caliber urethral or suprapubic catheter should be maintained for 5–7 days for simple fundal lacerations, and for two weeks for those closer to the trigone, the vaginal vault, or those that may be associated with significant thermal injury.

Intraoperative diagnosis of ureteric injury provides the opportunity for intraoperative management. Very limited damage may respond adequately to the passage of a ureteric stent for about 10 to 20 days. However, in most instances, repair is indicated. The principles should follow those previously established for open cases. While laparoscopically directed repair of ureteric lacerations and transections has been described (21, 51), such maneuvers should be practiced only by those with exceptional surgical skill and experience. Even in these cases it is advisable to consult intraoperatively with a specialist in urology.

When the diagnosis of ureteral injury is delayed until following surgery, the imperative is to establish drainage. Some obstructions or lacerations, if incomplete or small, may be successfully treated with either the retrograde or antegrade passage of a ureteral stent. Urinomas may be drained percutaneously. If a stent cannot be successfully manipulated across the lesion, a percutaneous nephrostomy should be created and plans should be made for operative repair.

NEUROLOGIC INJURY

The incidence of nerve injury associated with laparoscopy is unknown, but has been estimated at 0.5 per 1000 cases (5). Peripheral neurologic injury is usually related either to inappropriate positioning of the patient or occurs secondary to pressure exerted by the surgeon or assistants. During laparoscopy, nerve injury may happen rarely as a result of the surgical dissection.

In the lower extremity, the trauma may be direct, such as compression of the perineal nerve against stirrups. Alternatively, the femoral nerve or the sciatic nerve or its branches may be overstretched and damaged by inappropriate positioning of the hip or the knee joint (53–55).

Brachial plexus injuries may occur secondary to the surgeon or assistants leaning against the abducted arm during the procedure. Alternatively, if the patient is placed in steep Trendelenburg position, the brachial plexus may be damaged because of the pressure exerted on the shoulder joint (56).

Recognition

In most instances, the patient is found to have sensory and/or motor deficit as she emerges from the effects of the anesthesia. The diagnosis can usually be suspected by clinical examination. Injuries to the perineal nerve will be reflected by loss of sensation in the lateral aspect of the leg and foot together with a foot drop. Brachial plexus injuries may be variable, but usually involve damage to the C-5,6 roots manifesting in loss of flexion of the elbow and adduction of the shoulder. Electromyography can be used to further define the extent and location of the lesion by testing nerve conduction and recording the electrical potential for various muscles. This evaluation should be delayed for three weeks to allow for complete degeneration of injured nerves.

Risk Reduction

The incidence of brachial plexus injury can be reduced by placing the arms in an adducted position, which also facilitates the performance of pelvic surgery by allowing the surgeon to stand in a more comfortable position. Should it be necessary to leave the arm in an abducted position, adequate padding and support of the arms and shoulders are necessary and can be facilitated with the use of shoulder supports, preventing the slippage of the patient up the table when placed in Trendelenburg's position. Furthermore, in such a position, the surgeon may not lean on the patient's arm.

Sciatic and perineal nerve injury is minimized with the use of appropriate stirrups and careful positioning protocols. Those stirrups that combine both knee and foot support are probably best. Additional measures include simultaneous raising and lowering of the legs, flexion of the knees before flexion of the hips, and limitation of external rotation of the hip. Assistants should be admonished to avoid placing undue pressure on the inner thighs.

Injury to the obturator and genitofemoral nerves is uncommon but will likely increase as greater numbers of retroperitoneal dissections are performed. In such cases, it will be important to clearly understand the anatomy, maintain hemostasis, and to exert the utmost care in performing the dissections, carefully identifying the neural structures as they are encountered.

Management

Most injuries to peripheral nerves recover spontaneously. The time to recovery depends upon the site and severity of the lesion. For most peripheral injuries, full sensory-neural recovery occurs in three to six months. Recovery may be facilitated with physical therapy, appropriate braces, and electrical stimulation of the affected muscles. Transection of major intrapelvic nerves will require open microsurgical repair.

INCISIONAL HERNIA AND WOUND DEHISCENCE

While the incidence of laparoscopic incisional hernia is unknown, it is clear that the complication has been underreported. And, although the first case was described in 1967 (57), few such hernias had been reported in the gynecologic literature until 1994, when a survey of a large number of gynecologists uncovered over 900 laparoscopy associated defects (58). Further reports of incisional hernia have emanated from the urologic and general surgical literature as cholecystectomy and other procedures undergo conversion to laparoscopic technique (59–61).

These and other reports seem to indicate that while no incision is immune to the risk of herniation, those defects that are 10 mm or more in diameter are particularly vulnerable (58–61). The increasing number and size of the incisions, in combination with the surgeon's variable propensity to close them, will likely further contribute to the increasing incidence. Another important contributing factor may be the use of cannula anchoring devices that effectively increase the diameter of the incision by 2 to 3 mm.

One source of confusion in the literature is the lack of distinction among the terms evisceration, wound dehiscence, and true hernia, descriptions that seem to be used interchangeably. Indeed, the distinction may be rather moot as dehiscence of a laparoscopic wound may be irrelevant unless bowel or other intraperitoneal tissue herniates into and through the defect. One of the more sinister complications, involving only a portion of the bowel wall, is Richter's hernia, which is somewhat more difficult to diagnose and may result in perforation, peritonitis, and death.

Diagnosis

The most common hernia appears to occur in the immediate postoperative period where bowel or omentum passes through the unopposed or inadequately repaired defect. The patient may be asymptomatic or can present with any or a combination of pain, fever, periumbilical mass, obvious evisceration, and the symptoms and signs of mechanical bowel obstruction, often within hours and usually within the first postoperative week. Because the patients are usually discharged home shortly after surgery, the symptoms and signs usually manifest out of hospital with the presentation taking place by telephone. Consequently, the surgeon should take care not to casually disregard the patient who telephones with symptoms consistent with herniation.

Because Richter's hernias contain only a portion of the circumference of the bowel wall in the defect, the diagnosis is often delayed. It is likely that such lesions most commonly occur in incisions that are made away from the midline. The initial presenting symptom is usually pain, since the incomplete obstruction still allows the passage of intestinal content. Fever can present if incarceration occurs, and peritonitis may result from the subsequent perforation. The diagnosis is difficult to make and requires a high index of suspicion. Ultrasound or CT scanning may be useful in confirming the diagnosis (62).

While many defects likely remain asymptomatic, late presentation may occur if bowel or omentum becomes trapped (63). The symptoms and findings are similar to that described for earlier presentations.

Risk Reduction

There are a number of unproven but seemingly logical preemptive strategies. First, it is desirable to use the smallest possible cannulas whenever possible, recognizing that hernia has even been reported in conjunction with the use of 5-mm trocars (58–61). Second, the "Z-track" insertion method, particularly applied in the umbilicus, may be of value. This approach, described by Semm, offsets the skin and fascial incisions by entering the subcutaneous tissue, then sliding the conically-tipped trocar along the fascia for a short distance prior to penetrating it

(64). Such a track is purported to close like a curtain, reducing the incidence of hernia. However, evidence for this technique having prophylactic value is currently lacking. Third, all ancillary cannulas should be removed under direct vision to ensure that bowel is not drawn into the incision. Insertion of an obturator (or a laparoscope) into the cannula may further prevent suction from drawing bowel or omentum into the incision. Fourth, at least those incisions 10 mm or greater in diameter should undergo fascial closure under direct laparoscopic vision, thereby preventing incorporation of bowel. This may be accomplished by using a small caliber diameter laparoscope through one of the narrow cannulas to direct incisional closure. A narrow diameter, three-quarter round, needle (Ethicon UR-6; Davis & Geck TT-20; United States Surgical Corp. GU-46) facilitates such a closure, as does the use of one of the newer devices described in Chapter 11. Finally, the laparoscope cannula should be removed with the laparoscope in position, preventing accidental incorporation of bowel.

If the final incision is of sufficiently large diameter to require closure, blind insertion of needles may be avoided by prepositioning sutures. They are placed when the laparoscope is in another location and tied following removal of the final cannula. The sutures should be used to elevate the abdominal wall as the laparoscope and cannula are simultaneously removed, looking down the endoscope to ensure that bowel or omentum are not inadvertently drawn into the wound.

Management

Management of laparoscopic incisional defects depends upon the timing of the presentation and the presence or absence of entrapped bowel and its condition. Evisceration will always require surgical intervention. If the diagnosis is made in the recovery room, the patient may be returned to the operating room, the bowel or omentum replaced in the peritoneal cavity (provided there is no evidence of necrosis or suture incorporation), and the incision repaired, usually under laparoscopic guidance. However, if the diagnosis is delayed it is likely that the bowel is incarcerated and at risk for perforation. In such circumstances, resection will likely be necessary, usually via laparotomy. Most gynecologic surgeons should request general surgical consultation.

INFECTION

Wound infection following laparoscopy is rarely reported, making the incidence difficult to estimate. Early reports suggested an incidence of 1.2 to 1.7 per 1000 cases, most of which were minor skin abscesses that required no treatment or simple outpatient therapy (65, 66). However, these estimates reflected the era prior to the widespread use of operative laparoscopy when procedures were performed with only one or two incisions. In addition, potentially contaminating procedures such as culdotomy were not used. In the urologic and general surgical literature, wound infection rates seem to range from 5 to 6 per 1000 cases (67, 68). While the vast majority of wound infections are handled successfully with expectant management, drainage, or antibiotics, severe necrotizing fasciitis has been reported (69).

Other types of postlaparoscopy infection have been reported including bladder infection, pelvic cellulitis, and pelvic abscess (70–72). While bacteremia has been described, there have been no reports of disseminated infection following laparoscopic surgery (73). The incidence of infection following laparoscopic hysterectomy is difficult to assess, in part because of the absence of a large volume of studies, and in part because the use of prophylactic antibiotics has not been addressed in the published literature.

In summary, it seems that the risk of infection associated with laparoscopy is low; much lower than that associated with open abdominal or vaginal surgery. Nevertheless, until clinical studies dictate otherwise, it is prudent to continue to practice strict sterile technique and to offer appropriate prophylactic antibiotics to selected patients. These could include those with enhanced risk for bacterial endocarditis, as well as those who are to undergo procedures (e.g., laparoscopic hysterectomy), suspected of increasing the chance of wound or vault infection. Patients should be instructed to routinely take their temperature following discharge and to immediately report fever of 38° C or more to the health care provider team.

CONCLUSION

With care and adequate training, the incidence of complications associated with laparoscopy can be minimized. The outpatient nature of most of these procedures means that the presentation of adverse outcomes is frequently by telephone. Consequently, the patient must be adequately informed regarding the expected postoperative course, and know when to report unusual symptoms. The surgeon and colleagues have an obligation not to minimize these complaints. Remember, after laparoscopy the patient should feel better each day.

REFERENCES

1. Hulka JF, Soderstrom RM, Corson SL, Brooks PG. Complications committee of the American Association of Gynecologic Laparoscopists, First annual report. J Reprod Med 1973;10:310–316.
2. Cuschieri A. Laparoscopy in general surgery and gastroenterology. Br J Hosp Med 1980;24: 255–258.
3. Frenkel Y, Oelsner G, Ben-Baruch G, Menczer J. Major surgical complications of laparoscopy. Eur J Obstet Gynecol Reprod Biol 1981;12:107–111.
4. Riedel HH, Lehman-Willenbrock E, Conrad P, Semm K. German pelviscopic statistics for the years 1978–1982. Endoscopy 1986;18:219–222.
5. Peterson HB, Hulka JF, Philips JM. American Association of Gynecologic Laparoscopists 1988 membershhip survey in operative laparoscopy. J Reprod Med 1990;35:587–589.
6. Smith DC, Donohue LR, Waszak SJ. A hospital review of advanced gynecologic endoscopic procedures. Am J Obstet Gynecol 1994;170:1635–1640.
7. Lehmann-Willenbrock E, Riedel HH, Mecke H, Semm K. Pelviscopy/laparoscopy and its complications in Germany 1949–1988. J Reprod Med 1992;37:671–677.
8. Peterson HB, DeStefano F, Rubin GL, Greenspan JR, Lee NC, Ory HW. Deaths attributable to tubal sterilization in the United States, 1977 to 1981. Am J Obstet Gynecol 1982;146:131–136.
9. Brown DR, Fishburn JF, Robertson VD. Ventilation and blood gas changes during laparoscopy with local anesthesia. Am J Obstet Gynecol 1976;124:741–745.
10. Brady CE III, Harklerood LE, Pierson WP. Alterations in oxygen saturation and ventilation after intravenous sedation of peritoneoscopy. Arch Intern Med 1989;149:1029–1032.
11. Ishizaki Y, Bandai Y, Shimomura K, Abe H, Ohtomo Y, Idezuki Y. Safe intraabdominal pressure of carbon dioxide pneumoperitoneum during laparoscopic surgery. Surgery 1993;114:549–554.

12. Myles PS. Brady arrhythmias and laparoscopy: a prospective study of heart rate changes with laparoscopy. Aust NZ J Obstet Gynecol 1991;31:171–173.
13. Copeland C, WIng R, Hulka JF. Direct trocar insertion at laparoscopy: an evaluation. Obstet Gynecol 1983;62:655–659.
14. Burgatten L, Gruss L, Barad D, Kaali S. Direct trocar insertion versus Verres needle use for laparoscopic sterilization. J Repro Med 1990;35:891–894.
15. Byron JW, Fugiyoshi CA, Miyazawa K. Evaluation of the direct trocar insertion technique at laparoscopy. Obstet Gynecol 1989;74:423–425.
16. Kabukoba JJ, Skillern LH. Coping with extraperitoneal insufflation during laparoscopy: a new technique. Obstet Gynecol 1992;80:144–145.
17. Kent RB. Subcutaneous emphysema and hypercarbia associated with laparoscopy. Arch Surg 1991;126:1154–1156.
18. Bard PA, Chen L. Subcutaneous emphysema associated with laparoscopy. Anesth Analg 1990;71:101–102.
19. Doctor NH, Hussain Z. Bilateral pneumothorax associated with laparoscopy: a case report of a rare hazard and review of the literature. Anesthesiology 1973;28:75–81.
20. Kalhan SB, Reaney JA, Collins RL. Pneumomediastinum and subcutaneous emphysema during laparoscopy. Cleve Clin J Med 1990;57:639–642.
21. Gomel V, James C. Intraoperative management of ureteral injury during operative laparoscopy. Fertil Steril 1991;55:416–419.
22. Grainger DA, Soderstrom RM, Schiff SF, Glickman MG, DeCherney AH, Diamond MP. Ureteral injuries at laparoscopy: insights into diagnosis, management, and prevention. Obstet Gynecol 1990;75:839–843.
23. Corson SL. Electrosurgical hazards in laparoscopy. JAMA 1974;227:1261.
24. Engel T. The electrical dynamics of laparoscopic sterilization. J Reprod Med 1975;15:33–42.
25. Mintz M. Risks and prophylaxis in laparoscopy: a survey of 100,000 cases. J Reprod Med 1977;18:269–272.
26. Peterson H, Greenspan J, Ory H. Death following puncture of the aorta during laparoscopic sterilization. Obstet Gynecol 1981;59:133–134.
27. Bergqvist D, Bergqvist A. Vascular injuries during gynecological surgery. Acta Obstet Gynecol Scand 1987;66:19–23.
28. Baadsgarrd SE, Bille S, Egeblad K. Major vascular injury during gynecologic laparoscopy. Acta Obstet Gynecol Scand 1989;68:283–285.
29. Penfield AJ. How to prevent complications of open laparoscopy. J Reprod Med 1985;30:660–663.
30. Majeski JA. Rectus sheath abscess. South Med J 1986;79:1311.
31. Ryder RM, Hulka JF. Bladder and bowel injury after electrodesiccation with Kleppinger bipolar forceps: a clinicopathologic study. J Reprod Med 1993;38:595–598.
32. Yuzpe AA. Pneumoperitoneum and trocar injuries in laparoscopy, a survey on possible contributing factors and prevention. J Reprod Med 1990;35:485–490.
33. Cunanan RG Jr, Courey NG, Lippes J. Complications of laparoscopic tubal sterilization. Obstet Gynecol 1980;55:501–506.
34. Deziel DJ, Millikan KW, Economou SG, Doolas A, Sung-Tao K, Airan MC. Complications of laparoscopic cholecystectomy: a national survey of 4292 hospitals and an analysis of 77,614 cases. Am J Surg 1993;165:9–14.
35. Chi IC, Feldblum PJ. Laparoscopic sterilization requiring laparotomy. Am J Obstet Gynecol 1982;142:712–713.
36. Chi IC, Feldblum PJ, Baloh SA. Previous abdominal surgery as a risk factor in interval laparoscopic sterilization. Am J Obstet Gynecol 1983;145:841–846.
37. Franks AL, Kendrick JS, Peterson HB. Unintended laparotomy associated with laparoscopic tubal sterilization. Am J Obstet Gynecol 1987;157:1102–1105.
38. Reich H. Laparoscopic bowel injury. Surg Laparos Endos 1992;2:74–78.
39. Childers JM, Brzechfta PR, Surwit EA. Laparoscopy using the left upper quadrant as the primary trocar site. Gynecol Oncol 1993;50:221–225.
40. Wolfe BM, Gardiner BN, Leary BF, Frey CF. Endoscopic cholecystectomy; an analysis of complications. Arch Surg 1991;126:1192–1198.
41. CDC. Deaths following female sterilization with unipolar electrocoagulating devices. MMWR 1981;30:149.

42. AAGL. 1981 Board of trustees recommendations, June 11, 1981.
43. Levy BS, Soderstrom RM, Dail DH. Bowel injuries during laparoscopy: gross anatomy and histology. J Reprod Med 1985;30:168–172.
44. American Association of Gynecologic Laparoscopists News Scope 1985;4(1):1, 13.
45. Wheeless CR. Thermal gastrointestinal injuries. In: Phillips JM, ed. Laparoscopy. Baltimore: Williams & Wilkins, 1977:231–235.
46. Reich H, McGlynn F. Laparoscopic repair of bladder injury. Obstet Gynecol 1990;75:909–910.
47. Font GE, Brill AI, Stuhldreher PV, Rosenweig BA. Endoscopic management of incidental cystotomy during operative laparoscopy. J Urol 1993;149:1130–1131.
48. Steckel J, Badillo F, Waldbaum RS. Uretero-fallopian tube fistula secondary to laparoscopic fulguration of pelvic endometriosis. J Urol 1993;149:1128–1129.
49. Kadar N, Lemmerling L. Urinary fistulas during laparoscopic hysterectomy: causes and prevention. Am J Obstet Gynecol 1994;170:47–48.
50. Woodland MB. Ureter injury during laparoscopy-assisted hysterectomy with the endoscopic linear stapler. Am J Obstet Gynecol 1992;167:756–757.
51. Nezhat C, Nezhat F. Laparoscopic repair of ureter resected during operative laparoscopy. Obstet Gynecol 1992;80:543–544.
52. Nezhat C, Nezhat FR. Safe laser endoscopic excision or vaporization of peritoneal endometriosis. Fertil Steril 1989;52:149–151.
53. Loffler FD, Dent D, Goodkin R. Sciatic nerve injury in a patient undergoing laparoscopy. J Reprod Med 1978;21:371–372.
54. Hershag A, Loy RA, Lavy G, DeCherney AH. Femoral neuropathy after laparoscopy: a case report. J Reprod Med 1990;35:575–576.
55. al Hakin M, Katirjic B. Femoral neuropathy induced by the lithotomy position: a report of 5 cases with a review of the literature. Muscle Nerve 1993;16:891–895.
56. Reich H. Laparoscopic treatment of extensive pelvic adhesions, including hydrosalpinx. J Reprod Med 1987;32:736–742.
57. Levy M. A late complication of peritoneoscopy. Gastrointest Endosc 1967;14:117–119.
58. Montz FR, Holschneider C, Munro MG. Incisional hernia following laparoscopy: a survey of the American Association of Gynecologic Laparoscopists. Obstet Gynecol 1994;84:881–884.
59. Bloom DA, Ehrlich RM. Omental evisceration through small laparoscopy port sites. J Endourol 1993;7:31–33.
60. Plaus WJ. Laparoscopic trocar site hernias. J Laparoendo Surg 1993;3:567–570.
61. Kadar N, Reich H, Liu CY, Manko GF, Gimpleson R. Incisional hernias after major laparoscopic gynecologic procedures. Am J Obstet Gynecol 1993;169:1493–1495.
62. Maco A, Ruchman RB. CT diagnosis of post laparoscopic hernia. J Comp Ass Tomo 1991;15:1054–1055.
63. Bourke JB. Small intestinal obstruction from Richter's hernia at the site of insertion of a laparoscope. BMJ 1977;2:1393–1394.
64. Semm K. Operative manual for endoscopic abdominal surgery. Chicago: Year Book, 1987:142.
65. Chamberlain GVP, Carron-Brown J. Gynaecological Laparoscopy. London: Royal College of Obstetricians & Gynecologists, 1978.
66. Loffer FD, Pent D. Statistics. In: Phillips JM, ed. Laparoscopy. Baltimore: Williams & Wilkins, 1977:243–246.
67. Wolfe BM, Gardiner BN, Leary BF, Frey CF. Endoscopic cholecystectomy, an analysis of complications. Arch Surg 1991;126:1192–1198.
68. Capelouto CC, Kavoussi LR. Complications of laparoscopic surgery. Urology 1993;42:2–12.
69. Sotrel G, Hirsch E, Edelin KC. Necrotizing fasciitis following diagnostic laparoscopy. Obstet Gynecol 1982;62(suppl 3):675–695.
70. Levinson CJ, Daily HI, Marko ME, et al. Nonelectrical laparoscopic sterilization: experience with a Silastic band. Obstet Gynecol 1976;48:494–496.
71. Kumarasamy T, Hurt WG. Laparoscopic sterilization with silicone rubber bands. Obstet Gynecol 1977;50:351.
72. Glew RH, Pokoly TB. Tuboovarian abscess following laparoscopic sterilization with silicone rubber bands. Obstet Gynecol 1980;50:760–762.
73. Iwamura K, Ueno F, Itakura M, Sugimoto E. Evaluation of blood cultures following laparoscopy. Tokai J Exp Clin Med 1980;5:323–327.

Chapter 13

Chronic Pelvic Pain
Assessment and Treatment Guidelines for the Laparoscopic Surgeon
John F. Steege

Laparoscopy has without doubt vastly improved the gynecologist's ability to care for the woman with either acute or chronic pelvic pain (CPP). Although multiple factors may contribute to the development of CPP, as discussed below, the laparoscope is clearly the most reliable means available for diagnosing and treating the two forms of organic gynecologic pathology that are most often involved with CPP, and are the most difficult to accurately measure by pelvic examination: endometriosis and adhesions. This chapter will focus on the preoperative and postoperative diagnostic procedures that may augment the value of the laparoscopic findings in the overall care of the patient with CPP.

The surgically oriented gynecologist frequently conducts the clinical evaluation of CPP with the goal of finding "enough" pathology to explain the pain. This is often a frustrating and futile search. This same dilemma confronts those dealing with other chronic pain syndromes. Pain theorists have had to modify theories of pain perception in the attempt to explain this common clinical experience. A review of pain theory will provide an appropriate backdrop for the remainder of this chapter (1).

GENERAL PAIN THEORY

The Cartesian theory of pain perception suggested that dedicated pain fibers carried pain signals from the periphery to the brain. Pain was felt to be proportional to tissue damage or stimulation. This model reasonably explains clinical acute pain, but fails to explain the phenomena seen in chronic pain.

Chronic pain is qualitatively different from acute pain. It is a different illness, not just a warning signalling the presence of an illness. In acute pain, corroborative findings in laboratory or diagnostic tests are often present, while in chronic pain, the interpretation of diagnostic studies, including laparoscopy, is often problematic. In acute pain, it may be important to take the patient's personality and life situation into account in order to render thoughtful and effective care, but these factors will less often influence your choice of treatment (antibiotics, etc.). In chronic pain, understanding the patient's personality, affective state, family environment, etc. are critical to bringing about improvement in her pain.

Virtually all current theories of pain perception suggest that peripheral signals be termed "nociceptive," with the term "pain" being reserved for the central process of recognition of peripheral nociceptive signals (2). Down-regulation or up-regulation of signals may be under the control of higher centers in the brain and impinge upon the spinal cord directly. Multiple biochemical modulators may exist in the spinal cord, all of which serve to substantially alter the impact of nociceptive signals from the periphery. Thus, information travels in two directions between brain and spinal cord. Add to this the impact of individual experience, cultural and personal expectations, personality, etc., and you have a most complex mechanism responsible for recognizing and interpreting pain. The most widely recognized theory of pain perception, the Gate Control Theory (2) (Fig. 13.1), describes a framework for understanding pain that includes physical and psychological events in one coherent model.

In many instances of chronic pain, the intensity of the pain bears little or no relationship to the amount of tissue damage. Careful treatment of damaged tissue is an important component of care, but it is the clinician's clear responsibility to place such treatment in the overall context of the patient and her life. In other words, the clinician should proceed cautiously when, in addition to some evidence for organic pathology, the patient seems to present with elements of a "chronic pain syndrome."

A "chronic pain syndrome" can be psychologically and behaviorally defined (1). Although the need for further validating work is evident, the presence of the syndrome has been found to significantly predict the clinical outcome of laparoscopic adhesiolysis to relieve pain (3). The clinical diagnosis of a chronic pain syndrome is made when the patient fulfills four of the following criteria:

1. Pain has lasted six months or longer, for two weeks of each month.
2. Pain has not been relieved by analgesic medications.
3. Significant alteration of physical activity has occurred (recreation, household responsibilities, work, sexual life).
4. Vegetative signs of depression are present (sleep disturbance usually appears before appetite or weight changes).
5. Family roles have changed (care and discipline of children, decision-making processes, etc.) or the pain has become the most important problem the family faces.

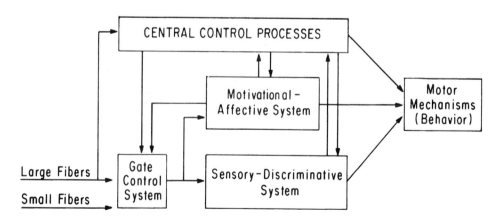

Figure 13.1. Conceptual model of the sensory, motivational, and central control determinants of pain, illustrating reciprocal interactions among the components of pain perception. (Adapted from Melzack R, Dennis SG. Neurophysiological foundations of pain. In: Sternbach RA. The Psychology of Pain. New York: Raven Press, 1978.)

When this constellation of findings is present, the physician should take care to prepare the patient and him/herself for a cautious interpretation of laparoscopic findings and the need for more broad-spectrum evaluation and treatment of the pain problem.

PREOPERATIVE ASSESSMENT

As with most clinical problems, a carefully performed history and physical examination will yield the vast majority of needed information. An adequate CPP history will elicit enough information to decide which of the criteria listed above are fulfilled. This should include a carefully elicited chronology of the pain's development.

CPP develops gradually, in increments. The woman with very focal pain of stable intensity that has not developed significant affective change or experienced any change of her roles within the family is very different from her opposite: the woman whose pain started out in one area and gradually came to include pain over a wider pelvic area as well as new bladder symptoms, low back muscular pain, altered bowel habit, feelings of depression, etc. Understanding the chronology of the pain while also asking about personal and family life events corresponding to the times at which new symptoms appeared may help both patient and physician gain insight into the psychosocial stressors involved in the gradual development of CPP. The process of documenting such a history conveys the message that multiple factors are important in the growth of CPP, hence multiple treatments might be necessary. This avoids the implication that surgical approaches are the only ones that really count.

Physical examination for CPP begins by observing the patient's posture: how she walks, sits, transfers from a sitting to a lying down position on the examining table, etc. Patients with lumbar muscle pain will walk slightly stooped or with increased lordotic posture. Those with levator plate and/or pyriformis spasm will sit with their weight primary resting on the buttock of the less symptomatic side, or will sit slumped forward in the chair if both sides are equally involved.

The abdominal examination should begin with systematic gentle palpation of the abdominal wall with a single finger tip, looking for possible trigger points (4). Their discovery is important for more complete treatment, as well as to avoid confusion during the bimanual portion of the pelvic examination, when pain from the abdominal wall may easily be mistaken for internal visceral pain. When a tender spot is found, ask the patient to elevate her head off the table while palpating the area. The resulting increased tension of the abdominal wall musculature will aggravate pain originating in the abdominal wall, while usually causing internal visceral pain to diminish.

During the pelvic examination, a simple stepwise technique will help identify specific symptomatic areas. Start with gentle palpation of the vaginal vestibule (looking for vestibulitis (5)), then ask for contraction and relaxation of the introitus (vaginismus (6)). Palpate each levator plate (pelvic floor tension myalgia (7)), and the piriformis muscle on each side (pyriformis syndrome (8)). Pain from this latter muscle may be elicited by palpating the muscle transvaginally while asking the patient to externally rotate the ipsilateral thigh against resistance.

Then palpate the urethra and the bladder base. Trigonitis is often diagnosed by palpation, although cystoscopic confirmation is useful and can be done at the same time as a laparoscopy if indicated. Continue by reaching back to palpate the sacrum and coccyx. With the index finger of the vaginal hand on the coccyx, position the external hand at the tip of the coccyx and try to flex it anteriorly: this maneuver will reproduce the pain of coccydynia.

Having completed a palpatory survey of the "non-gynecologic" organs of the pelvis, then proceed with the traditional maneuvers to detect cervical, uterine, or adnexal pathology, i.e., motion of the cervix in four directions, sequential palpation of the broad ligament and ovarian areas, and rectovaginal examination of the cul-de-sac and adnexal areas. The uterosacral ligaments may be more clearly defined by displacing the cervix with the vaginal index finger while palpating the ligaments with the rectal middle finger. When trying to determine if pain is originating in the abdominal wall or the pelvic viscera, during the bimanual examination it is most informative to separate the motions of your two hands instead of pressing simultaneously with both.

WHEN TO USE LAPAROSCOPY

Ideally, if the development of the pain problem has been observed over time, it may be best to pursue the examination described above and to consider laparoscopy before the stigmata of the chronic pain syndrome become painfully evident.

At this point in the evaluation, there is usually a fairly good idea about the probability of finding organic pathology at laparoscopy. Before proceeding, the following should be considered: if you did not have the option of doing surgery, what other methods of treatment would you employ? If the answer includes any of the methods used to treat chronic pelvic pain (bowel management, bladder symptom control, physical therapy for mechanical and musculoskeletal components, antidepressants, psychotherapy, support group therapy, sexual counseling, trigger point injection, massage therapy, acupuncture, family therapy, etc.), it is well worthwhile to introduce and possibly implement these ideas before proceeding to the operating room. The bottom line: surgery is just one of the things that can be done, and makes observable organic pathology take its place among the many possible contributing factors in CPP. Emphasize to the patient and her family that regardless of what the laparoscopic findings and procedures may turn out to be, she may still have to work on the other components of the pain problem.

THE DIAGNOSTIC LAPAROSCOPY FOR PAIN

A word about preoperative preparation. Many laparoscopic procedures now being performed are by no means "minor" procedures. The patient should receive the same level of general medical assessment and review of anesthetic considerations as if she were having an abdominal hysterectomy. If any degree of adhesive disease or endometriosis is expected (especially in the cul-de-sac), a full mechanical bowel preparation is indicated, in the form of a gallon of polyethylene glycol solution (or equivalent) by mouth starting in the late afternoon before surgery, followed by a Fleet's enema later that evening. (If the thought of a bowel preparation even crosses your mind, you should probably order one.)

The Procedure

In the case of CPP, the laparoscopy should be carried out with the goal of searching for as many of the potential causes as possible, both gynecologic and otherwise. Endometriosis and pelvic adhesions are at the top of the list from the standpoint of prevalence. The presence of these abnormalities by no means proves their causal role in the patient's pain. Given the well-known powerful placebo effect of any surgical intervention, even a positive therapeutic result after laparoscopic treatment of such problems must be interpreted with a critical clinical eye and a well-considered grain of salt.

A careful laparoscopic review of the pelvic peritoneum should be done at close range, with the laparoscope no more than 1–2 cm from the tissue. Begin in the anterior cul-de-sac and review as much of the pelvis as possible before you start manipulating organs with a probe; probing often produces petechiae, which can be mistaken for endometriosis. Anteversion of the uterus with an intrauterine manipulator (the author prefers the Zumi) allows a no-touch review of most of the pelvis. The ovarian fossae are best seen by passing the tip of the laparoscope behind each ovary and tube, entering the ovarian fossa from its cephalad end and nudging the ovary medially with the tip of the laparoscope. Decrease the light intensity as the laparoscope is withdrawn from the ovarian fossa in order to view the lateral side of the ovary atraumatically.

Next, introduce a second probe and be sure that all the pelvic organs move freely, especially the adnexae. Filmy adhesions suggestive of old infection may at times lie flat against structures, only becoming evident when such structures are put on stretch. Finally, put enough irrigant solution (the author prefers Ringer's lactate, which is less acidic than normal saline) in the cul-de-sac to allow flotation of the tubes to observe the delicacy of fimbrial architecture.

The evaluation of the pelvic floor should be very thorough, especially in the person complaining of midline or cul-de-sac pelvic pain. For example, recent work (9) has emphasized that in 10–20% of cases of endometriosis, implants may hide beneath the peritoneum of the pelvic floor, betraying their presence with only the most minimal visible change. These nodules may be suspected when performing preoperative examination during menses. They can also be demonstrated during laparoscopy by performing rectovaginal examination with one hand while palpating the pelvic floor with a smooth laparoscopic probe held in the other hand. Carefully trace over the entire cul-de-sac, uterosacral ligaments, anterior rectum and the areas between the uterosacrals and the ureters.

The most common gynecologic pathologic findings in women with chronic pelvic pain will be adhesions and endometriosis. A more comprehensive list of occasional findings should be evaluated during the laparoscopic pelvic and abdominal survey:

1. The appendix: Move the cecum and terminal ileum until a complete view of the appendix is obtained, noting its diameter, attachments, and any signs of inflammation or pigmentation suspicious of endometriosis. (Of all bowel implants of endometriosis, about 10% are on the appendix.)
2. The terminal ileum: On occasion, stiffness and thickening of the terminal ileum may betray the presence of Crohn's disease. In all fairness, most cases

having this much pathology will have been suspected clinically and diagnosed radiologically prior to laparoscopy.
3. The internal inguinal rings: The round ligaments exit the abdomen via the internal inguinal ring on each side. An indirect inguinal hernia (the most common type) may be diagnosed simply by viewing the hernia sac surrounding the round ligament. A clinical judgment must then be made concerning the significance of the herniation and its relevance to the patient's complaints.
4. The femoral canal: A femoral hernia is much less common than an inguinal hernia. Clinical diagnosis is difficult, and many times surgical exploration is undertaken to look for a hernia when none can be found. A femoral hernia is easily diagnosed laparoscopically by observing the area of the femoral canal. The location can be confirmed by external palpation while looking through the laparoscope.
5. The paracolic gutters: The peritoneal investment of the cecum, ascending colon, and sigmoid colon is highly variable. In many instances, these peritoneal attachments can look very much like adhesions, especially when they are put on stretch in Trendelenberg position. If the folds of tissue are continuous all the way out to the abdominal sidewalls and have an even pattern of vessels throughout, they probably represent normal anatomy. Actual adhesions are usually discontinuous and vary in density and vascularity from place to place.
6. The anterior abdominal wall: Rarely, hernias may occur along the lateral margins of the rectus muscle (spigelian hernias).
7. The intestines: It is not really possible to "run" the bowel in the traditional sense, but often enough loops can be isolated and inspected to reduce the possibility of loop-to-loop adhesions or a Meckel's diverticulum.
8. The liver and gallbladder: The tip of the gallbladder can be visualized and its size noted. The surface of the liver should be observed for signs of cirrhosis, masses, or post-pelvic inflammatory disease (Fitz-Hugh-Curtis) adhesions between the liver and the sidewall.
9. The diaphragm: On rare occasions, endometriosis may implant on the diaphragm, which can be diagnosed and treated laparoscopically.

The Operative Report

Most importantly, having completed this survey, the operative note should be dictated immediately. List the positive findings in a separate section, and be sure to list all pertinent negatives. Emphasize that the pelvic surfaces have been examined at very close range in a careful step-by-step fashion. This indicates that a thoroughly complete diagnostic laparoscopy was undertaken. This is very useful information for anyone who may be involved in the patient's future care.

Most laparoscopy suites now have the capacity to make still photos of the surgery. Make several copies, for the medical record, office files, and for the patient. Use these when talking with the family and the patient.

The Postoperative Talk with the Family

Obtain permission from the patient to talk with her family immediately after the surgery. Ideally, you will have had the opportunity to meet at least one member of the family before surgery and have used that opportunity to educate the family about the nature of chronic pain. That talk will have laid the groundwork for the postoperative discussion.

Postoperatively, the family will have been waiting for several hours. They are most concerned with their loved one's safety, but they are also hoping that you will discover a single cause and perform a curative procedure. They will also have been talking among themselves about how difficult the pain has been for your patient to bear. Collectively, they will be in a state of heightened emotional vulnerability. All the feelings they may have about the pain problem will be closer to the surface: worry, frustration, sympathy, anger, etc. At that moment they may be more willing than at any other time to share their concerns and offer their perspective on your patient's coping skills, pain behaviors, and emotional condition. This is the best opportunity, in the case of the more difficult chronic pain problem, to help them understand the need to simultaneously address all the components of the pain, and the need to approach pain relief as a longer-term rehabilitative task. This will help the patient by assisting the family in giving her appropriate support and understanding your therapeutic approach. It will also reinforce a more realistic set of expectations of any surgical benefit.

TREATING PATHOLOGY FOUND AT LAPAROSCOPY FOR PAIN

Endometriosis

Pain associated with endometriosis has long been mysterious in nature. There is a growing consensus that the location of pain will most often correspond reasonably well to the location of the endometriosis. The intensity of the pain, however, cannot be correlated with the extent of disease (10, 11). It has often been said that those with a little endometriosis will have a lot of pain, while those with larger amounts of disease may have little pain. Cases exist that fit this rule, and are recalled because they don't conform to the (now outdated) expectation that pain should be proportional to the amount of organic pathology. When examined systematically, there is simply no correlation between the extent of disease and the degree of pain. One possible exception to this rule is the deep implant of endometriosis, most typically found in the cul-de-sac, which may be more reliably associated with pain and dyspareunia the larger and deeper it is (9).

There is considerable debate concerning the best way to treat endometriosis once it is discovered. Removal by excision, laser vaporization, or electrocautery is associated with more rapid conception, although the ultimate cumulative pregnancy rate over time may be no greater than that accomplished through expectant management (12). Similar studies of pain relief by medical versus surgical management have not been performed. A recent study showed that laparoscopic treatment resulted in relief of pain in 62.5% of patients overall. More puzzling is the observation that pain relief at 6 months was inversely related to anatomic stage: 38% in Stage I, 69% in Stage II, and 100% in Stage III. The study was limited by the absence of biopsies in early stage disease and the small number ($n = 3$) of patients with Stage III disease (13).

There are several explanations for this apparent anomaly. Possibly, early stage endometriosis is a biologically different form of the disease than the later stages that involve large endometriomas and gross anatomic distortion of pelvic organs. Qualitative and quantitative differences may exist in the production of various chemical mediators of pain: cytokines, prostaglandins, substance P, etc. It may be that the coelomic metaplasia theory and Sampson's theory of the etiology of endometriosis both have merit, and that the clinical course and symptomatology may vary with the etiology. Finally, the meaning of the disease to the patient may play a role.

The patient afflicted with endometriosis often quickly learns that the disease has a highly variable rate of progression in different women, and is treatable but not curable, short of hysterectomy and oophorectomy. (She soon hears about the cases in which hysterectomy and bilateral oophorectomy are ineffective.) She also learns that the noninvasive means for monitoring the progression of disease are very inaccurate, i.e., pelvic examination, vaginal ultrasound, computerized tomography, and magnetic resonance imaging. This leaves laparoscopy as the only truly accurate way of monitoring the success or failure of medical and surgical therapy—that is, except for her pain level. Her pain therefore becomes the primary barometer by which she judges the likelihood of further uncomfortable and expensive medical therapies, extirpative surgery, impaired sexual function, and loss of fertility.

Having endometriosis thus has tremendous impact on a woman's life and can cause severe levels of emotional stress. The longer this continues, the more likely it is that this impact will include both diminished pain threshold and pain tolerance. The location of the pain may also spread, as sleep is disturbed, musculoskeletal pains develop, bowel function deteriorates, deconditioning becomes a problem as activity decreases, and marital strife occurs. A chronic pain syndrome has developed.

Laparoscopic management of endometriosis may have its best effects when conducted in the context of a thorough understanding of these factors by the patient, her family, and her physician.

During the laparoscopy itself, after a careful survey of the pelvis has been performed, any implants of endometriosis should be treated. If endometriosis implants are found in the anterior cul-de-sac, they should be treated first. This avoids the problem of producing petechiae by the blunt trauma of a probe and then later misinterpreting these "lesions" as endometriosis. The remainder of the pelvic peritoneum should be inspected at close range, and lesions treated. Larger endometriomas should be left for last, as treating them first may again result in confusing peritoneal trauma.

The energy source used to destroy lesions of endometriosis should be the surgeon's choice, as comfort and skill with a given type of energy are probably more important. Bipolar electrocautery scissors or forceps avoid the risk of capacitance injury that is present with monopolar instruments, but the surgeon well familiar with monopolar physics can certainly use these instruments with safety. The CO_2 laser may be somewhat safer than the KTP or Nd:YAG sources due to its shallower tissue penetration, but again, the familiarity of the user with the nature of the energy source is probably more important.

Regardless of the energy source, the basic principles of surgery apply: exposure, traction-countertraction, and working from an area of known anatomy toward the unknown. Easily treated areas should be excised or destroyed to the point of seeing normal retroperitoneal fat beneath. Lesions sitting over vital structures such as the ureter can be isolated by pulling the peritoneum to one side or elevating it before applying the energy source. If the ureter appears to travel with the overlying peritoneum, then the peritoneum should be opened in a nearby uninvolved area (start with the "known") and the ureter peeled off the back side of the peritoneum containing the endometriosis.

When treating lesions over the bowel or bladder, great care must be taken regardless of the energy source used. Turn the CO_2 laser down to 5–10 watts of superpulse and work slowly, irrigating off char as soon as it forms, then proceeding a bit farther. Users of electrocautery sources suggest that higher wattages may actually be safer when used carefully, as tissue destruction will be more precisely localized and collateral thermal damage that is invisible may be minimal. The time of contact needs to be carefully controlled when using higher wattage electrocautery. The author's view is that the CO_2 laser is easier to control, and therefore safer to use in this type of situation.

Lesions of the pelvic floor require special comment. Koninckx (9) has described several types of endometriotic lesions that can occur, including the mostly-hidden lesion that presents with only a small visible part on the peritoneal surface. After discovering such a lesion by the method described above, ablation can be carried out using basically the same maneuvers. Here again, the author feels that the laser offers a more controlled energy source in this type of tight corner, but others feel comfortable using cautery. The advocates of cautery suggest, when working with deep lesions in the cul-de-sac, that the surgeon should basically excise the entire lesion, first freeing up the rectosigmoid in order to retract it out of the way. If such retraction proves impossible, then the more aggressive (and experienced) laparoscopic surgeon can perform an intrafascial dissection down the posterior margin of the cervix, enter the rectovaginal septum, free the rectosigmoid from its lateral attachments close to the uterosacral ligaments, and then excise the endometriosis lesion. At this point the rectosigmoid is sufficiently freed up so that if serosal or muscular bowel injury should take place, it can be oversewn with interrupted absorbable sutures placed laparoscopically. Although traditionally surgical teaching would hold that a large bowel enterotomy should be treated with a diverting colostomy and open repair, a few surgeons have reported repairing complete enterotomies laparoscopically without complications (PR Koninckx, personal communication, 1994). As mentioned, whenever substantial cul-de-sac disease is suspected, a thorough mechanical bowel preparation should be done the evening before surgery.

Ovarian endometriomas are yet another area of controversy in the laparoscopic surgical literature. When removed by laparotomy, the traditional approach has been to incise the ovarian cortex over the lesion, shell out the entire lining of the endometriotic cyst, then close the ovary in one of a variety of ways with absorbable suture. When seen at subsequent surgery, ovaries treated in this manner are most often covered with adhesions (14). Three laparoscopic approaches have been used: simple drainage, drainage followed by destruction of the lining with laser or cautery, or removal of the entire cyst lining and leaving the ovary open. Direct comparison has so far not demonstrated a clear advantage of any one method over the others (15), although most operators feel that removal of the entire cyst lining should be done in the attempt to reduce the risk or rapidity of recurrence. Most feel that the ovary should be left open to heal on its own.

Pelvic Adhesions

Here again, the basic principles of surgery apply: exposure, traction-countertraction, and work from a place where the anatomy is clear toward the areas that are unclear. Extensive adhesiolysis can be carried out with minimal risk and minimal blood loss when done properly. Adhesiolysis is usually done with the hope that they will not re-form. It is useful to recall the factors that are felt to promote adhesion formation: bleeding, foreign bodies such as sutures, infection, and tissue abrasion, desiccation, or necrosis. Incise those that appear avascular first. This often allows the more difficult areas to simplify. Use blunt dissection carefully. An area that seems to come away easily with blunt dissection often looks quite bloody within another minute as multiple small bleeders appear. If you isolate what looks like a blood vessel running through an adhesion, coagulate it before cutting it with scissors or laser, or use cautery scissors. Start with the easy areas first, or to use a basketball/football metaphor, "take what the defense gives you."

Special care must be taken when dealing with bowel adhesions. Use good atraumatic graspers from lateral ports to retract the loop or loops you are working with, using scissors through another port or the laser through the laser laparoscope to cut the adhesions. A flexible measuring probe (Wisap) amputated to a length of 2.5 cm on the part that hinges, makes an excellent retractor and a backstop for the CO_2 laser beam. The most common sites of concern with bowel adhesions are on the pelvic organs themselves, the pelvic sidewalls, and the anterior abdominal wall. Because the uterus is red, the boundary lines between the bowel and the uterus are not usually difficult to see, even when adhesions are dense. Adhesiolysis in these areas usually goes smoothly unless bleeding is encountered. When this happens, the surgeon must make the considered judgment of whether to abandon further lysis and secure hemostasis as simply as possible, or to continue with lysis in the hope that further dissection will simplify the anatomy enough to allow the re-establishment of hemostasis and thus permit the procedure to safely go ahead.

When bowel loops are densely adherent to the ovary or pelvic sidewall, progress can be more difficult. In this situation, there may be little color or texture difference between bowel and ovary. The surgeon should therefore proceed slowly, frequently moving the bowel tissue to and fro and "palpating" with graspers or suction-irrigator to determine the location of the bowel margin. On the pelvic sidewall, in most cases you can still see a "white line" of the margin of the parietal peritoneum, thus easily allowing dissection between this and the bowel. Again, traction is important. Be aware that pelvic sidewall structures, most notably the ureter, can be retracted medially with ease. When significant fibrosis exists, such as in cases of endometriosis, the "white line" may not be present, and the ureter can easily enter your field of dissection without being recognized.

Two methods, used individually or simultaneously, may help in this circumstance. First, follow the principle of working from the known to the unknown. Enter the retroperitoneal space lateral to the ureter and more cephalad to the area of adhesions, starting in an area not involved with the adhesions. Isolate the ureter and peel it away from the area of adhesions. Having simplified the anatomy, then proceed with the adhesiolysis. Second, many surgeons find that a ureteral stent facilitates this dissection by making it always possible to locate the ureter quickly and to more easily recognize when it is being pulled medially with traction.

On many occasions, small bowel loops and omentum are adhered to the anterior abdominal wall. This occurs more often when a patient has had one or more laparotomies. The adhesions are usually most dense in the midline. The frequency of peritoneal adhesions may be no different whether the peritoneum was closed or not, but it is the author's opinion that when it is left open, small bowel loops may become adhered to rectus muscle and fascial layers, thus taking up a position anterior to the plane of the peritoneum across the uninvolved anterior abdominal wall. This makes dissection especially difficult, as the limits of the bowel are quite difficult to determine. This is a situation in which the author feels especially strongly that the CO_2 laser, using a small spot size and superpulse mode with the power turned down to 5–10 watts, provides the best controlled energy source for this kind of difficult dissection.

How do you know when you're in trouble? A through-and-through enterotomy will usually be obvious, as the bowel mucosa will roll out around the edges of the wound like an opening flower. Proceeding slowly, there is another warning sign prior to a complete enterotomy when the tissue being dissected starts to show parallel lines, looking "stringy," like a piece of celery having some of its strands pulled away. The bowel muscularis is being dissected. Again, this is more likely when the bowel is attached above the plane of the anterior parietal peritoneum. When this is seen, stop, reassess the anatomy, and try to redirect the dissection more anteriorly to get above the bowel. Once the bowel is completely freed, the mucosal layer will protrude beyond the plane of the uninjured bowel in the area of muscularis injury, forming a "blister" much like that seen on the sidewall of an automobile tire that is about to have a blowout. Double layer repair is appropriate, as described below.

Another occasional mishap is the appearance of a possible bowel injury from cautery. When monopolar or bipolar cautery is used very close to the bowel, a gray area of tissue damage may be seen. It is very tempting to mobilize denial mechanisms and assume this will heal without incident. In fact, the area is dead tissue, and depending on the depth of the injury and other factors, the bowel will perforate within one to seven days. Primary repair is preferable, even in the suboptimally prepared bowel.

HANDLING BOWEL COMPLICATIONS

In the case of the complete enterotomy, the injury is obvious and will be repaired. When the injury is partial, keep in mind another "Golden Rule" of surgery: when a complication occurs, recognize it and fix it. Downplaying its significance or hoping that further complications will not occur is a disservice to the patient and will create a deeper ethical and medicolegal hole for the surgeon.

When a complete enterotomy occurs, stop and reassess. If the bowel preparation is good and minimal soilage is taking place, then fill the pelvis with a large amount of your irrigant solution (Ringer's lactate) to dilute the effect of any further spillage, and continue the dissection as much as you can. Be careful to keep the enterotomy within easy view so that it can be found later. If substantial spillage occurs, then an immediate judgment must be made whether to attempt laparoscopic repair or convert the procedure to a laparotomy. Whether the bowel is repaired by the primary surgeon or the gynecologic oncologist or a general surgeon, will depend on the level of experience and the resources (politics?) of that institution.

In the case of a thermal injury of the bowel (either by electrocautery or laser) without an obvious hole, resect the gray tissue sharply, avoiding further cautery as much as possible. Most often, the lesion will extend into the muscularis, but not through the mucosa. In this case and in the case of mechanical muscularis ("celery stalk") injury described above, repair it with one layer of interrupted absorbable suture and a second layer of either absorbable or permanent suture, again in interrupted fashion. On the large bowel, having a larger diameter, the direction of the suture line does not matter. In the small bowel, all but the smallest of injuries should have the axis of the suture line perpendicular to the axis of the bowel.

LAPAROSCOPY UNDER LOCAL ANESTHESIA

Assume a careful history and physical examination have been completed and all the functional components of the pain problem have been treated optimally. The levator spasm is improved, bowel function is normal, and a good sleep pattern has been restored. The patient still complains of pain that inhibits function in a variety of ways. Contemplating laparoscopy, there are two concerns: either intrinsic pelvic pathology is likely to be minimal, or the clinical importance of highly probable pathology is uncertain.

In this situation, much can be learned from a laparoscopic examination done under local anesthesia. In the appropriate (less anxious) patient, this may be accomplished with the office laparoscopy technique being developed currently, using a miniature (1.7–2.0 mm) laparoscope. The more typical chronic pain patient may require the reassurance of an operating room setting, where more complete analgesia or anesthesia may be safely administered if the procedure should prove too uncomfortable.

The procedure itself is simple and uses techniques well established for tubal sterilization procedures done under local anesthesia. Under intravenous analgesia with intravenous narcotic and sedative-hypnotic agents, the patient can be made comfortable for the entire procedure. Local injections of 0.5% bupivacaine or 1% xylocaine are then placed in the umbilicus and in a second site in the midline suprapubic area. After nitrous oxide insufflation, a 5-mm umbilical port may be quickly placed after warning the patient that she will feel increased discomfort for a count of 5. Once a successful insertion is documented, a second 5-mm probe is placed suprapubically in similar fashion. Two-mm ports can be used and cause less discomfort. Having previously educated the patient about the plan, she is asked to rate, on a 1 to 10 scale, the tenderness of various areas touched. Using a smooth-tipped probe, touch all the pelvic organs in sequence and then put each on traction in all directions possible. When adhesions are present, tug on them with the probe or an atraumatic grasper and ask if this reproduces the pain she feels on a day-to-day basis.

To date this method of examination has not been systematically reported. Anecdotal experience suggests that it is especially useful in two situations: (*a*) the ovary that is tender on pelvic and transvaginal ultrasound examination but is normal in size, shape, and mobility, and (*b*) the pelvis with postoperative adhesions of uncertain importance in producing pain. In the first case, intraovarian lesions such as endometriosis will (rarely) occur even in the absence of other pelvic lesions; the ovary itself will be tender. If the ovary is not unusually tender, palpation of the sigmoid colon may reproduce the pain, suggesting a bowel source. The abdominal wall may be intrinsically tender to palpation, suggesting a myofascial, trigger point, or traumatic neuroma origin. In some instances, abdominal wall pain may be a sign of dermatomally distributed pain from a vertebral facet syndrome. In the second instance (adhesions), it is often possible to decide if tugging on the adhesions reproduces that pain adequately, or if there is intrinsic abdominal wall pain near the adhesions. The author has seen a number of patients in whom repeated adhesiolysis procedures had been done with transient benefit each time. During laparoscopy under local anesthesia, tugging the adhesions did not reliably reproduce the pain. Once educated about the findings, the patients put more effort into medical and behavioral management and reached significant levels of improvement. Perhaps as importantly, they were spared further surgeries that would be unlikely to help.

POSTOPERATIVE MEDICAL AND BEHAVIORAL MANAGEMENT

There is an almost overwhelming temptation to hope that the reassurance of a normal laparoscopy will relieve the pain, and sometimes it does. Nevertheless, this is a good time to repeat the preoperative caution: the patient will need to continue to work on the other contributing factors. When significant pathology has been found, a similar temptation exists; the same cautionary comments should be offered. By including the operative procedure as but one of several elements of treatment, your words and behavior are "modeling" for the patient and her family the model of pain perception described above.

WHEN TO REPEAT LAPAROSCOPY

As laparoscopy has become more accepted, and as office laparoscopy is being developed for diagnostic applications, a problem has emerged. The author has seen a number of patients who have had as many as ten or fifteen laparoscopies in as many years. In most such cases, insufficient attention has been paid to multiple contributing factors in the pain problem. The patient going through this process gets the strong message that surgery is the only thing that really counts, and she comes to expect multiple repeat procedures over time. At some point in this process, the responsible clinician has to call a halt and either reorient the therapy process him/herself or get consulting help to accomplish this goal.

Reevaluation, and possibly relaparoscopy, should be contemplated under the following circumstances: (*a*) new organ system involvement appears, e.g., new bladder or bowel symptoms refractory to medical management; (*b*) new symptoms appear despite optimal medical management, e.g., dyspareunia; or (*c*) new physical examination findings are evident, e.g., cul-de-sac nodularity or increased adnexal pain with increasingly limited ovarian mobility. In some women (and couples) dealing with endometriosis, the fear of the disease can become as disabling as the disease itself. A repeat laparoscopy one to three years after the first one at which the diagnosis was established is sometimes useful in the anxious patient to provide some reassurance regarding the degree of biological aggressiveness present in her particular case of the disease.

SUMMARY

The role of diagnostic and operative laparoscopy in the management of chronic pelvic pain is undisputedly substantial. Paradoxically, its greatest value is realized when its importance is played down, and the surgery is integrated into a plan that takes the whole patient into account. The physician must understand the complexities of pain perception, apply this understanding to the diagnostic and treatment process, and play a key role in educating the patient to play an important active role in her own rehabilitation.

REFERENCES

1. Steege JF, Stout AL, Somkuti SG. Chronic pelvic pain: toward an integrative model. Obstet Gynecol Surv 1993;48:95–110.
2. Melzack R. Neurophysiologic foundations of pain. In: Sternbach RA, ed. The Psychology of Pain. New York: Raven Press, 1986:1–24.
3. Steege JF, Stout AL. Resolution of chronic pelvic pain following laparoscopic adhesiolysis. Am J Obstet Gynecol 1991;165:278–281.
4. Slocumb J. Neurological factors in chronic pelvic pain: trigger points and the abdominal pelvic pain syndrome. Am J Obstet Gynecol 1984;149:536–543.
5. Friedrich EG Jr. Vulvar vestibulitis syndrome. J Reprod Med 1987;32:110–114.
6. Lamont J. Vaginismus. Am J Obstet Gynecol 1978;131:633–636.
7. Sinaki M, Merritt JL, Stillwell GK. Tension myalgia of the pelvic floor. Mayo Clin Proc 1977;52:717–722.
8. King PM, Myers CA, Ling FW, Rosenthal RH. Musculoskeletal factors in chronic pelvic pain. J Psychosom Obstet Gynecol 1991;12(suppl):87.
9. Koninckx PR, Meuleman C, Demeyere S, Lesaffre E, Cornillie FJ. Suggestive evidence that pelvic endometriosis is a progressive disease, whereas deeply infiltrating endometriosis is associated with pelvic pain. Fertil Steril 1991;55:759–765.
10. Fedele L, Parazzini F, Bianchi S, et al. Stage and localization of pelvic endometriosis and pain. Fertil Steril 1990;53:155–158.
11. Stout AL, Steege JF, Dodson WC, et al. Relationship of laparoscopic findings to self-report of pelvic pain. Am J Obstet Gynecol 1991;164:73–79.
12. Olive DL, Schwartz LB. Endometriosis. N Engl J Med 1993;328:1759–1769.
13. Sutton CJG, Ewen SP, Whitelaw N, Haines P. Prospective, randomized, double-blind, controlled trial of laser laparoscopy in the treatment of pelvic pain associated with minimal, mild, and moderate endometriosis. Fertil Steril 1994;62:696–700.
14. Brumsted JR, Deaton J, Lavigne E, Riddick DH. Postoperative adhesion formation after ovarian wedge resection with and without ovarian reconstruction in the rabbit. Fertil Steril 1990;53:723–726.
15. Fayez JA, Vogel MF. Comparison of different treatment methods of endometriomas by laparoscopy. Obstet Gynecol 1991;78:660–665.

Chapter 14

Laparoscopic Pelvic Denervation Procedures

John F. Steege

Pelvic denervation procedures have been used since the beginning of the 20th century for the treatment of pelvic pain. Developed primarily to treat dysmenorrhea prior to the widespread performance of hysterectomy, they soon were employed for other purposes. Their popularity for the treatment of pelvic pain has waxed and waned; the possibility of performing these procedures laparoscopically has stimulated renewed interest. They are perhaps most frequently combined with other procedures performed toward the same end, such as lysis of adhesions or treatment of endometriosis. It is difficult to document the clinical efficacy of these procedures due to subjective endpoints and numerous confounding variables, such as the simultaneous performance of other procedures that may relieve pain.

Following discussion of the history of denervation procedures, this chapter will continue with a brief review of general pain theory, the relevant anatomy and physiology, and a discussion of the preoperative evaluation of women for whom a laparoscopic denervation procedure is being considered. The surgical techniques and clinical results for each technique will then be discussed.

PELVIC DENERVATION PROCEDURES

Historical Background

Presacral Neurectomy

Jaboulay of France and the Italian physician Ruggi first performed pelvic sympathectomy in 1899, but the operation was not generally accepted. Beginning in 1924, Cotte of France revived the procedure and promoted it vigorously over the subsequent 25 years, performing over 1500 such operations (1).

While the procedure was first developed for the treatment of dysmenorrhea, Cotte and others soon theorized that this and many other disorders were the result of "hyperexcitability" of the sympathetic nervous system, and therefore used sympathectomy (presacral neurectomy) to treat "dyspareunia, vaginismus, cystalgia, sensation of burning on urination, tenesmus ani, vaginal pain, pruritus vulvae, (and) sexual hyperexcitability" (2). The report of this series claims 98% success in relieving pain, with virtually no significant sexual, intestinal, or urinary tract complications.

Black (3) reviewed the work of 72 authors who reported retrospective clinical series totalling an additional 2,516 cases from 1936 through 1963, including the work of well-known investigators such as Joe V. Meigs and Louis E. Phaneuf. In the literature series, Black's personal series of 43 cases, and in 7,378 cases reported in his questionnaire survey of physicians, dysmenorrhea was relieved in from 62 to 83% of cases. Primary dysmenorrhea was somewhat more often relieved than secondary dysmenorrhea. Constipation and mild urinary retention problems were acknowledged by many authors to occur in 5 to 15% of cases, although the criteria used to define such complications were not specified. Changes in sexual functioning were either denied or not addressed.

Following the development of oral contraceptives, and later, nonsteroidal antiinflammatory drugs (NSAIDs), denervation procedures were virtually abandoned for a number of years. With recognition of a 10 to 15% failure rate for these medical therapies of dysmenorrhea, surgical denervation approaches re-emerged. Finally, with the advent of operative laparoscopy, both uterosacral interruption (usually by electrocautery or Laser Uterosacral Nerve Ablation (LUNA)) (4) and presacral neurectomy (5) have joined the growing list of laparoscopic gynecologic surgical procedures performed.

Laparoscopic Uterosacral Nerve Ablation (LUNA)

Surgical interruption of the uterosacral ligaments for the purpose of relieving pelvic pain began in the 1950s. Doyle (6) reasoned that since the bulk of both sympathetic and parasympathetic innervation of the uterus traverse the uterosacral ligaments, transection should relieve dysmenorrhea. In a series of 73 patients, he either excised a portion of the ligaments or transected them, then reapproximated the cut ends in side-by-side fashion, being careful to interpose a flap of viable peritoneum between the severed ends of uterosacral ligaments. Half the cases were performed transvaginally, and half via laparotomy, the latter route being selected when significant pelvic pathology required additional surgical attention. He reported complete relief in 86% and partial relief in 8% of patients. Doyle felt that by interrupting both sympathetic and parasympathetic fibers, his procedure avoided "imbalance" between the two systems that he felt might be responsible for the instances of menorrhagia reported by some authors to follow some cases of presacral neurectomy. Further, Doyle reported that by carrying the dissection sufficiently deep to interrupt Frankenhäuser's uterovaginal plexus, lateral pelvic pain was ameliorated in some cases.

Interruption of uterosacral nerve supply to the uterus was perhaps one of the earliest operative laparoscopic procedures to be widely performed following the introduction of the CO_2 laser. Reports of the effectiveness of the LUNA procedure are few. Several clinical observational studies report significant relief of dysmenorrhea in 60–75% of patients (7, 8), while the only prospective study in the literature, by Lichten and Bombard (4), reports only 45% of patients treated with LUNA to have persistent relief of dysmenorrhea 1 year after the operation. Since one is often performing other surgical interventions along with the LUNA, it is difficult to measure benefit specifically attributable to the LUNA procedure.

GENERAL PAIN THEORY

As described previously, pain perception is a complex phenomenon. Multiple factors may contribute to the pain experience, and hence may influence the outcome of denervation procedures.

Early reports of pelvic denervation would occasionally attribute failure to psychiatric causes (otherwise undefined), but virtually none of the literature undertakes any form of behavioral or psychiatric evaluation. Given the chronic and debilitating nature of the pain experienced by women usually subjected to denervation procedures, multiple variables become relevant (see Chapter 13).

Given the level of neurologic redundancy present in the pelvis, it seems unlikely that any procedure will result in complete and total denervation. Hence, some afferent, and probably nociceptive, signals will no doubt persist in many circumstances. The factors listed may serve to augment the impact of such persistent nociceptive signals, thus accounting for instances of partial or complete failure of the procedure even when clearcut psychiatric disorders cannot be documented.

PREOPERATIVE EVALUATION

Denervation procedures should be undertaken only when careful clinical assessment and management have dealt with confounding factors, both gynecological and nongynecological. Some of the syndromes potentially contributing to pelvic pain in the absence of laparoscopically visible pathology are described in Chapter 13.

Clinically, the most common problems encountered are irritable bowel syndrome, depression, and musculoskeletal problems. These may be primary disorders or they may develop secondarily after a long time of putting up with pelvic pain. Nevertheless, they often attain a life of their own, and if left untreated may persist despite the most meticulous surgical technique. The patient will be better prepared for surgery and her results will be better if treatment for these problems is at least begun, if not well established, prior to going to the operating room. (See Chapter 13 for further discussion.)

Patients should be cautioned that the interruption of the superior hypogastric plexus should only be expected to relieve deep central pelvic pain. Discomfort in the adnexal areas, the intestines, the vagina, and the vulva is not relieved by this procedure.

Anatomy and Physiology

Sympathetic sensory afferent fibers from the uterus form the inferior hypogastric plexus lateral and inferior to the uterosacral ligaments, then traverse the uterovaginal plexus of Frankenhäuser on each side before traveling cephalad to unite in the superior hypogastric plexus. The precise course of these fibers is highly variable (Fig. 14.1) (9) as they cross the common iliac vessels and ascend anterior and lateral to the aorta before entering spinal cord segments T_{10} through L_1.

Traditional teachings maintain that parasympathetic branches from the upper vagina and cervix travel to their S_2 through S_4 origins partly independently and partly via Frankenhäuser's plexus. Bonica (10), on the basis of extensive work with a variety of segmental, regional, and local blocks administered during labor, has challenged this formulation, suggesting that sacral fibers to the lower uterus and cervix are motor rather than sensory. This assertion is supported by the observation that uterosacral interruption may not add to the effectiveness of presacral neurectomy for relief of pelvic pain, but does not explain the apparent effectiveness of the LUNA procedure in some cases.

The adnexae are innervated largely by the ovarian nerves, which travel

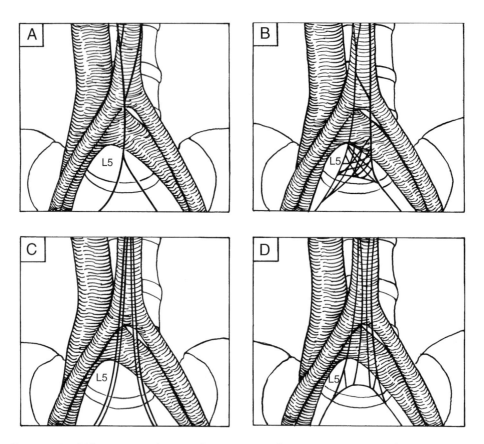

Figure 14.1. Different types of presacral nerves. **A.** Single nerve type, 24%. **B.** Plexus type, 58%. **C.** Parallel type, 16%. **D.** Arc-shaped type, 2%.

predominantly with the arterial supply of the ovaries. Although one report (11) suggests that transection of the infundibulopelvic ligament will relieve adnexal pain without compromising ovarian function, subsequent corroboration is lacking. Pelvic denervation should therefore be expected to relieve only central pelvic pain.

Motor function of the lower large intestine is mediated by sacral parasympathetics and to some extent by sympathetic supply via the inferior mesenteric plexus. Motor function for the bladder is mediated both by sacral parasympathetics, as well as by some sympathetic output from the inferior hypogastric plexus. Given the multiple levels of enervation, it follows that partial interruption of the nerve supply to these structures may partially interfere with their function. In most instances these changes can be accommodated without clinically significant deficit. The literature supports this notion in reporting constipation as a complication of presacral neurectomy in 0–30% of cases. Inhibition of bladder function, manifested by mild urinary retention, is also noted anecdotally. Neither of these complications has received either careful observational reporting or physiologic investigation in the form of bowel motility studies or urodynamic studies.

Another area of potential concern is sexual response. The two major physiologic components of this response are vasocongestion, thought to be primarily parasympathetically mediated, and contraction of uterine and vaginal musculature, which appears to be sympathetically mediated. Early reports on denervation procedures either did not mention changes in sexuality at all, or specifically denied adverse effect. However, these observations took place prior to the time when these neurologic pathways were understood. Cultural norms of sexual behavior may have influenced the reports: recall that Cotte performed presacral neurectomy to "treat. . . . sexual hyperexcitability." (Frank reported (12) that 11% of happily married women complain of reaching orgasm too quickly, but the author respectfully doubts that this was the condition being treated in the Cotte (2) series.) More recent reports are anecdotal at best with regard to this matter, and certainly none have undertaken serious investigation. It is curious that on the one hand, some laparoscopists are advocating supracervical hysterectomy in order to preserve cervical innervation and thereby conserve sexual response, while others are suggesting that thorough denervation of these structures does not alter sexual response.

The superior hypogastric plexus can be blocked by the translumbar injection of local anesthetic. This technique would seem attractive as a way of preoperatively assessing the likelihood of benefit of sympathectomy in the patient with a normal pelvis. It would not, of course, tell you if presacral neurectomy would provide relief beyond that attainable by thorough treatment of all pelvic pathology.

Surgical Technique

Presacral Neurectomy

The surgical approach to sympathectomy requires opening the retroperitoneal space in a triangular area bordered by the iliac vessels, (the interiliac trigone), with the apex of the triangle at the bifurcation of the aorta. All retroperitoneal tissue anterior to the sacrum and iliac vessels must be excised, proceeding from the ureter on the right and to the root of the sigmoid mesentery on the left. Some sympathetic branches may emerge from between the left common iliac artery and vein.

The traditional transabdominal approach is through a midline incision, although it can be accomplished via a Pfannenstiel incision in some patients. The peritoneum is incised in the midline over the body of L_5 for a distance of 6–8 cm and retracted laterally to the base of the sigmoid mesentery on the left and the ureter on the right. Care must be taken as one approaches the base of the sigmoid mesentery, as the location of this structure is highly variable, and large mesenteric vessels may be encountered close to the margin of the base of the mesentery. Especially in the patient with more retroperitoneal fat tissue, the middle sacral artery and vein should be isolated and avoided with great care. Perforating veins emerging from the periosteum of the vertebral bodies can pose a hazard if the dissection is not gentle.

The bundle of fatty tissue containing nerves that lies anterior to L_5 and S_1 vertebrae may then be isolated by blunt dissection as a unit. Proximal and distal ligatures are placed around the bundle before it is excised and sent for pathologic examination. The peritoneum has traditionally been closed, but current practice would suggest that it need not be reapproximated.

The laparoscopic approach is fundamentally identical, simply being accomplished with longer instruments (Fig. 14.2). It is most often performed in conjunction with other laparoscopic procedures, which may dictate initial trocar diameter choices and placements. With the patient placed in modified lithotomy position (thighs horizontal, knees flexed) and in steep Trendelenburg position, the presacral area may be viewed either via the umbilical trocar or through a low midline trocar, with the operator standing between the patient's legs (Fig. 14.3). In the latter case, it is best to move the video monitor cephalad, so the monitor view is from the operator's perspective. A right lower quadrant probe is needed for retraction of small bowel, and a left lower quadrant port for a sigmoid colon retractor. The base of the sigmoid mesentery and the right ureter must be clearly identified before beginning. Again, the root of the sigmoid mesentery takes a highly variable course across the presacral area, sometimes crossing from left to right as high as S_2.

From this point on, the difficulty of the procedure depends entirely upon two factors: hemostasis and bowel retraction. When extra ports are needed to accomplish retraction, the procedure can begin to look cumbersome, but when this is efficiently accomplished, as it usually is in the thinner patient, the procedure is much more straightforward. Similarly, the blunt dissection of the presacral tissue is more easily accomplished in the patient with less retroperitoneal fat. The author prefers to use bipolar cautery scissors, although others may prefer monopolar scissors or the Nd:YAG laser. Kleppinger forceps should be available, although they are often insufficient to stabilize the venous bleeding from periosteal perforators. The vessels cannot be exposed sufficiently to allow placement of clips, and other methods of hemostasis such as the argon coagulator have not had wide laparoscopic applica-

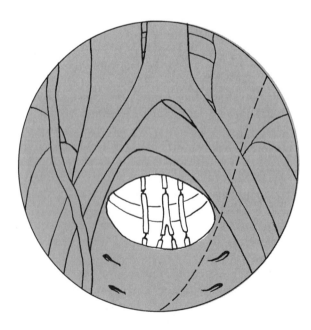

Figure 14.2. The laparoscopic approach to the presacral neurectomy.

Chapter 14: Laparoscopic Pelvic Denervation Procedures 299

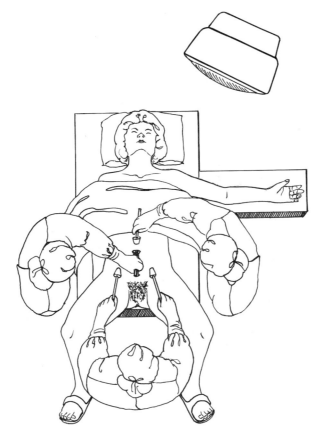

Figure 14.3. Position of the patient for operative laparoscopy.

tion for this particular purpose. The bundle of fatty tissue in front of the lower L_5 and S_1 vertebral bodies containing the presacral nerves may be transected with cautery scissors or laser in two places, freeing the intervening tissue for removal and pathologic examination. Again, the peritoneum need not be closed.

Despite the proximity of the great vessels to the area of dissection, reports of significant hemorrhage during or following this procedure are very infrequent in the literature. The middle sacral artery and vein are perhaps greater hazards, as they may be obscured by fat and have a very variable course through the interiliac trigone and hence down the anterior sacrum. Presacral veins, which perforate the periosteum, are more of a problem at the S_{2-3} level, which should be caudad to the main area of dissection. If such perforators are encountered, hemostasis is most easily accomplished by pressing stainless steel thumbtacks directly into the sacrum (13). Methods are currently being developed to apply thumbtacks via a laparoscopic instrument.

Given the variability in the course of sympathetic nerves as described, it is tempting to sever them at a higher level (where they are more concentrated) in hopes of achieving better relief of pelvic pain. However, the closer the dissection is to the inferior mesenteric artery, the greater the potential risk of bowel compromise.

Laparoscopic Uterosacral Nerve Ablation (LUNA)

Two basic approaches have been in wide use, although statistics are not available concerning the relative popularity of each one:

1. Complete transection: Those who favor electrocoagulation instruments have grasped each uterosacral ligament close to the uterus and coagulated it through its full thickness, then severed it with scissors or laser. This amounts to the Doyle procedure without the interposition of an intact layer of peritoneum between the severed ends.
2. Partial ablation: Those favoring the CO_2 laser have generally laser-ablated the medial two-thirds of each uterosacral ligament over a distance of approximately 1 cm just adjacent to the uterus. If ablation of the lateral third of the ligament is done, a small artery is encountered, which will not be rendered hemostatic by the laser. The unipolar needle electrode, the Nd:YAG laser, and other energy sources may be equally effective.

Regardless of the technique chosen, clear identification of the uterosacral ligaments and ureters is critical. In women with attenuated ligaments this may not be easy. The thickness of the ligament can be better appreciated by tucking the tip of a probe (usually the suction/irrigation cannula) on the lateral margin of the uterosacral ligament close to the uterus and pushing medially (Fig. 14.4). If the ligament cannot be clearly identified, then the procedure should not be done. As

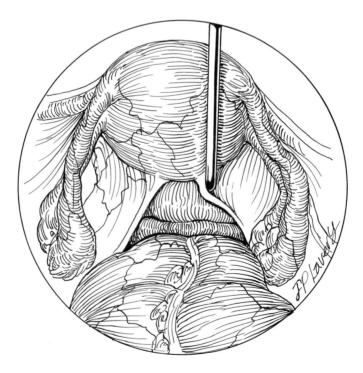

Figure 14.4. Tucking the laparoscopic probe behind the uterosacral ligament to facilitate laparoscopic uterosacral nerve ablation.

with any ablative procedure, it is useful to rinse and rub away all charred tissue with the tip of the suction/irrigator. This gives a better idea of how much of the ligament has been removed and will prevent future laparoscopists from mistaking residual carbon particles for recurrent endometriosis.

Many surgeons, including Lichten and Bombard (4) also either cauterize or laser-ablate a line of tissue between the uterosacral ligaments at the level of the uterocervical junction, in order to interrupt sympathetic fibers traversing this area on their way from the superior to the inferior hypogastric plexus. The impact of this logical step has not been separately evaluated.

Aside from bleeding from the ligament or unlikely straying of the laser or cautery instrument to neighboring organs, there are only two significant possible complications:

1. Ureteral injury: The course of the ureter is quite regular, usually passing about 1.5 to 2 cm lateral to the insertion of the uterosacral ligament into the uterus. On rare occasions, the ureter may follow an anomalous course, passing just underneath the uterosacral ligament. At times the ureter may pass closer to the uterus than it usually does due to contraction of endometriotic or postcesarean section scarring. In any event, the cautious surgeon will take care to visualize the ureter prior to ablating the uterosacral ligaments.

2. Rectosigmoid injury: This injury has not been reported in the literature, but there have been anecdotal rumors of such injuries in medicolegal circles. When the cul-de-sac is partially or completed obliterated by scarring from endometriosis, the rectum may be pulled anteriorly to a substantial degree, taking up a position adjacent to the uterosacral ligaments. Ordinarily one can easily visualize the end of the linear white teniae of the colon, marking the margin of the true cul-de-sac. When one fails to see this landmark, or the retroperitoneal space is so infiltrated with fat that the landmarks may be obscured, then the operator should exercise even greater caution. The peritoneal covering over the bowel may appear as an uninterrupted surface all the way up to the uterosacral ligaments. In this case, it is useful to perform double-gloved rectovaginal examination with one hand while manipulating a laparoscopic probe with the other in order to more clearly outline the anatomy. This method also may help define more obscure uterosacral ligaments as well as identify retroperitoneal implants of endometriosis in the cul-de-sac (Fig. 14.5).

SUMMARY OF RESULTS

Presacral Neurectomy

The clinical literature includes a total of over 12,000 cases reported over the last 70 years. There is general internal consistency in the reports in that pain relief is reported in approximately 70–80% of women. These percentages apply to early populations of women without pelvic pathology in whom the procedure was done for dysmenorrhea alone, as well as later series, which included mixed populations of women with and without significant pelvic pathology.

With the advances in medical therapies for primary dysmenorrhea, a more current dilemma is to investigate the value of presacral neurectomy in women

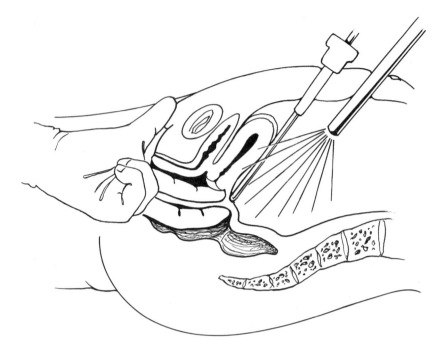

Figure 14.5. Simultaneous laparoscopy and rectovaginal examination to examine the posterior cul-de-sac and pelvic floor.

having conservative pelvic surgery for such disorders as endometriosis and pelvic adhesions. Unfortunately, the literature offering a valid comparison between conservative surgery versus conservative surgery plus presacral neurectomy is extremely limited. Candiani (14) reported a series of 71 patients with Stage III or IV endometriosis, 36 of whom were randomized to conservative surgical resection only, while 35 were randomized to surgery plus presacral neurectomy (via laparotomy). Careful pain assessments were performed on the approximately 50% of the population who reported pain preoperatively. The authors were careful to evaluate dyspareunia, dysmenorrhea, and daily pain as separate categories. Quite dramatic improvement was obtained in both groups in the study, thus failing to demonstrate a significant additional benefit attributable to presacral neurectomy. Unfortunately, since only a portion of the population had pain preoperatively, the total number of patients with pain who were subjected to randomization is relatively small, thus limiting the statistical power of the study. Tjaden et al. (15), after initial positive clinical experience with presacral neurectomy in conjunction with conservative resection of Stage III and IV endometriosis, randomized eight women to conservative resection with or without presacral neurectomy. The four allocated to presacral neurectomy obtained good relief, while the other four did not. At that point, the institutional review board mandated discontinuation of the study, as the statistical significance level chosen had been reached. The authors went on to report good results in 15 of 17 patients in a subsequent clinical series.

Denervation procedures for pain relief in other areas of the body are often followed by the re-emergence of enervation, and therefore pain. The time course for re-enervation is usually 12–18 months or more, suggesting that adequate follow-up for pelvic denervation should be at least that long. Sympathetic denervation procedures for vascular compromise of the lower extremities occasionally fail after this length of time, although the natural re-enervation process seems less successful in autonomic denervations than it does in somatic procedures. The literature on pelvic sympathectomy in general has reported a range of follow-up times, seldom offering a mean and uniformly failing to report the number of patients followed for over two years.

By the same token, potential bladder, bowel, and sexual complications of presacral neurectomy need to be examined on a far more rigorous basis than they have been in the past, and on a large series of patients.

It might be argued that if the question of benefit remains unsettled, that the presacral neurectomy and LUNA should still be performed in view of the apparently low incidence of complications. However, ureteral injuries are reported anecdotally with an unknown frequency following the LUNA procedure, and two cases of uterine prolapse were reported to occur soon after the LUNA procedure (15). A more extensive clinical follow-up of the LUNA procedure would be a substantial addition to the literature, as would a detailed pre and postoperative physiologic study of women undergoing presacral neurectomy.

While the LUNA procedure is apparently of some demonstrable value and is relatively safe to perform, the laparoscopic presacral neurectomy involves considerably greater hazard and should remain the province of the more experienced operative laparoscopist. The capability of performing a sympathectomy procedure should not tempt the enthusiastic surgeon to "short-circuit" his/her attention to the multiple factors that often contribute to the total distress of the chronic pain patient. Patients should continue to be carefully chosen, rather than simply including presacral neurectomy as part of a surgical laparoscopic procedure with several components.

Finally, technology is currently available to accurately describe bladder and bowel contractility and diagnose dysfunctions. These methods should be used preoperatively and postoperatively to more carefully evaluate the impact of denervation on autonomic functions.

REFERENCES

1. Cotte G. Technique of presacral neurectomy. Am J Surg 1949;78:50–53.
2. Cotte G. Resection of the presacral nerve in the treatment of obstinate dysmenorrhea. Am J Obstet Gynecol 1937;33:1034–1040.
3. Black WT. Use of presacral sympathectomy in the treatment of dysmenorrhea. Am J Obstet Gynecol 1964;89:16–20.
4. Lichen EM, Bombard J. Surgical treatment of primary dysmenorrhea with laparoscopic uterine nerve ablation. J Reprod Med 1987;32:37–41.
5. Perez JJ. Laparoscopic presacral neurectomy. J Reprod Med 1990;35:625–630.
6. Doyle JB. Paracervical uterine denervation by transection of the cervical plexus for the relief of dysmenorrhea. Am J Obstet Gynecol 1955;70:1–16.
7. Daniell JF: Fiberoptic laser laparoscopy. Baillieres Clin Obstet Gynaecol 1989;3:545–562.
8. Sutton C, Hill D: Laser laparoscopy in the treatment of endometriosis. Br J Obstet Gynaecol 1990;97:181–185.

9. Elaut L. The surgical anatomy of the so-called presacral nerve. Surg Gynecol Obstet 1932;23: 581–589.
10. Bonica JJ. The management of pain. 2nd ed. Malvern, PA: Lea & Febiger, 1990.
11. Brown OD. A survey of 113 cases of primary dysmenorrhea treated by neurectomy. Am J Obstet Gynecol 1949;57:1053.
12. Frank E, Anderson C, Rubinstein D. Frequency of sexual dysfunction in "normal" couples. N Engl J Med 1978;299:111–115.
13. Timmons MC, Kohler MF, Addison WA. Thumbtack use for control of presacral bleeding, with description of an instrument for thumbtack application. Obstet Gynecol 1991;78:313–315.
14. Candiani GB, Fedele L, Vercellini P, Bianchi S, DiNola G. Presacral neurectomy for the treatment of pelvic pain associated with endometriosis: a controlled study. Am J Obstet Gynecol 1992;167: 100–103.
15. Tjaden B, Schlaff WD, Kimball A. The efficacy of presacral neurectomy for the relief of midline dysmenorrhea. Obstet Gynecol 1990;76:89–91.
16. Good MC, Copas PR, Doody MC. Uterine prolapse after laparoscopic uterosacral transection. J Reprod Med 1992;37(12):995–996.

APPENDIX
LAPAROSCOPIC SUTURING EQUIPMENT

The following appendix is composed of three sections. The first section contains descriptive tables of needle drivers and knot manipulators that are divided into groups with similar types of handles and end effectors. All of these instruments are pictured in the second section and are referenced by number. The manufacturers' information is contained in the third section.

NEEDLE DRIVERS
HANDLES: INLINE

Handle	Shaft	End Effector	Description/Cat #	Manufacturer
#1	Diameter: 5 mm Length: 30 cm	#33	Nonlocking, spring, inline 006698-935	Cabot Medical
#2	Diameter: 5 mm Length: 30 cm	#32	Locking, spring, inline 006699-935	Cabot Medical
#3	Diameter: 5 mm Length: 32 cm	#32 #25 #26 #27	Castro-vieho ratcheted	Jarit
#4	Diameter: 5 mm Length: 30 cm	#36	Castro-vieho ratcheted 6668-3	Reznik
#5	Diameter: 5 mm Length: 30 cm	#36	Inline Classic ratcheted 708-511	Reznik
#6	Diameter: 5 mm Length: 36 cm (curved shaft not pictured)	#29	Cuschieri needle holder 26173 SK straight shaft 26173 NB curved shaft	Karl Storz
#7	Diameter: 5 mm Length: 33 cm	#24 #23	Ratcheted locking handle 26173-SD 26173-SC	Karl Storz

305

NEEDLE DRIVERS
HANDLES: OFFSET

Handle	Shaft	End Effector	Description/Cat #	Manufacturer
#8	Diameter: 5 mm Length: 30 cm	#37	Ratcheted handle 6668-5	Reznik
#9	Diameter: 5 mm Length: 30 cm	#30	Ratcheted handle rotating shaft	Ethicon
#10	Diameter: 5 mm Length: 30 cm	#22	Spring closure and ratcheted handle (interchangeable) rotating shaft MP 7828	Marlow
#11	Diameter: 5 mm Length: 33 cm	#31	Spring closure 600-275	Jarit
#12	Diameter: 5 mm Length: 33 cm	#35 #22	Spring closure and ratcheted handle (interchangeable) MP 7681	Marlow
#13	Diameter: 5 mm Length: 36 cm	#28	Spring closure 26173 MS	Storz
#14	Diameter: 3 mm Length: 33 cm	#45	Spring closure rotating 5-mm adaptor MP 7681	Marlow
#15	Diameter: 3 mm Length: 33 cm	#38	Spring closure rotating 5-mm adaptor #600-273	Jarit
#16	Diameter: 3 mm Length: 36 cm	#40	Spring closure rotating 5-mm adaptor 26173 LS	Storz
#18	Diameter: 3, 5 mm Length: 30 cm	#43 #42	Spring-loaded handle J-ENH-033100 (3 mm) J-ENH-053100 (5 mm)	Cook
#20	Diameter: 5, 10 mm Length: 30 cm	#40	Pistol, grip, locking handle 87510—10 mm 87515—5 mm	Sharpe

SEMIAUTOMATED NEEDLE DRIVER

End Effector	Shaft	Handle	Description/Cat #	Manufacturer
#44	Diameter: 10 mm Length: 37 cm	#56	Endostitch Passes and grasps double-ended needle with a variety of USSC sutures	USSC
#45	Diameter: 10 mm Length: 26 cm	#21	Drives an Ethicon CT-2, SH-2 or equivalent needle #ND2600	Laurus

NEEDLE DRIVERS
END EFFECTORS: ALLIGATOR CURVED/ANGLED

End Effector	Shaft	Handle	Description/Cat #	Manufacturer
#22	Diameter: 5 mm Length: 30 cm	#10	Reddick-Saye Heaney type double hinged Right-handed—M4101S Left-handed—M4102S Universal—M4100S	Marlow
#23	Diameter: 5 mm Length: 33 cm	#7	Parrot-jawed needle holder 26173-SC	Storz
#24	Diameter: 5 mm Length: 33 cm	#7	Flamengo needle holder 26173-SD	Storz
#25	Diameter: 5 mm Length: 32 cm	#3	Appel up-angle carb-bite 600-255	Jarit
#26	Diameter: 5 mm Length: 32 cm	#3	Appel carb-bite left curved 600-250	Jarit
#27	Diameter: 5 mm Length: 32 cm	#3	Appel micro needle holder carb-bite left curved 600-264	Jarit

NEEDLE DRIVERS
END EFFECTORS: ALLIGATOR STRAIGHT

End Effector	Shaft	Handle	Description/Cat #	Manufacturer
#28	Diameter: 5 mm Length: 36 cm	#13	26173 MS	Storz
#29	Diameter: 5 mm Length: 36 cm	#6	Straight and curved shaft straight (26173 SK) curved (26173 NB)	Storz
#30	Diameter: 5 mm Length: 30 cm	#9	Rotating shaft #1002	Ethicon
#31	Diameter: 5 mm Length: 36 cm	#11	#600-275	Jarit
#32	Diameter: 5 mm Length: 32 cm	#3	Appel carb-bite 600-260	Jarit
#33	Diameter: 5 mm Length: 30 cm	#1	Nonlocking 006698-935	Cabot
#34	Diameter: 5 mm Length: 30 cm	#2	Locking 006699-935	Cabot
#35	Diameter: 5 mm Length: 33 cm	#12	MP 7861	Marlow
#36	Diameter: 5 mm Length: 30 cm	#4 #5	#6668-3 #6668-4	Reznik
#37	Diameter: 5 mm Length: 30 cm	#8	Convex/concave alligator jaw 6668-5	Reznik
#38	Diameter: 3 mm Length: 33 cm	#15	5-mm adaptor #600-273	Jarit
#39	Diameter: 3 mm Length: 33 cm	#14	5-mm adaptor MP 768	Marlow
#40	Diameter: 3 mm Length: 36 cm	#16	5-mm adaptor 26173 LS	Storz

NEEDLE DRIVERS
END EFFECTORS: SIDE-LOADING

End Effector	Shaft	Handle	Description/Cat #	Manufacturer
#41	Diameter: 5, 10 mm Length: 30 cm	#20	10 mm 87510 05 mm 87515	Sharpe
#42	Diameter: 3, 5 mm Length: 30 cm	#18	Right-angle load 03 mm J-ENH-033100 05 mm J-ENH-053100	Cook
#43	Diameter: 3, 5 mm Length: 30 cm	#18	45° right- or left-handed load 3 mm—RH J-ENH-033130 3 mm—LH J-ENH-033120 5 mm—RH J-ENH-053130 5 mm—LH J-ENH-053120	Cook

KNOT MANIPULATORS
TYPE I (OPEN)

End Effector	Shaft	Handle	Description/Cat #	Manufacturer
#46	Diameter: 5 mm Length: 29 cm	N/A	Clarke ligator Reddick-Saye style 19° offset 5-0 and larger MP-783	Marlow
#47	Diameter: 4 mm Length: 29 cm	N/A	Clarke-Reich ligator 5-0 and larger MP-782 6-0 and smaller MP-781	Marlow
#48	Diameter: 5 mm Length: 35 cm	N/A	Levine open-ended guide #6664	Reznik
#49	Diameter: 4 mm Length: 32 cm	N/A	600-289	Jarit
#50	Diameter: 4 mm Length: 33 cm	N/A	Semm knot tier right-angled or linear right-angled 26596 T linear 26596 R (not pictured)	Storz
#51	Diameter: 5 mm Length: 30 cm	N/A	Disposable open-ended guide #174510	Auto Suture

KNOT MANIPULATORS
TYPE II (CLOSED)

End Effector	Shaft	Handle	Description/Cat #	Manufacturer
#52	Diameter: 5, 10 mm Length: 40 cm	N/A	Appel Knot Pusher 10 mm 600-285 5 mm 600-287	Jarit
#53	Diameter: 5 mm Length: 29 cm	N/A	M4503P	Marlow
#54	Diameter: 5, 7, 10 mm Length: 30 cm	#17	Endoassit knot pusher 5 mm—87025 7 mm—87005 10 mm—87000	Sharpe

LIGATURE CARRIERS

End Effector	Shaft	Handle	Description/Cat #	Manufacturer
#55	Diameter: 5, 10 mm Length: 33 cm	#19	Retractable, straight carrier 5 mm—87525 10 mm—87520	Sharpe

312 GYNECOLOGIC ENDOSCOPY: Principles in Practice

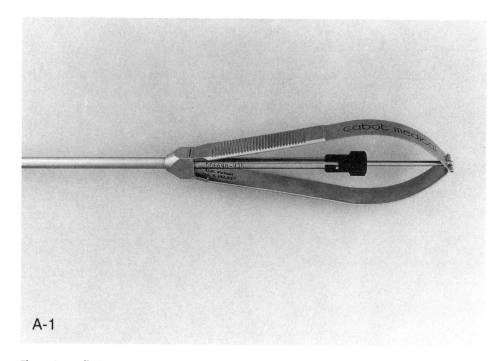

Figure Appendix 1

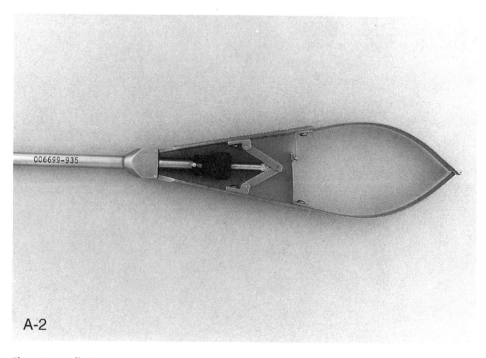

Figure Appendix 2

Appendix 313

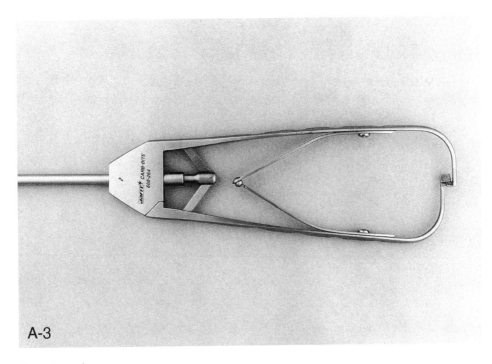

Figure Appendix 3

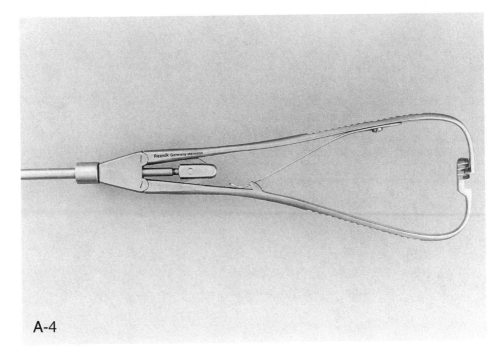

Figure Appendix 4

314 GYNECOLOGIC ENDOSCOPY: Principles in Practice

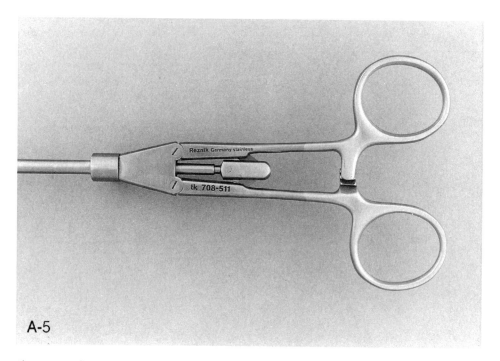

Figure Appendix 5

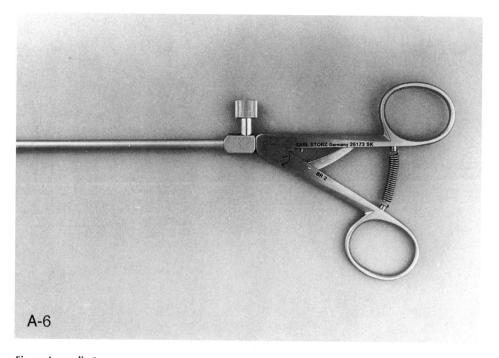

Figure Appendix 6

Appendix 315

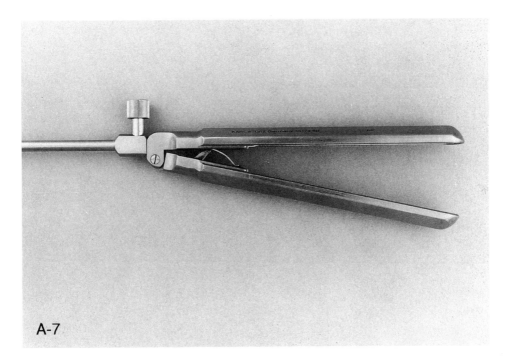

Figure Appendix 7

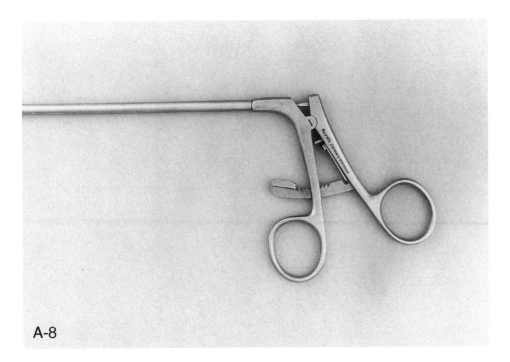

Figure Appendix 8

316 GYNECOLOGIC ENDOSCOPY: Principles in Practice

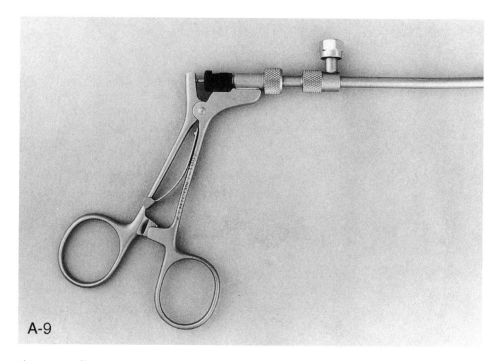

Figure Appendix 9

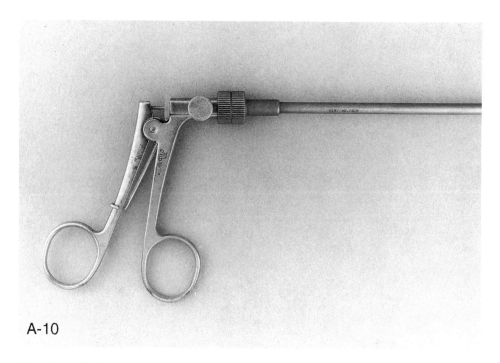

Figure Appendix 10

Appendix 317

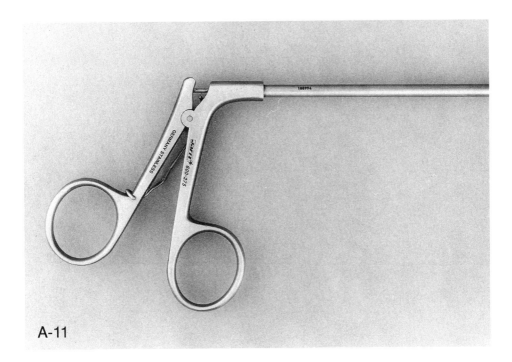

Figure Appendix 11

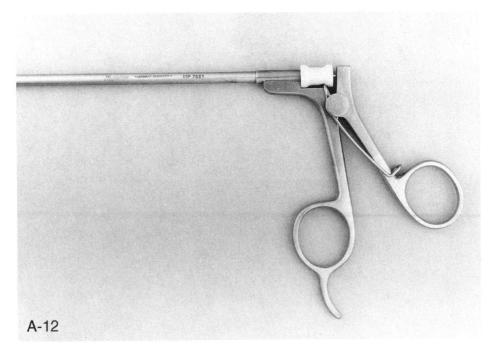

Figure Appendix 12

318 GYNECOLOGIC ENDOSCOPY: Principles in Practice

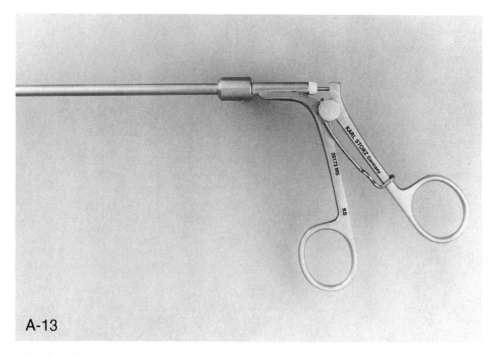

Figure Appendix 13

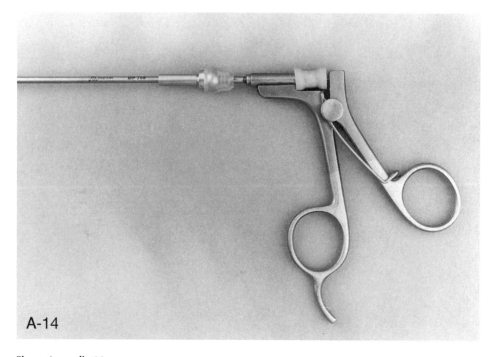

Figure Appendix 14

Appendix 319

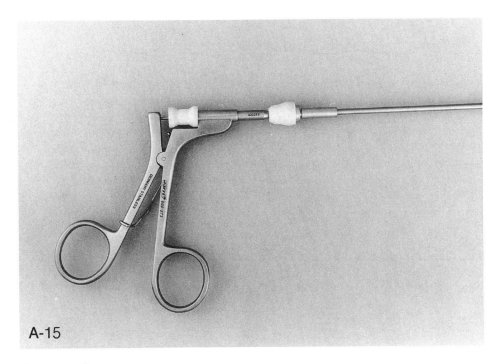

Figure Appendix 15

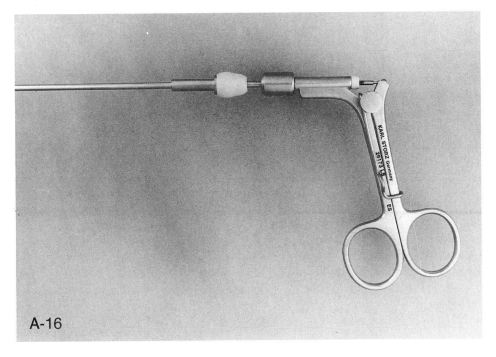

Figure Appendix 16

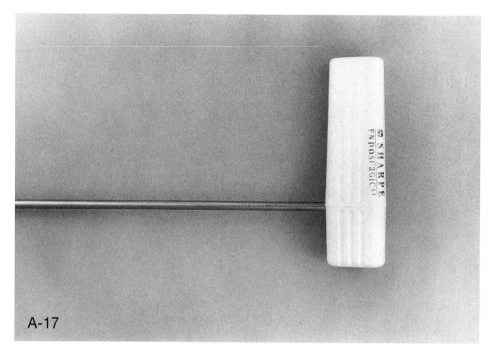

Figure Appendix 17

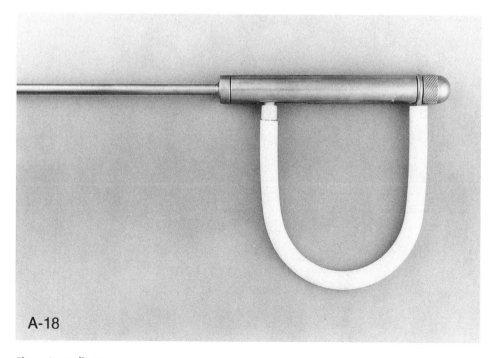

Figure Appendix 18

Appendix 321

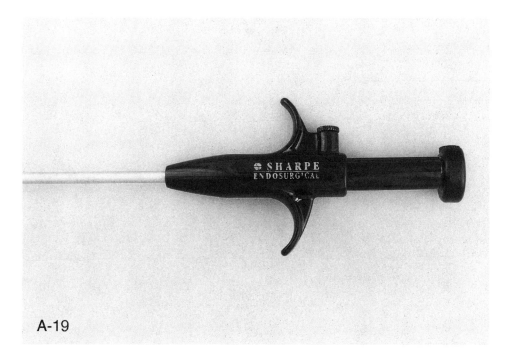

Figure Appendix 19

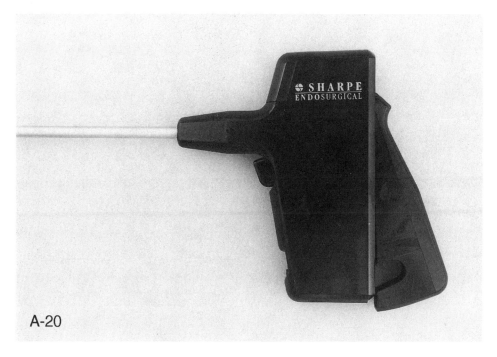

Figure Appendix 20

322 GYNECOLOGIC ENDOSCOPY: Principles in Practice

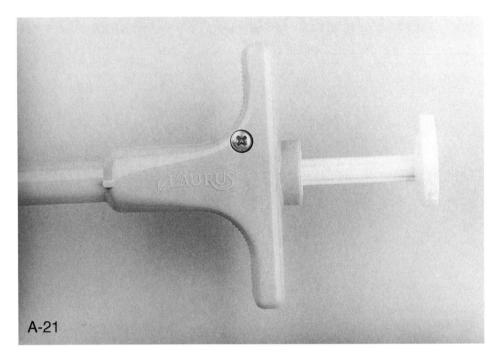

Figure Appendix 21

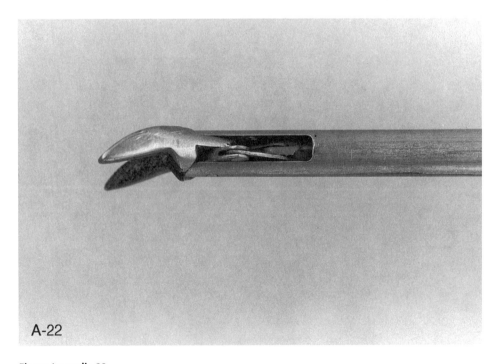

Figure Appendix 22

Appendix 323

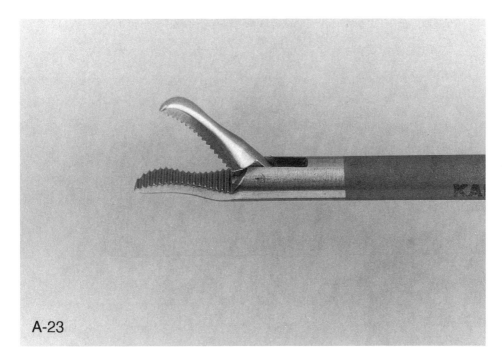

Figure Appendix 23

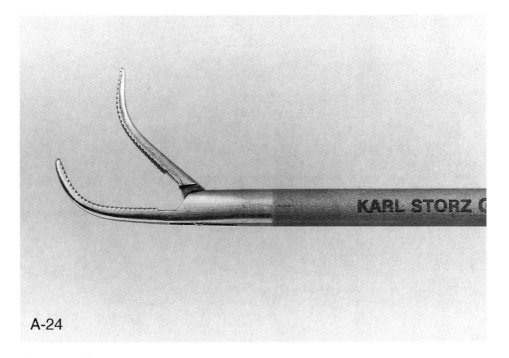

Figure Appendix 24

324 GYNECOLOGIC ENDOSCOPY: Principles in Practice

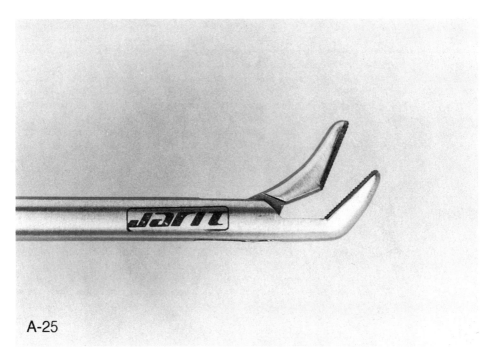

Figure Appendix 25

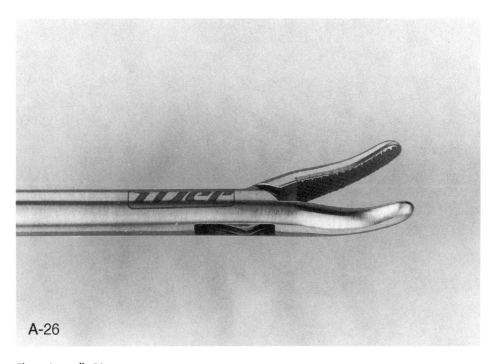

Figure Appendix 26

Appendix 325

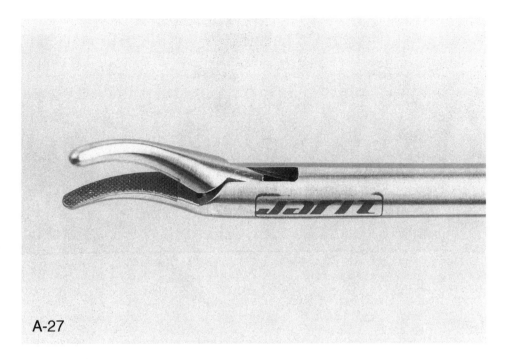

Figure Appendix 27

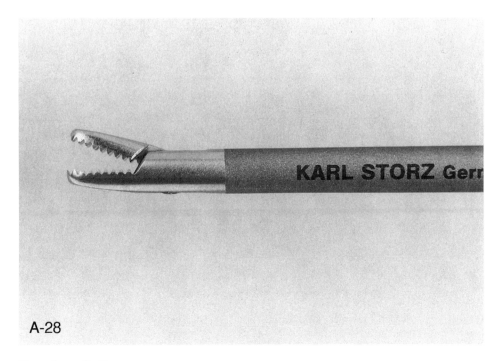

Figure Appendix 28

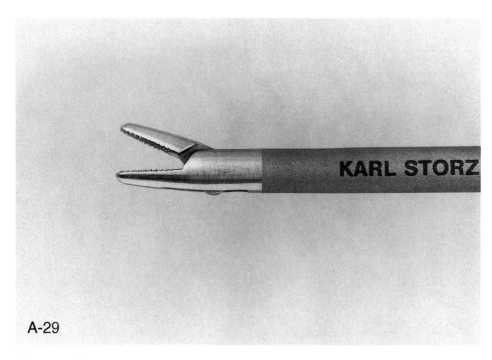

Figure Appendix 29

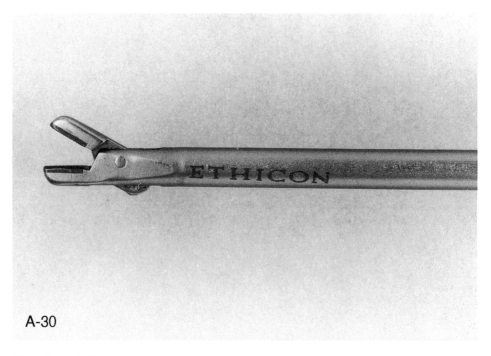

Figure Appendix 30

Appendix 327

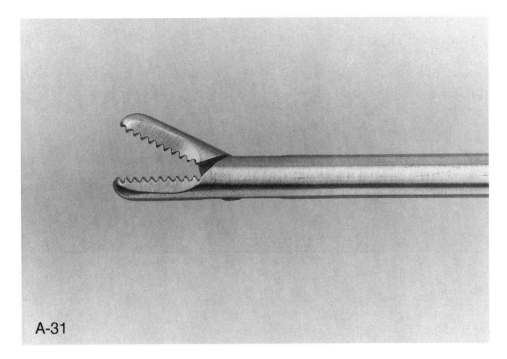

Figure Appendix 31

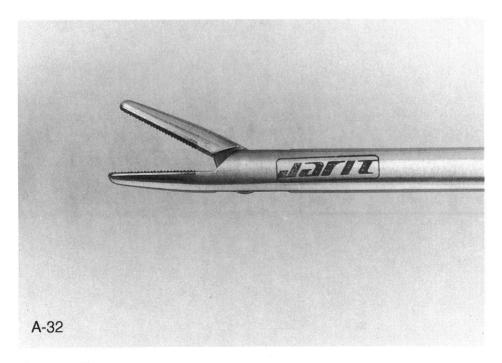

Figure Appendix 32

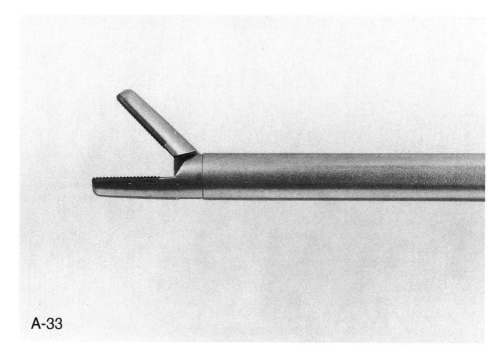

Figure Appendix 33

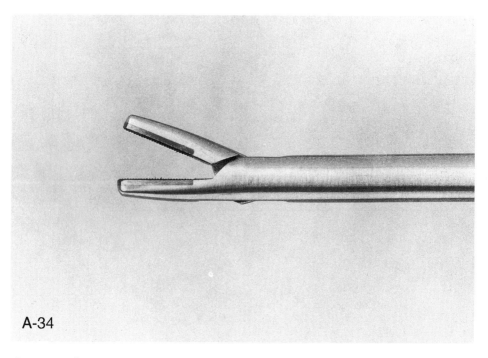

Figure Appendix 34

Appendix 329

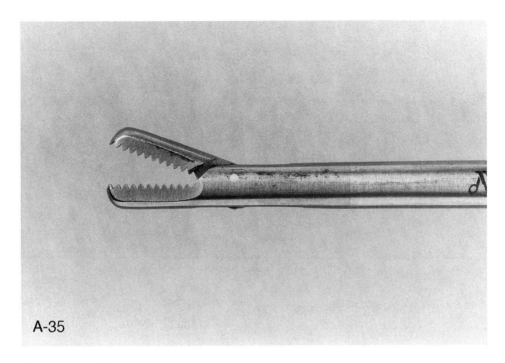

Figure Appendix 35

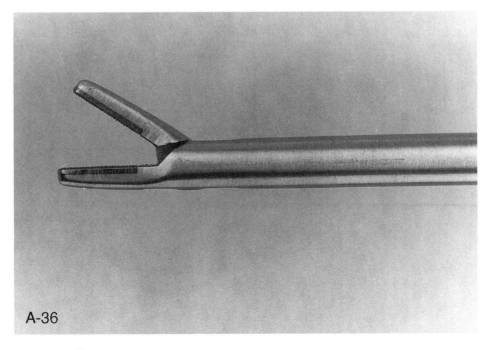

Figure Appendix 36

330 GYNECOLOGIC ENDOSCOPY: Principles in Practice

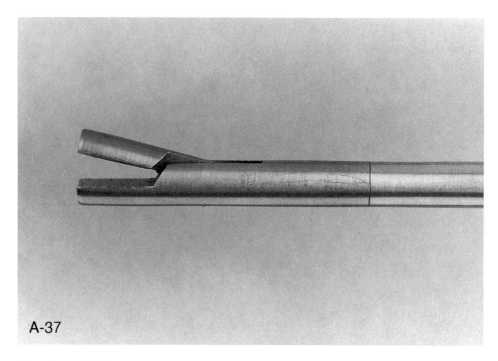

Figure Appendix 37

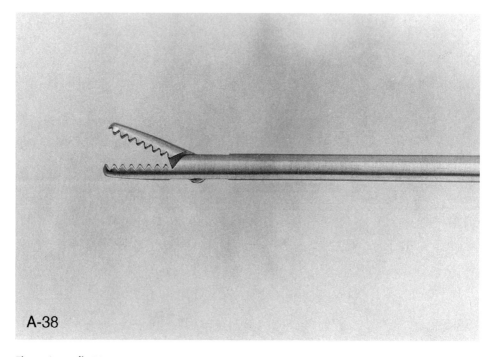

Figure Appendix 38

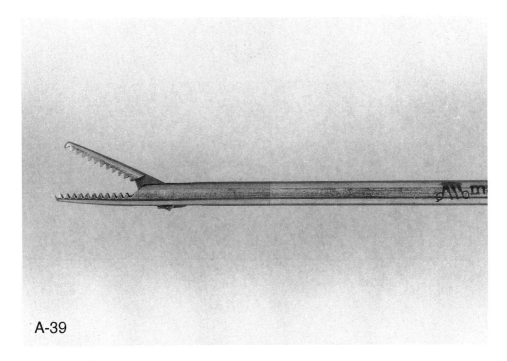

Figure Appendix 39

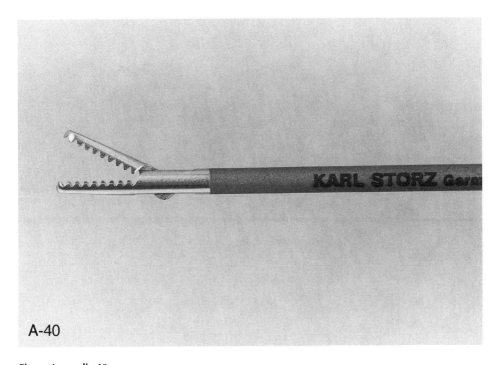

Figure Appendix 40

332 GYNECOLOGIC ENDOSCOPY: Principles in Practice

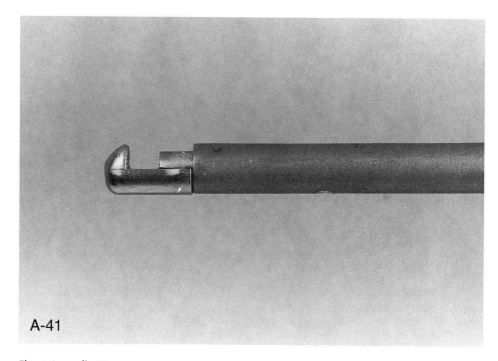

Figure Appendix 41

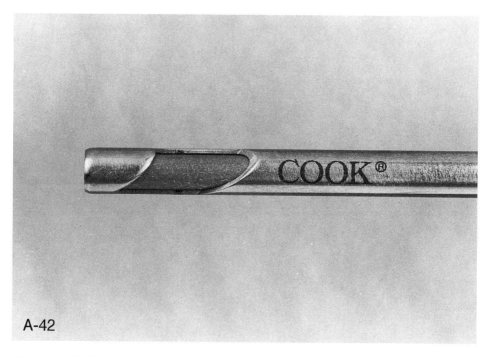

Figure Appendix 42

Appendix 333

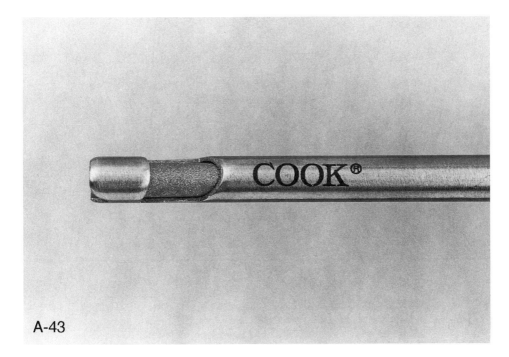

Figure Appendix 43

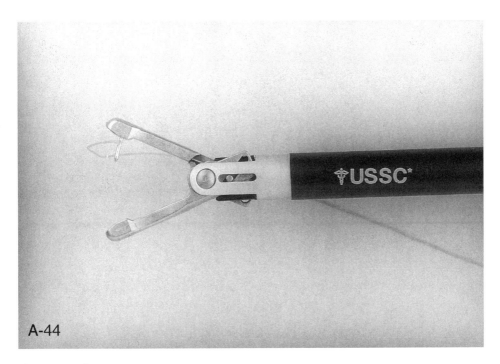

Figure Appendix 44

334 GYNECOLOGIC ENDOSCOPY: Principles in Practice

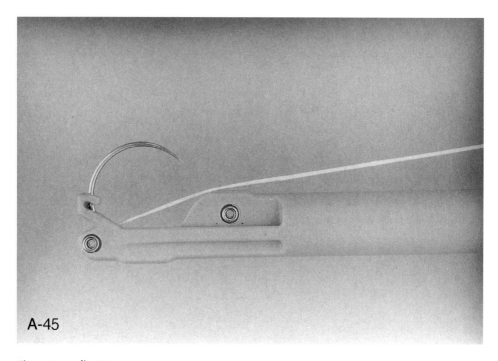

Figure Appendix 45

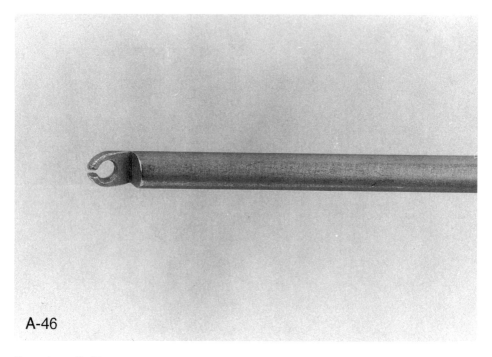

Figure Appendix 46

Appendix 335

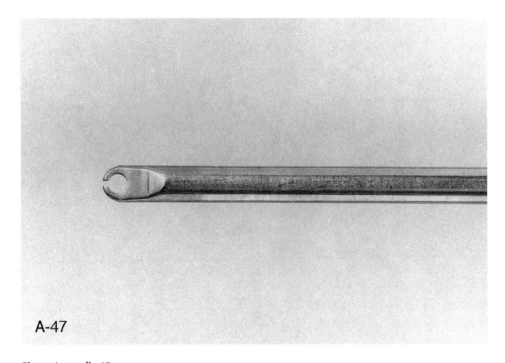

Figure Appendix 47

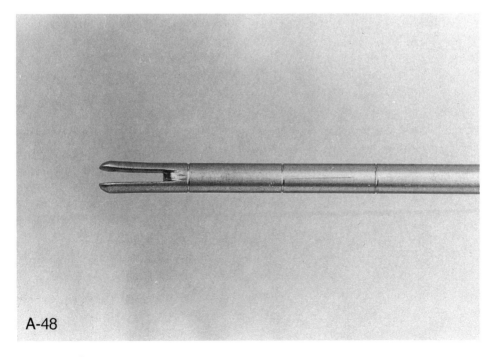

Figure Appendix 48

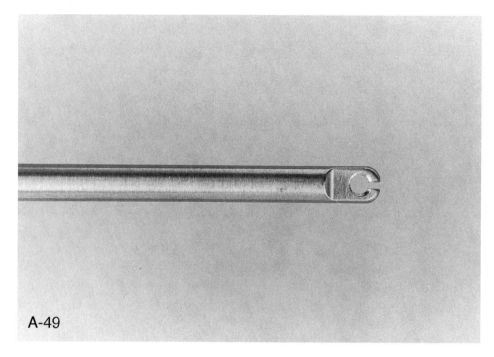

Figure Appendix 49

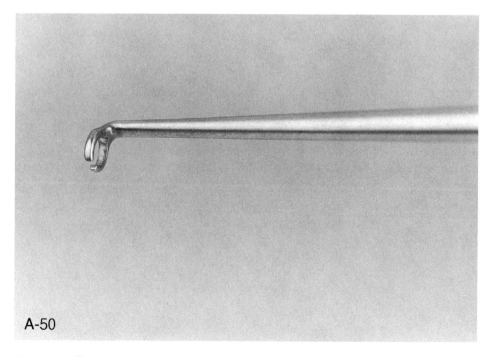

Figure Appendix 50

Appendix 337

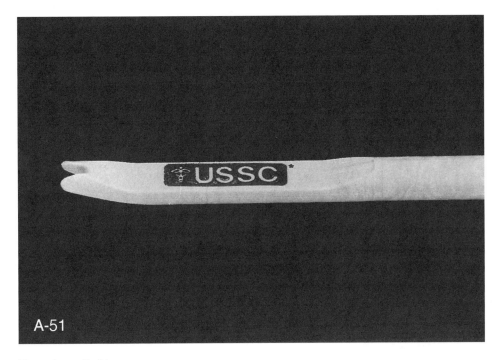

Figure Appendix 51

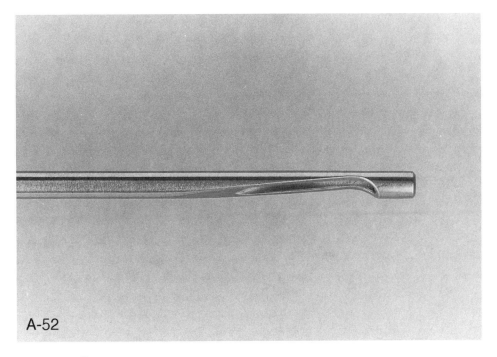

Figure Appendix 52

338 GYNECOLOGIC ENDOSCOPY: Principles in Practice

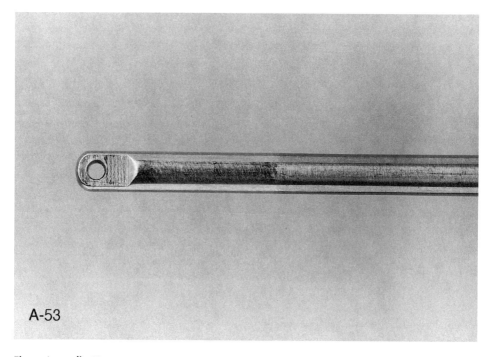

Figure Appendix 53

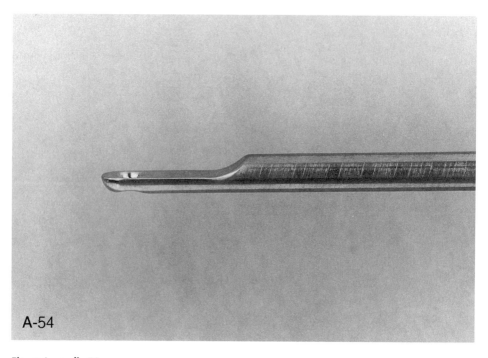

Figure Appendix 54

Appendix 339

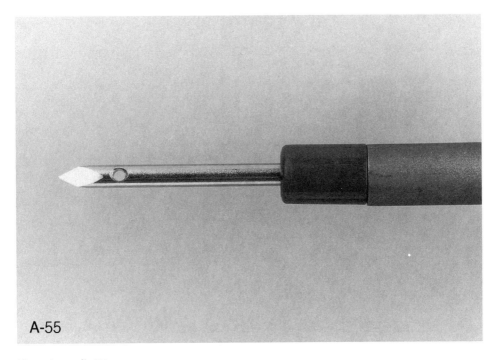

Figure Appendix 55

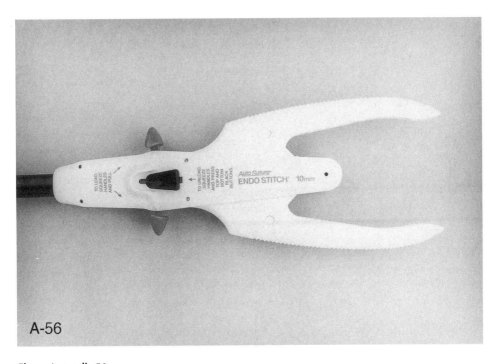

Figure Appendix 56

MANUFACTURERS

Cabot	Cabot Medical 2021 Cabot Blvd., West Langhorne, PA 19047 (215) 752-8300 (800) 523-6078
Cook	Cook OB/GYN 1100 West Morgan St. P.O. Box 271 Spencer, IN 47460 (812) 829-6500 (800) 541-5591
Ethicon	Ethicon, Inc., Customer Service 4545 Creek Rd. Cincinnati, OH 45242 (800) 438-4426
Jarit	J. Jamner Surgical Instruments, Inc. 9 Skyline Drive Hawthorne, NY 10531 (914) 592-9050
Laurus	Laurus Medical Corporation 30 Hughes St., #202 Irvine, CA 92718 (714) 859-6002 (714) 859-2109
Marlow	Marlow Surgical Technologies, Inc. 1811 Joseph Lloyd Parkway Willoughby, OH 44094 (216) 946-2453 (800) 992-5581
Reznik	Reznik Instrument, Inc. 7337 N. Lawndale Ave. Skokie, IL 60076 (708) 673-3444
Sharpe	Sharpe Endosurgical Instruments, Inc. 3750 Annapolis Lane, Suite 135 Minneapolis, MN 55447 (612) 557-1143 (800) 238-3484
Storz	Karl Storz Endoscopy-America, Inc. 10111 West Jefferson Blvd. Culver City, CA 90232-3578 (310) 558-1500 (800) 421-0837
USSC	Auto Suture Company 150 Glover Ave. Norwalk, CT 06856 (203) 845-1000

# Index

Page numbers followed by "f" denote figures; those followed by "t" denote tables.

Abdominal ectopic pregnancy
  laparoscopy for, 13–14
  laparotomy for, 12–13
Abdominal wall
  suturing of, 240–243. (see also Suturing, of abdominal wall)
  vessels of, anatomy of, 262, 265f
Accessory instruments, 176–177
Adenocarcinoma, hysteroscopic identification of, 58
Adenomyosis, hysteroscopic identification of, 58
Adhesiolysis
  of bowel, 288–290
  complications during, 72–73, 289–290
  hysterosalpinogogram preparation for, 71, 72
  laparoscopic guidance in, 71, 72
  outcome following, 71
  of pelvic floor, 288–289
  sound dilator in, 72, 72f
  synechiae classification for, 71t, 71–72
  termination of, 72–73
Adhesions (synechiae)
  hysteroscopic identification of, 58
  pelvic, 288–289
  training model for, 147, 153f
Adnexal mass, 37–49
  adnexectomy of, 42f, 42–44, 43f, 44f, 45f
  assessment of abdominal cavity for, 39
  laparoscopic management of
    literature review of, 30–32, 31t
  in menopausal women
    literature review of, 31–32
  oophorocystectomy for, 40–41, 41f
  operative laparoscopy of
    equipment for, 37–39
    procedure selection for, 39–40
    safety of, 47–48
  preoperative procedure and, 39
  removal of, 44–48, 46f, 47f, 48f
    via colpotomy incision, 45–47, 47f, 48f
    via suprapubic incision, 45, 46f
  size of
    risk for malignancy and, 27–28, 28t
Adnexal structure(s)
  training models of
    adhesion, 147, 153f
    hydrosalpinx, 146, 150f
    ovarian, 146–147, 151f, 152f
    ovarian cyst, 147, 152f

    tubal, 144–145, 147f, 148f
    tubal ectopic pregnancy, 145, 149f
Adnexectomy, 42f, 42–44, 43f, 44f, 45f
Age, pelvic malignancy and, 27, 27t
Amenorrhea, post endometrial ablation, 89
Analgesia
  for hysteroscopy
    office-based, 56
  intravenous
    local anesthesia with, 129t, 290
Anesthesia. (see also Local anesthesia)
  complications with
    carbon dioxide embolus, 247–248
    Trendelenburg position and, 246
  for hysteroscopy
    office-based, 56
  for live animal training, 156t
  for sterilization, 129t
Artery(ies)
  epigastric. (see also Epigastric vessel(s))
    suture ligation of, 240
  middle sacral
    in presacral neurectomy, 297
  ovarian
    in adnexectomy, 43, 44f
  uterine
    staple ligation of, 107–108, 110f
Aspiration, of ovarian cyst, 157–158, 160–161, 163f

Barium enema, in evaluation of pelvic mass, 26
Bipolar electrosurgery
  description of, 184–185
  limitations of, 185–186
Bladder
  endometriosis lesions over, 287
  laceration of, 270
    treatment of, 271–272
  perforation of, 114
  suturing models of, 148, 154f
Bladder flap development, in laparoscopically assisted vaginal hysterectomy, 105, 106f
Blade (knife) electrode, effects with, 186, 187
Bowel
  adhesiolysis of, 288–290
  injury to
    in electrocoagulation sterilization, 119
    in laparoscopically assisted vaginal hysterectomy, 114

341

Bowel (continued)
    literature review of, 189–190
    mechanical, 269
    perforation of, 188
    thermal, 268–269, 290
    rectosigmoid injury and
        in laparoscopic uterosacral nerve ablation, 301, 302f
    suturing model of, 148–149, 155f
    trocar injury to, 267–268
Brachial plexus injury, 272–273
Bupivacaine
    for laparoscopy, 290
    in tubal ligation, 125–126
        for field block, 129, 129t
Burns
    alternate ground site, 252
    from dispersive electrodes, 255, 257, 257f

CA-125
    in malignancy prediction for pelvic mass, 30, 30t
    in nongynecologic tumors, 30
    in pre- versus perimenopausal women, 30
Cancer, stage I endometrial, laparoscopically assisted vaginal hysterectomy for, 103
Cannula, uterine, 176
Capacitance, in monopolar electrosurgery, 183f, 183–184, 185f
Carbon dioxide insufflation, for diagnostic hysteroscopy, 56
Cardiac arrhythmias, 248
CASH (Classic Abdominal S.E.M.M. [Serrated Edged Macro-Morcellated] Hysterectomy), for laparoscopic hysterectomy, 111
Cervix, septate, 68, 69f
Chromopertubation
    risks with, 128
    for tubal patency assessment, 127–128
Chronic pelvic pain (CPP), 279–292. (see also Local anesthesia; Pain)
    laparoscopy for
        in endometriosis, 285–287
        local anesthesia for, 290–291
        operative report following, 284
        in pelvic adhesions, 288–289
        postoperative talk with family and, 284–285
        preoperative preparation, 282
        procedure, 283
        repetition of, 291–292
        survey in, 283–284
    pain theory and, 279–281
    preoperative assessment of, 281–282
Classic Abdominal S.E.M.M. (Serrated Edged Macro-Morcellated) Hysterectomy (CASH), for laparoscopic hysterectomy, 111
Clip ties, 219f, 232, 234f, 236f
Clips and clip applicators, 195, 212, 219f
Collection bag
    in adnexectomy, 45, 46f, 47f
    in endometrial ablation, 83f
    training with for removal of ovarian cyst, 160–161, 165f, 166, 166f
Collection pouch, training with for removal of ovarian cyst, 164f, 165f–166f, 166
Colpotomy incision, in adnexectomy, 45–47, 47f, 48f
Complication(s)
    anesthetic, 246–247
    carbon dioxide embolus, 247–248
    cardiac arrhythmias, 248
    electricity-associated, 251–259. (see Electricity, complications associated with)
    extraperitoneal gas (subcutaneous emphysema), 249–250
    gastric reflux, 248–249
    gastrointestinal, 265–269. (see also Gastrointestinal complications)
    hemorrhagic, 259–265. (see also Hemorrhage)
    hypotension, 246–247
    incisional hernia and wound dehiscence, 273–275
    infection, 275–276
    neurologic, 272–273
    urologic, 269–272
Cost
    of anesthesia
        in laparoscopic tubal ligation, 129
    comparison of laparoscopically assisted vaginal hysterectomy
        with total abdominal hysterectomy, 100
        with total vaginal hysterectomy, 102
    of methotrexate therapy versus surgery, 1–2
CPP. (see Chronic pelvic pain (CPP); Pain)
Cuff salpingostomy, (Bruhat technique), 157, 162f
Current diversion
    complications from, 252–255
        alternate ground site burns from, 252
        capacitance coupling, 254–255, 256f
        from detached dispersive electrode, 253f
        direct coupling, 253–254, 255f
        from insulation defects, 253, 254f

Danazol (Danocrine), for endometrial suppression, 77
Dessication (cut mode)
    cut waveform in, 181, 181t
    fulguration versus, 182, 182f

description of, 181, 183f
occurrence of, 182, 183f
Distension
  uterine
    agents for, 77–78
    inadequate, 58–59
Doderlein hysterectomy, laparoscopic, 111
Duncan loop knot, 220

Ectopic pregnancy
  following tubal ligation, 6
  laparoscopic management of, 3–23
    abdominal, 12–14
    interstitial, 16
    ovarian, 14–16
    preoperative preparation for, 3–5
    procedure selection in, 5–6
    proficiency development in, 16–21
    risks in, 16
    salpingectomy in, 6, 7f, 8, 21
    salpingostomy in, linear, 8–12, 18–19, 19f
    segmental resection in, 12, 13f, 14f–15f, 19–21, 20f
    tubal, 145, 149f
  laparoscopy versus laparotomy for, 2–3
  luteal phase, 126
  methotrexate treatment of, 1–2, 12
  persistent, 16
Electricity
  complications associated with
    from current diversion, 252–255, 253f, 254f. (see Current diversion)
    dispersive electrode burns, 255, 257, 257f
    electrode trauma, 251–252
    prevention with electrode shields and monitors, 257, 258f
Electrocoagulation
  in sterilization
    bipolar, 117–118, 118f
    current in, 119
    failure with, 127
    unipolar, 118–119
Electrode(s)
  blade (knife), 186, 197
  for endometrial ablation, 79, 80f
  exercises in use of, 186–187
  grounding of, 146f
  loop, 80f
  rollerball, 79, 80f, 82
  rollerbar, 80f
  thermal injury from, 251–252
Electrosurgery, 179–191
  of adnexal mass, 37–38
  basic electricity in, 180
  biologic behavior of, 180–183
    blend, 181

    coagulation (fulguration), 181–182, 182f
    cut (dessication), 181, 183f
    waveforms in, 181t
  bipolar, 184–186
  complications in
    literature review of, 189–190
  development of, 179
  electrophysics definitions in, 180, 180t
  electrophysics in
    in hysteroscopy, 188–189
    in laparoscopy, 187–188
  exercises in applications of, 186–187
  monopolar, 183f, 183–184, 184f, 185f
  unipolar current in, 38
Electrosurgical generator, 175
Encephalopathy, hyponatremic, 90–91
Endocoagulation, Semm, in sterilization, 123–124
Endometrial ablation, 75–96. (see Nd:YAG [neodymium:yttrium-aluminum-garnet] laser)
  alternatives to, 92
  cancer following, 91–92
  complications of, 89–92
  contraindications to, 76
  electrodes in, 79, 80f, 82, 188
  electroresection for, 85–86
  electrosurgery in, 188–189
  experience development in
    didactic, 92–93
    with equipment, 93
    laboratory exercises for, 94–95
    practical, 92
  history of, 75–76
  indications for, 76
  instrumentation in, 78f, 78–79, 79f, 80f, 81f, 82
  Nd:YAG laser in, 86–89, 87f, 94–95
  operating room setup for, 82f, 83f, 84f, 85f
  patient preparation for, 76–77
  postoperative care and, 89
  results of, 89
  rollerball technique in, 82–85
  sow bladder demonstration of, 153–154
  uterine distension for, 77–78
Endometrioma, ovarian, 287
Endometriosis
  laparoscopically assisted vaginal hysterectomy for, 102–103
  pain with, 285
  treatment of, 285–287
Endometrium, hyperplastic, hysteroscopic identification of, 58
Enterotomy, during adhesiolysis, 289–290
Epigastric vessel(s)
  deep, 261–264
  inferior, 261–262

Epigastric vessel(s) *(continued)*
    laceration of, 261–264, 263f
    superior, 262–263
Extraperitoneal gas, 249

Fallopian tubes, local anesthesia of, 125–126
Fever, post lapariscopically assisted vaginal
        hysterectomy, 113
Field block, umbilical, for tubal ligation, 129,
        129t
Filshire clip, for tubal occlusion, 123, 123f,
        124f
Finishing knot, 231–232
    Aberdeen, 233f
Fluid absorption
    in endometrial ablation, 90–91
    in office-based hysteroscopy, 58
Forcep(s)
    atraumatic grasping, 5, 5f
    bipolar, 4, 4f
Fulguration (coagulation mode)
    description of, 181–182, 182f
    versus dessication, 182, 182f
    smoke management in, 187–188

Gas source, for endoscopy, 174
Gastric reflux, 248–249
Gastrointestinal complication(s)
    dissection and thermal injury, 268–269
    insufflation needle injury, 265–266
    trocar injuries, 266–268
Glycine
    in electrocoagulation, 187–188
    fluid absorption with, 90, 91
    for uterine distension, 77–78
GnRH agonists, for endometrial suppression, 77
Granny knot, 130
    description of, 214–215, 220f
    tying of, 231
Grasping device
    in hysteroscopic myoma removal, 65, 65f
    in suturing of abdominal wall, 242f–243f
Great vessel injury
    anatomic relationships and, 260f, 261
    causes of, 261
    recognition of, 259
    risk reduction and, 259–261

Half hitch knot
    description of, 213, 220f
    extracorporeal, 234–235, 238–240
        passing ligature around pedicle, 235,
            236f
        sequential, 238
        tying, transferring, securing, 235, 237f, 238f
    intracorporeal, 229
    tying of, 235, 236f, 238–240

Hemorrhage, 259–264
    in ectopic pregnancy, 16
    following endometrial ablation, 90
    from intraperitoneal vessel injury, 264–265
    in lapariscopically assisted vaginal hysterectomy, 113
    with peritoneal entry, 259–264
        and abdominal wall vessel injury, 261–264,
            263f
        and great vessel injury, 259–261, 260f
Hemostasis, in electrosurgery, 38
Hulka clip, in segmental tubal resection, 12
Hulka-Clemens clip, for tubal occlusion, 123,
        123f, 124f
Hydrosalpinx model
    for intracorporeal knot tying, 169
    for laparoscopy, 146, 150f
Hypomenorrhea, post endometrial ablation, 89
Hyponatremia, endometrial ablation and, 90–91
Hypotension, 248
Hyskon, in hysteroscopy, office-based, 56, 57, 59
Hysterectomy
    for ectopic pregnancy, 5–6
    laparoscopically assisted vaginal. (*see*
        Laparoscopically assisted vaginal hysterectomy (LAVH))
    prevalence of, 97
    supracervical (subtotal) laparoscopic, 109,
        111, 113t
    total abdominal, 99–101
    total vaginal, 101–102
Hysteroscope(s)
    continuous flow system, 53, 54f, 79f
    for endometrial ablation, 78f, 78–79
    flexible, 53, 55, 55f
    for office hysteroscopy, 53–55
    panoramic with sheath and scissors, 53, 55f
Hysteroscopy
    electrophysics in, 188–189
    intrauterine
        myoma in, 153, 160f, 162f
    office, 51–60. (*see also* Office hysteroscopy)
    operative, 61–96. (*see also* Operative
        hysteroscopy)
    resectoscope box in training for, 154, 161f
    sow urinary bladder training for, 151,
        153–154, 159f
        disadvantages of, 153–154
        myoma in, 153, 160f

Infection, after endometrial ablation, 91
Institutional Animal Care and Use Committee
    policies of, 142t
    principles of, 142t
Insufflation needle
    positioning of, 251–252
    in stomach trauma, 265

Insufflators
    for endoscopy, 174
    for hysteroscopy
        carbon dioxide 53, 54f
Interstitial pregnancy, 16
Intrauterine training model(s)
    resectoscope box, 154, 161f, 162f
    sow urinary bladder, 151, 153–154, 159f, 160f
Intravenous pyelogram (IVP), in evaluation of pelvic mass, 26
Introducer sleeves, 211–212, 219f
IVP (intravenous pyelogram), in evaluation of pelvic mass, 26

Keith needle, in suturing of abdominal wall, 240
Kleppinger bipolar forceps, study of, 189
Knot manipulators, Type 1 (open), 311t, 334f, 335f, 336f, 337f, 338f, 339f
Knot tying
    board for, 150, 159f
    extracorporeal (overhand), 167, 169f, 170f, 234–235, 238–240
        half hitches and surgeon's, 235, 236–238
        slip knots, 239–240
    intracorporeal, 167, 172–173, 229
        clip ties, 219f, 232, 235f–236f
        finishing, 231–232, 233f
        granny, 230
        half hitch and variations, 230–231
        hydrosalpinx model for, 169
        instruments for, 169
        mechanical impediments to, 215f
        noose, 231, 232f
        overhand, 231f
        twist technique, 171f–173f
Knot(s), 212–220
    overhand, 212–215
        granny, 214–215, 220f
        half hitch, 213–214, 220f
        square, 214, 220f
        surgeon's, 215, 220f
        traction when securing, 221f
    slip, 215–220, 222f

Laboratory studies, in evaluation of pelvic mass, 26
Laparoscopic ureterosacral nerve ablation (LUNA)
    complete transection in, 300
    complications of, 301, 302f
    history of, 294
    partial ablation in, 300
    ureterosacral ligament identification in, 300–301
Laparoscopically assisted vaginal hysterectomy (LAVH), 97–116
    classification systems for, 111–112, 112t, 113t
    comparative studies of, 99–102
        total abdominal hysterectomy and, 99–101
        total vaginal hysterectomy and, 101–102
    complications of, 112–114
        literature study of, 189
    contraindications to, 103, 104
    early experiences with, 98–99
    indications for, 102t, 102–104
    techniques for
        CASH procedure, 111
        Doderlein, 111
        standard, 104–109, 110f
        supracervical (subtotal), 109–111, 113t
        total, 112t
    training and credentialing for, 114–115
Laparotomy
    for abdominal ectopic pregnancy, 12–13
    for adnexal mass, 39
    laparoscopy versus
        in ectopic pregnancy, 2–3
LAVH. (see Laparoscopically assisted vaginal hysterectomy (LAVH))
Leiomyomas. (see also Myomectomy)
    operative hysteroscopy of, 61–67
Leuprolide (Lupron), for endometrial suppression, 77
Ligature carriers, 210, 217f
    in abdominal wall suturing, 217f, 240, 241f, 242f, 243f
    design of, 211, 216f, 217f
    in suturing of abdominal wall, 217f, 240, 241f
    technique with, 228, 229f
Ligatures
    absorption of, 197–198, 198f
    caliber of, 196f, 196–197
    composition of, 197
    construction of, 197, 198–199
    selection of
        for extracorporeal ties, 199
        for intracorporeal ties, 199, 201
    training models for
        knot tying training board, 150, 159f
        vessel ligation, 149–150, 157f
Light source, for endoscopy, 174
Live animal training
    approved anesthetics for, 156t
    basic equipment and instruments for, 158t
    pig, 155, 158t
    potential problems with, 157
    species in, 155, 156t
Local anesthesia. (see also Anesthesia)
    for hysteroscopy
        office-based, 57

Local anesthesia. *(continued)*
   laparoscopy under, 290–291
   in sterilization, 125–126, 128t, 128–129, 129t, 130f
LUNA. *(see* Laparoscopic ureterosacral nerve ablation [LUNA])

Malignancy, pelvic, risk factors for, 27–30
Mechanical clips
   in tubal occlusion, 122–123, 123f
     application of, 123, 124f
     failure with, 126
Medical complications, 246–249
Medroxyprogesterone acetate (Provera), for endometrial suppression, 77
Mesosalpinx, injection of, 11f, 17–18, 18f
Methotrexate
   for ectopic pregnancy, 1–2, 12
     cost savings with, 1–2
     in lieu of excision, 12
     patient eligibility for, 1
   for ovarian pregnancy, 15
Metroplasty
   hysteroscopic, 67–70
     for complete uterine septum with septate cervix, 68, 69f
     follow-up of, 69–70
     laparoscopic guidance in, 68
     postoperative medications and, 69
     scissors and laser fibers in, 68
     for septate uterus, 67–68
     for subseptate uterus, 68, 70f
   retroscopic, 70–71
Monopolar electrosurgery
   capacitance in
     description of, 183f, 183–184
     increase in, 184, 185f
     injury prevention and, 184, 185f
Morcellation
   intraperitoneal, 167
   orange peel technique, 167, 168f
   of ovarian cyst, 167
   training exercises in, 167
Myoma. *(see* Myomectomy)
   hysteroscopic identification of, 58
   model of (raw potato), intrauterine, 154, 160f, 162f
Myomectomy
   hysteroscopic, 61–67
     antibiotic prophylaxis and, 67
     fluid status and, 67
     GnRH antagonists and, 67
     instruments for, 62t, 63f
     in intramural leiomyoma, 61–62, 63f
     in intrauterine myoma, 62
     Nd:YAG laser in, 67
     in pedunculated leiomyoma, 62, 64f, 65f
     in sessile myoma, 64–65, 66f
     technique in, 64–67, 66f

Nd:YAG (neodymium:yttrium-aluminium-garnet) laser
   in endometrial ablation, 75
     disadvantages of, 89
     laboratory exercises in, 94–95
     nontouch technique, 87, 88f, 94
     operating sheath for, 86, 87f
     versus rollerball technique, 88–89
     touch technique, 86–87, 88f, 95
   in intrauterine myoma removal, 75, 86–89, 87f
Needle drivers, 202–209
   alternatives to
     ligature carriers, 210, 217f
     mechanical suturing devices, 210, 217f
   end effector of, 204–205
     alligator curved/angled, 308t, 322f, 323f, 324f, 325f
     alligator jaw, 204–207, 213f
     alligator straight, 309t, 325f, 326f, 327f, 328f, 329f, 330f, 331f
     microsurgical needle holder, 214f
     side loading, 207, 209, 216f, 310t, 332f
   handles of, 203–204, 209f
     alignment of, 209f
     inline, 209f, 210f, 211f, 305f, 322f, 323f, 326f, 315f
     locking mechanism of, 204
     offset, 209f, 212f, 306t, 315f, 316f, 317f, 318f, 319f
   performance of, 206
   selection of, 220, 224
   semiautomated, 307t
     end effector of, 333f, 334f
     handle of, 332f, 339f
   shaft of, 209
Needle electrode, exercises with, 186, 187
Needle(s)
   curved, 200f, 225f
     insertion of, 223, 224f
   insertion of, 223, 224f, 225f
   insufflation
     injury from, 265–266
     placement of, 249–250
   manipulation of, 226, 228
   pneumoperitoneum, 176
   selection of, 220, 224
   ski-tipped, 200f
   straight, 200f, 224f
     insertion of, 223, 224f
Neodymium:yttrium-aluminum-garnet (Nd:YAG) laser. *(see* Nd:YAG (neodymium:yttrium-aluminum-garnet [Nd:YAG] laser)

Neosalpingostomy, (Bruhat cuff technique), 157, 162f
Noose knot
　description of, 220, 222f, 231
　pretied, 232f
　tying technique, 229–231

Office hysteroscopy, 51–60
　complications of, 58–59
　contraindications to, 51–52
　endometrial anatomy and pathology in, 57–58
　equipment for, 52–53, 53f, 54f, 55f, 55–56
　indications for, 51–52
　sterilization in, 56
　technique in, 56–57
　training in, 59
Oophorocystectomy, 40–41, 41f
Operative endoscopy
　instruments for
　　accessory, 176–177
　　basic, 174–176
　learning, 135–177
　　basic equipment for, 137t
　　exercises in, 157–167
　　hysteroscopic models in, 150–155
　　instruments for, 174–177
　　knot tying exercises in, 167–173. (see also Knot tying)
　　laparoscopic models in, 139–150. (see also Training model(s))
　　live animal models in, 155–157
　　pelvic trainers in, 136-141 (see also Pelvic trainer(s))
Operative hysteroscopy, 61–96
　for endometrial ablation, 75–96. (see also Endometrial ablation)
　for leiomyomas, 61–67. (see also Myomectomy)
　for septums, 67–71. (see also Metroplasty, hysteroscopic)
　for synechiae (adhesions), 71–73. (see also Adhesiolysis)
Orange peel technique, for morcellation, 167, 168f
Ovarian cyst
　removal without spillage
　　aspiration of, 158, 163f, 169
　　endoscopic pouch/bag collection in, 160–161, 165f–166f, 166
　　morcellation exercise in, 167
Ovarian mass, 25, 25t
　laparoscopic management of
　　literature review of, 31
　　malignant, 27
　　intraoperative rupture of, 32–33
Ovarian pregnancy, 14–16
　cystectomy in, 15
　oophorectomy in, 15
　wedge resection in, 15
Ovaries
　arteries of
　　coaptation of, 43, 44f
　　skeletonization of, 43, 44f
　benign versus malignant lesions of
　　transvaginal-color Doppler ultrasound for, 29, 29t
　cancer of, stage 1,
　　intraoperative tumor spill in, 32–33
　endometrioma of, 289
　training model of, 146–147, 152f, 515f

Pain. (see also Chronic pelvic pain [CPP])
　acute versus chronic, 279–280
　criteria for chronic, 280
　model of determinants of, 280f
　pelvic denervation and, 294–295. (see also Pelvic denervation procedure(s))
　up- and down-regulation of, 279–280
Pelvic denervation procedure(s), 293–304. (see also named procedure, e.g., Presacral neurectomy)
　laparoscopic uterosacral nerve ablation, 294
　pain theory and, 294–295
　preoperative evaluation, 295
　presacral neurectomy, 297–299, 301–303
　results with, 301–303
Pelvic floor, endometriosis lesions on, 287
Pelvic mass, 25–36
　diagnostic evaluation of, 26
　differential diagnosis of, 25t, 25–26
　laparoscopic management of
　　literature review of, 30–32, 31t
　risk factors for malignancy of
　　age, 27, 27t
　　size of mass, 27–28, 28t
　　tumor markers and, 29–30, 30t
　　ultrasound characteristics of, 28t, 28–29, 29t
　tumor spill in stage 1 ovarian malignancy and, 32–33
Pelvic trainer(s)
　hard top, opaque, 136–137, 137f
　　disadvantages of, 137
　positioning with, 138–139, 141f
　simplified, 138, 140f
　soft top, opaque, 138, 138f
　totally encased, insufflated, 138, 139f
Perforation
　of bladder, 114
　of bowel, 267–268
　　in electrosurgery, 188
　during endometrial ablation, 89–90
　of stomach, 265

Perineal nerve injury, 273
Pneumoperitoneum
    with carbon dioxide or nitrous oxide, 129
    needles for, 176
    subcutaneous emphysema from, 249
Pomeroy tubal ligation, laparoscopic, 124–125, 125f
Ports, in electrosurgery, 38–39
Power, in endometrial ablation, 84–85, 86
Pregnancy. (*see* Ectopic pregnancy)
Presacral neurectomy
    history of, 293–294
    laparoscopic approach in, 300f, 300–301
        position for, 302f
        potential complications of, 299
    results with, 303
    transabdominal approach in, 297
Probes, irrigation/dissection, in electrosurgery, 39
Prostaglandins
    for ovarian pregnancy, 15
    for tubal pregnancy, 12

Resectoscope
    continuous flow, 81f
    for endometrial ablation, 75-76, 78, 78f, 80f
Resectoscope box, 154, 161f, 162f
Retroperitoneal space
    access to, 42f, 42–43
    dissection of, 43, 43f
Richter's hernia, 274
Roeder loop knot, 216, 219
Rollerball electrode
    effects with, 186–187
    electroresection versus, 85–86
    in hysteroscopy, 188
    Nd:YAG laser versus, 88–89

Salpingectomy
    exercise for, 21
    techniques for, 21
    for tubal pregnancy
        procedures for, 6, 7f, 8
Salpingo-oophorectomy, for ovarian pregnancy, 8
Salpingostomy
    contraindications to, 8
    electrocoagulation in, 9, 10f, 11f
    laparoscopic, 10, 12
    linear
        exercise for, 18–19, 19f
        procedure, f, 9, 10f, 11
        salpingectomy versus, 9
    microscissors in, 9, 11f
    postoperative care and, 9
    vasopressin injection of mesosalpinx in, 9, 11f
Segmental resection, exercise for, 19–21, 20f

Septums, 67–68, 67–71, 70f. (*see also* Metroplasty, hysteroscopic)
    with septate cervix, 68, 69f
Silastic rings
    in tubal occlusion
        complications in, 121–122
        versus electrocoagulation, 129
        failure with, 126–127
        knuckle absoprtion following, 121, 121f
        placement of, 120f, 120–121
        Yoon three-grasp technique in, 121, 122f
Slip knot(s), 215–220, 220f
    Duncan loop, 220
    noose, 222f, 231
    Roeder loop, 216, 219
    tying of, 235, 238–240
    Weston, 220
Smoke, glycine reduction of, 187–188
Sorbitol
    fluid absorption with, 90, 91
    for uterine distension, 77–78
Spillage, prevention in adnexal mass removal, 44–45, 46f, 47f, 49
Square knot, description of, 214, 220f
Staplers, in electrosurgery, 38
Stapling, in laparoscopically assisted vaginal hysterectomy, 107, 108f, 109f, 110f
Steam, from dessication technique, 187
Sterilization, 117–133
    electrocoagulation for, 117–119
    endocoagulation for, 123–124
    failures in
        chromoperturbation for prevention of, 127–128
        from failed tubal occlusion, 126–127
        luteal phase pregnancy, 126
        technical, 127
    laparoscopic Pomeroy tubal ligation for, 124–125, 125f
    local anesthesia in
        advantages and disadvantages of, 128, 128t
        agents for, 129t
        diamond field block for, 129, 130f
        of fallopian tubes, 125–126
        versus general anesthesia, 128
    mechanical clips for, 122–123, 123f, 124f
    silastic rings for, 120f, 120–122, 121f, 122f
    teaching modules for, 130–131
    tubal
        bipolar electrosurgery for, 187
Stomach
    insufflation needle injury to, 265
    trocar injury to, 266
Subcutaneous emphysema
    diagnosis of, 249
    management of, 250
    risk reduction and, 250–251

Supracervical (subtotal) hysterectomy
  laparoscopic, 109–111
    classification system for, 113t
    versus transabdominal, 110–111
Suprapubic incision, in adnexectomy, 45, 46f
Surgeon's knot, 215, 220f
Suture
  for extracorporeal knot tying, 167
  selection of, 226
Suturing, 193–244
  of abdominal wall, 240–243
    grasping device for, 242f, 243f
    Keith needle in, 240
    ligature cariers for, 217f, 240, 241f
    vessel ligation, 240
  in adnexectomy, 43
  general considerations in, 194–195
  historical perspective, 193–194
  instruments and supplies for, 196–220. (see also Knot(s)); named instrument, e.g. Needle driver(s)
    clips and clip applicators, 212
    introducer sleeves, 211–212
    knot manipulators, 201–202
    knots, 211–220
    needle driver alternatives, 210–211
    needle drivers, 202–209
    needles and ligatures, 196–201
  selection of suture, needle, needle driver, 220–221
  techniques, 220–228
    knotting, 230–241. see also Knot tying
    ligature carriers in, 228, 229f, 240, 241f, 242
    needle insertion into peritoneal cavity, 223–224, 224f, 225f
    needle manipulation, 226, 227f, 228
    preparation and tissue orientation, 221–222
    triangulation of instruments, 223f
  training and practice in, 194
    endoscopic simulator for, 195f
Synechiae (adhesions).(see Adhesiolysis; Adhesions)

TAH. (see Total abdominal hysterectomy (TAH))
Telescopes, 175
Thermal injury
  from current diversion, 252, 253f
  from direct coupling, 254f, 255f
  from electrode, 251–252
  to ureter, 270
Total abdominal hysterectomy (TAH)
  laparoscopically assisted vaginal hysterectomy comparison with
    advantages of, 100
    cost of, 99
    patient selection for, 100–101
Total vaginal hysterectomy (TVH)
  laparoscopically assisted vaginal hysterectomy comparison with
    costs of, 102
    duration of surgery in, 101
    pain following, 101, 102
Training model(s), 139–144
  for adnexal structures, 144–145, 147–150
  endoscopic pouches and bags
    exercises in use of, 160–161, 164f, 165f, 166, 166f
  grounding of, 143–144, 146f
  hysteroscopic, 150–151, 154–154. (see also Hysteroscopy, training models for)
  ligature, 149–150, 157f
  live animal, 140, 142t, 155–157
  nontissue, 140–141, 142t
  suturing, 148–149, 154f, 155f
    bladder, 148, 154f
    bowel, 148–149, 155f
    uterine, 141–143
      creation of, 143f, 143–144, 144f, 145f
Trocar sleeves, in electrosurgery, 39
Trocars, 176
  bowel injury from, 267–268
  complications from
    in laparoscopically assisted vaginal hysterectomy, 113
  gastrointestinal injury from, 266–268
Tubal ligation, ectopic pregnancy following, 6
Tubal occlusion
  failure of
    from incorrect site, 128
    from misidentification of tube, 126
  incomplete
    with electrocoagulation, 127
    with mechanical clips, 126
    with silastic rings, 126–127
Tubal resection
  segmental
    dessication in, 12, 13f
    Hulka clip in, 12
    suture technique, 12, 14f–15f
TVH. see Total vaginal hysterectomy (TVH)

Ultrasound
  in evaluation of pelvic mass, 26
  in benign versus malignant ovarian lesions
    findings of, 28t, 28–29, 29t
    transvaginal-color Doppler of, 29, 29t
Ureterovaginal fistula, 270
Ureters
  identification of, 107f
  injury to, 270–271

Ureters (continued)
   laceration, 270
   in laparoscopic ureterosacral nerve ablation, 301
   in laparoscopically assisted vaginal hysterectomy, 114
   thermal, 270
   treatment of, 272
Uterine cannula, 176
Uterine training model(s). (see also Intrauterine models)
   creation of, 143–144
      pear, 143, 144f
      placental, 143, 145f
      sock, 143, 143f

Uterus
   septate, 67–68
   subseptate, 68, 70f

Vesicovaginal fistula, 270
Video systems, 175
   for electrosurgery, 38
   learning general principles of, 136

Waveforms, 181t
   coagulation mode, 181–182, 182f
   cut mode, 181, 183f
   in electrosurgery, 000
   in endometrial ablation, 84
Weston knot, 220